Colorectal Cancer in Clinical Practice

Second Edition

Colorectal Cancer in Clinical Practice

Prevention, Early Detection and Management

Second Edition

Paul Rozen, MD
Department of Gastroenterology, Tel Aviv Medical Center and Tel Aviv University, Israel

Graeme P Young, MD
Flinders Centre for Innovation in Cancer, Flinders Medical Centre, Adelaide, Australia

Bernard Levin, MD
Division of Cancer Prevention and Population Sciences, University of Texas MD Anderson Cancer Center, Houston, Texas, USA

Stephen J Spann, MD
Department of Family and Community Medicine, Baylor College of Medicine, Houston, Texas, USA

informa
healthcare

New York London

First published in 2002 by Martin Dunitz.
Second edition published in 2006 by the Taylor & Francis Group.

This edition published in 2011 by Informa Healthcare, Telephone House, 69-77 Paul Street, London EC2A 4LQ, UK.

Simultaneously published in the USA by Informa Healthcare, 52 Vanderbilt Avenue, 7th Floor, New York, NY 10017, USA.

Informa Healthcare is a trading division of Informa UK Ltd. Registered Office: 37–41 Mortimer Street, London W1T 3JH, UK. Registered in England and Wales number 1072954.

A CIP record for this book is available from the British Library.

Library of Congress Cataloging-in-Publication Data available on application

ISBN-13: 9781841844558

Orders may be sent to: Informa Healthcare, Sheepen Place, Colchester, Essex CO3 3LP, UK
Telephone: +44 (0)20 7017 5540
Email: CSDhealthcarebooks@informa.com
Website: http://informahealthcarebooks.com/

For corporate sales please contact: CorporateBooksIHC@informa.com
For foreign rights please contact: RightsIHC@informa.com
For reprint permissions please contact: PermissionsIHC@informa.com

Contents

Preface to the second edition

Four years ago we published the first edition of this book, which aimed to provide the practicing clinician with an easy-to-read update on colorectal cancer. We believe that this objective was reached and the volume received complimentary and positive reviews in prestigious journals (Pignone M, Book review. *Gastroenterology* 2003; 125: 549; Nelson H, Book review. *New England Journal of Medicine* 2002; 347: 71). The first edition is now also available as an ebook (http://www.ebookstore.tandf.co.uk).

Unfortunately, colorectal cancer is still a major malignancy in countries with a westernized lifestyle and is becoming so in countries that adopt this lifestyle. With the increasing industrialization and resulting affluence of non-Western countries, colorectal cancer has become a major medical problem in Eastern Europe, and in areas of Asia and Latin America. Together with the increasingly aging population of these countries, these lifestyle risk factors have made colorectal cancer one of the most common malignancies worldwide.

Since preparing the first edition, there has been progress in identifying these risk factors, both lifestyle and genetic factors. This has led to a better understanding of the dietary and lifestyle preventive actions that need to be implemented from early life. Recognition of the genetic pathways to neoplasia helps us understand how to timely recognize families at risk and offer clinical intervention, including chemoprevention, when appropriate. Screening for colorectal cancer is being accepted as good and standard medical practice in more and more countries. Screening methodology has become more sophisticated, sensitive, and specific, with the large-scale introduction of quality controlled, automated developed quantitative immunochemical fecal occult blood tests, and endoscopy screening programs.

The last few years have seen the development of new colorectal cancer therapies that significantly prolong survival. These are now based on a better understanding of the biologic pathways of carcinogenesis and metastasis.

For all the above reasons, we believe it is timely to update the first edition. We do not regard this as a reference tome, but as a book that the practicing clinician can refer to for updated information on colorectal cancer in all its aspects. The text has been updated and so have the references. These are not intended to be all-inclusive, but to provide recent publications for extra information and back references. We have kept the language and layout straightforward and added tables and figures to illustrate points made in the text.

We hope that readers will find the information and advice they need in this book.

Paul Rozen, Graeme P Young,
Bernard Levin, Stephen J Spann

Preface to the first edition

A wise man has great power and a man of knowledge increases strength.
Proverbs 24:5.

(New International Version)

Colorectal cancer is one of the major malignancies afflicting westernized societies, both in terms of incidence and cause of cancer mortality. In many Western countries, the individual's lifetime risk for this neoplasm is about 5–6%, and approximately half will be long-term survivors.

However, *colorectal cancer is a preventable and treatable disease.* Other than tobacco-related lung cancer, it is the malignancy that has been most extensively studied and understood. Its etiology is complex and multifactorial, including both diet and inherited susceptibility. The pathogenesis of cancer from pre-existing dysplastic lesions, usually adenomas, has been well described. Its relatively easy accessibility to radiologic and endoscopic diagnosis facilitates early detection and even non-surgical therapy by polypectomy. Polypectomy itself will reduce the cancer incidence, while if cancer is detected in the asymptomatic and usually pre-invasive stage, then a surgical cure is possible in almost 90% of the cases.

In spite of this excellent outcome, most westernized countries have not systematically and actively promoted primary and secondary preventive policies for their general population. This is in contrast to the status of breast cancer screening, which has both emotional appeal and, most importantly, political support. Even so, at national levels, we have examples of the health services of Japan, the United States, Israel, and Germany providing large-bowel screening programs *for those who request it.* In addition, nationally budgeted pilot population screening studies have been initiated in the UK and Australia.

However, recently, the national media, key role-model personalities, professional medical societies, medical insurance organizations, individual physicians, and individuals at risk are promoting and demanding preventive medical practices. In the United States, this has led to the inclusion of colorectal cancer screening in the Medicare Program.

In 1996, three of us edited a multi-authored book that brought together the scientific evidence and knowledge relevant to colorectal cancer prevention: Young GP, Rozen P, Levin B (eds), *Prevention and Early Detection of Colorectal Cancer.* London: WB Saunders. This has been well received by general physicians, as well as specialists, as a reference volume. As new information is being acquired and preventive medicine (including chemoprevention, changes in diet and lifestyle) is being promoted, we feel that it is important to provide the clinician in practice with an easy-to-read and up-to-date guide on the primary and secondary prevention of large-bowel neoplasia. This includes primary care physicians such as family physicians and internists, as well as surgeons, gastroenterologists, oncologists, and public health personnel.

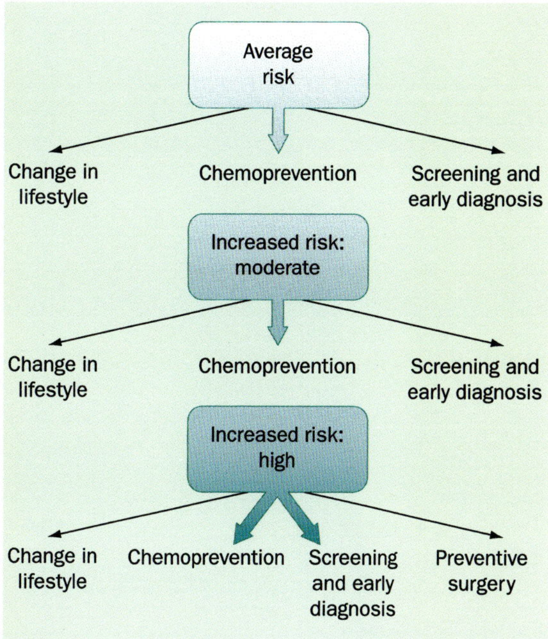

Figure *Algorithm of preventive medical strategies for persons at average or increased risk for colorectal cancer.*

The chapters in this volume provide an up-to-date précis of knowledge and also emphasize the practical preventive

Table *Colorectal cancer: its prevention and management*

- The size of the problem
  - How it might present
- How cancer develops
- Risk factors
  - Diet and chemoprevention
  - Familial risk
  - Premalignant conditions
- Screening
  - Follow-up of high-risk conditions
  - Average-risk screening
- Cancer management
- Public health aspects

steps that can be taken to reduce morbidity and mortality from colorectal cancer (see the Table and Figure). For those who want more information, we have provided recent references and indicated review or general articles on the topics discussed.

We hope that this volume will become a guide for the clinician who has both the first and the ongoing contact with the general population, as well as with those at increased risk.

Paul Rozen, Graeme P Young, Bernard Levin, Stephen J Spann

Acknowledgments

This book is dedicated to our wives Etta, Joan, Ronnie, and Nancy, for their love, support, and patience. Without the excellent help of our secretaries Sally Zimmerman, Fiona Bertrand, Rosanne Lemon, and Sherry Franovich, it would not have been possible to compile this book – to them we are extremely grateful.

We are also very grateful to Dr John Skibber, Associate Professor of Surgical Oncology, University of Texas, MD Anderson Cancer Center, for his contribution to Chapter 9. Finally, we wish to acknowledge our constructive working relationship with the Publishers.

The Authors

Dr Paul Rozen is a gastroenterologist and internist who is a Professor of Medicine (Emeritus) at the Tel Aviv University and is also at the Department of Gastroenterology, Tel Aviv Medical Center, Tel Aviv and Beilinson Hospital, Petach Tikvah (Israel). He has received research grants relevant to this publication from Boehringer Mannheim (Germany), SmithKline Diagnostic and Beckman Coulter (California), Alfa Wasserman (Milan), and Eiken (Japan). He is Chairman of the World Organization for Digestive Endoscopy (OMED) Colorectal Cancer Screening Committee. His address is: Department of Gastroenterology, Tel Aviv Medical Center, 6 Weizmann St, Tel Aviv 64239, Israel; Fax: +972–3–6474622; E-mail: rozen@tasmc.health.gov.il.

Dr Graeme P Young is a gastroenterologist who is Professor of Gastroenterology at Flinders University of South Australia and the Academic Head of Gastrointestinal Services at Flinders Medical Centre, Adelaide, South Australia. He has been in receipt of research funds from commercial entities relevant to the prevention of bowel cancer: Kellogg's Australia, Uncle Toby's Australia, Starch Australasia, Meadow Lea Corporation Sydney, SmithKline Diagnostics Inc. Sunnyvale, Beckman Coulter Primary Care Diagnostics Palo Alto, and Enterix Pty Ltd, Sydney. He has also served as a consultant or advisory board member for the following: Starch Australasia, Sanitarium Health Food Corporation Sydney, Enterix Pty Ltd, Boehringer Mannheim, Germany, Encore Pharmaceuticals Los Angeles, and SmithKline Diagnostics Inc. His address is: Department of Gastroenterology and Hepatology, Flinders Medical Centre, Bedford Park (Adelaide), South Australia 5042, Australia; Fax: +61–8–8204–3943; E-mail: graeme.young@flinders.edu.au.

Dr Bernard Levin is a gastroenterologist and internist who is a Professor of Medicine and Vice President of Cancer Prevention at the University of Texas MD Anderson Cancer Center. He is the recipient of the Betty B Marcus Chair in Cancer Prevention. He is the Chair of the United States National Colorectal Cancer Roundtable. He has served as a consultant to Enterix and to Pfizer in the area of chemoprevention of colorectal neoplasia. His address is: Bernard Levin, MD, Division of Cancer Prevention, University of Texas MD Anderson Cancer Center, 1515 Holcombe Boulevard, Box 203, Houston, TX 77030, USA; Fax: +713–792–0629; E-mail: blevin@mdanderson.org.

Dr Stephen J Spann is a family physician who is Professor and the Richard M Kleberg Sr Chair of the Department of Family and Community Medicine at Baylor College of Medicine. His address is: Stephen J Spann, MD, Department of Family and Community Medicine, Baylor College of Medicine, 3701 Kirby, Houston, TX 77098, USA; Fax: +713–798–7778; E-mail: sspann@bcm.tmc.edu.

1 Colorectal cancer: how big is the problem, why prevent it, and how might it present?

Stephen J Spann, Paul Rozen, Graeme P Young, Bernard Levin

The size of the problem

Colorectal cancer is one of the most commonly diagnosed cancers, and a leading cause of cancer deaths, around the world.[1] The high-incidence countries include all of North America, Western and Eastern Europe, Japan, Israel, Singapore, Australia, and New Zealand. They also include areas of Brazil and Argentina, Hong Kong, and the southern industrialized and affluent areas of China and Malaysia. The relative incidence of different cancers varies with that country's level of economic development, affluence, and westernization of lifestyle (Figures 1.1 and 1.2). In the developed regions of the world, colorectal cancer is the third most common malignancy in males after prostate and lung cancer, and the second most common in women after breast cancer (Tables 1.1 and 1.2). However, in terms of national health burden, mortality reflects not only prevalence but also availability of diagnostic services, adequate therapy, and comorbidity due to pre-existing conditions that influence survival. As can be seen in Figures 1.3 and 1.4, mortality from colorectal cancer is very high throughout Eastern Europe and the former Soviet Union, as well as in most of the other countries mentioned above. In 2002, it was the fourth most common cancer diagnosed and the fourth most common cause of cancer mortality in men worldwide; and the third most common cancer diagnosed and the fourth most common cause of cancer mortality in women.[1] In the United States, for example, colorectal cancer is the fourth most commonly diagnosed cancer across both genders, with an estimated 146 940 new cases in 2004; it is the second leading cause of cancer mortality there, accounting for an estimated 56 730 deaths in that year.[2] Even so, the United States is one of the few countries now demonstrating a reduction in colorectal cancer mortality (Figures 1.3b and 1.4b). The costs of treating patients with colorectal cancer are significant. It is estimated that in the United States in 2001 these costs approached $6.5 billion per year. This was second in cancer treatment costs only to breast cancer, at $7 billion per year.[3]

Time trends

In some developed countries, notably in the United States, both the incidence and mortality rates for colorectal cancer have been stable and even declining.[4] Declining incidence rates may reflect the preventive effects of a change in lifestyle as well as earlier detection and treatment of adenomatous polyps and non-invasive cancers, before they advance to metastatic carcinomas. Declining mortality rates are felt to reflect both the decreasing incidence of disease and the earlier detection of treatable disease. In the US population, the greatest reduction in incidence and mortality has occurred in white women (Figure 1.5). But, in the corresponding period, there was actually an increased mortality in African-American men of 21% and women of 7%.[2]

In other countries that have an improving socio-economic status and a westernizing lifestyle, there has been a parallel rising incidence of large bowel neoplasia.[1,5] These include countries from diverse regions such as Eastern Europe, Asia, and Latin America.

Many of these 'high-risk' countries are undergoing aging of their indigenous populations. With their decreasing birthrate and increasing affluence and availability of medical services, the proportion of 'healthy elderly' in their populations is ever increasing. As about 50% of colorectal cancer is identified in people over 65 years old, its prevalence is even increasing in those countries (Figure 1.6), and it will present an ever-increasing financial burden for the younger, but diminishing, community.

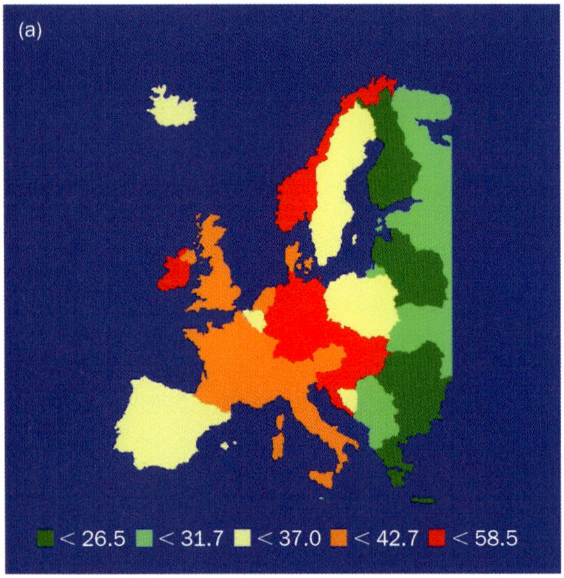

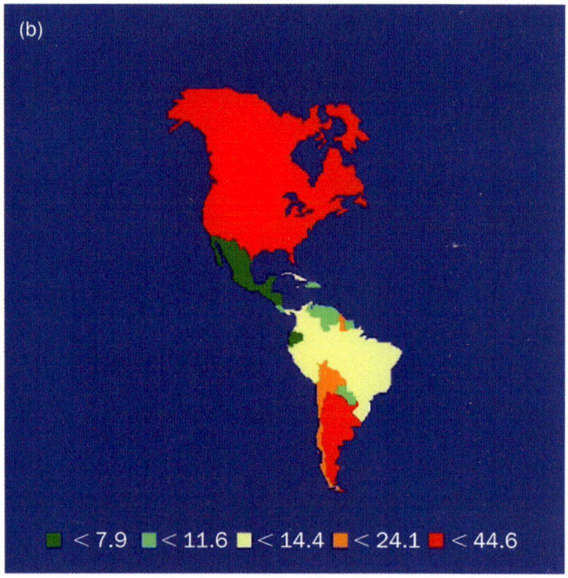

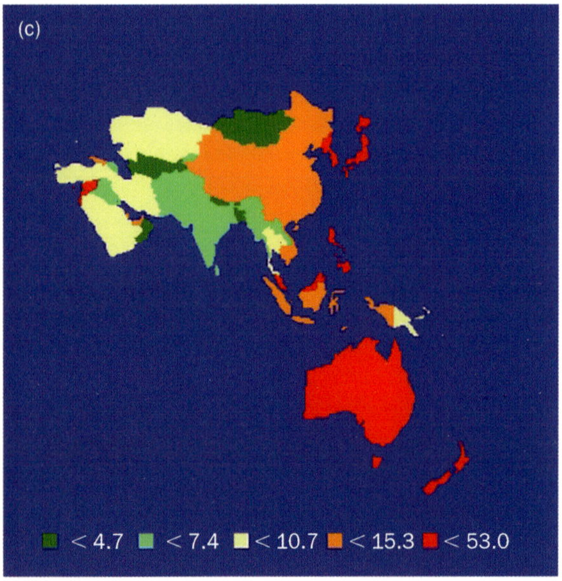

Figure 1.1 *Colorectal cancer incidence in males for 2002 in (a) Europe, (b) the Americas, and (c) Asia and Oceania, derived from GLOBOCAN 2002*[1] *and prepared by Ms S Bayua and Dr A Zauber, New York.*

Risk factors for colorectal cancer

A number of factors appear to increase an individual's risk for colorectal cancer, including older age, male gender, diet and exercise habits, a personal history of inflammatory bowel disease, certain genetic syndromes, and a family history of colorectal cancer or adenomatous polyps (see Chapters 2, 4 and 6). Adenomatous polyps are the precursors of most colorectal cancers; removal of these polyps significantly lowers the incidence of subsequent colorectal cancer.[6]

Stage at diagnosis and mortality

Colorectal cancer survival is closely related to the clinical and pathologic stage of the disease at diagnosis. The commonly used classifications of staging are given in

Table 1.1 *Age-standardized rates of cancer incidence (per 100 000) for males by site: select regions, 2002*[a]

	Esophagus	Stomach	COLON/ RECTUM	Liver	Lung	Prostate
Northern Africa	2.1	4.4	**5.1**	4.2	12.0	5.8
Western Africa	19.7	8.2	**11.3**	7.0	23.1	40.5
Central America	2.2	15.2	**7.9**	4.9	16.1	30.6
South America (tropical)	7.1	24.2	**16.4**	3.7	23.7	47.0
North America	5.8	7.4	**44.4**	5.3	61.2	119.9
Eastern Asia: China	27.4	41.4	**13.6**	37.9	42.4	1.6
Eastern Asia: Japan	10.0	62.1	**49.3**	23.1	38.1	12.6
South central Asia	8.1	6.9	**4.7**	2.6	11.9	4.4
Western Europe	7.6	12.8	**42.9**	6.2	50.9	61.6
Australia/New Zealand	5.5	9.9	**48.2**	3.9	39.1	79.9

[a] Adapted from reference 1.

Table 1.2 *Age-standardized rates of cancer incidence (per 100 000) for females by site: select regions, 2002*[a]

	Esophagus	Stomach	COLON/ RECTUM	Liver	Lung	Breast	Cervix
Northern Africa	1.4	2.5	**4.0**	2.2	2.2	23.2	12.1
Western Africa	7.0	3.7	**8.9**	2.5	6.9	33.4	38.2
Central America	0.9	10.8	**7.4**	4.9	6.5	25.9	30.6
South America (tropical)	2.0	12.2	**14.8**	2.8	7.6	46.0	28.6
North America	1.3	3.4	**32.8**	1.9	35.6	99.4	7.7
Eastern Asia: China	12.0	19.2	**9.2**	14.2	19.0	18.7	6.8
Eastern Asia: Japan	1.3	26.1	**26.5**	7.6	12.3	32.7	8.0
South central Asia	5.9	3.6	**3.5**	1.4	2.4	21.8	26.2
Western Europe	1.4	6.6	**29.8**	1.7	12.0	84.6	10.0
Australia/New Zealand	2.3	4.2	**36.9**	1.3	17.4	84.6	7.4

[a] Adapted from reference 1.

Table 1.3. The 5-year survival is approximately 90% in patients with cancers limited to the bowel wall, compared with 68% in those with lymph node involvement, and 9% in patients with metastatic disease at the time of diagnosis (Table 1.3).[7] This emphasizes that if colorectal cancer is detected at an early, asymptomatic stage, we should expect decreased morbidity and mortality from the disease (secondary prevention) (see Chapter 8).

Table 1.3 *Relationship between 5-year survival and stage at diagnosis*[a]

Stage at diagnosis			
	Dukes (modified)	**TNM**	**5-year survival rate (%)**
Limited to bowel wall	A and B	Stage 1	90%
Regional node involvement	C	Stages 2 and 3	68%
Distant metastates	D	Stage 4	9%

[a] Adapted from reference 7.

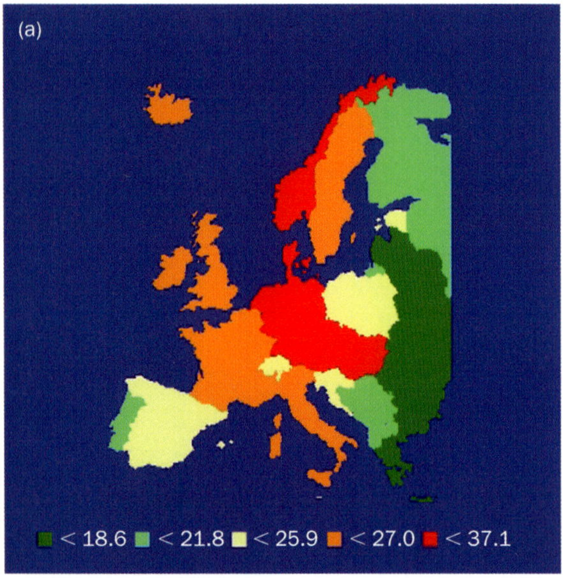

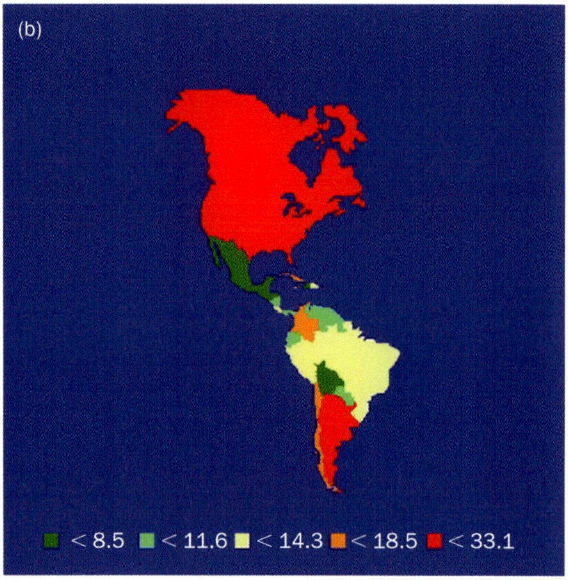

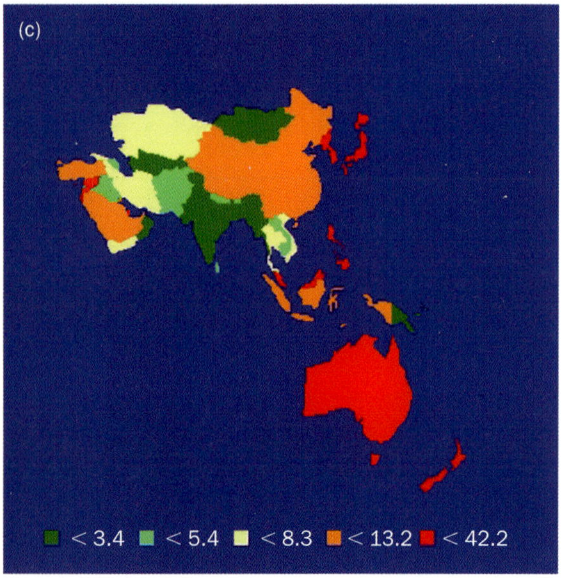

Figure 1.2 *Colorectal cancer incidence in females for 2002 in (a) Europe, (b) the Americas, and (c) Asia and Oceania, derived from GLOBOCAN 2002[1] and prepared by Ms S Bayua and Dr A Zauber, New York.*

Screening for cancer and the terminology used

Secondary prevention, which is offered to an entire population at average risk for a given disease, is called 'screening' for that disease. When secondary prevention is targeted at individuals who have one or more risk factors for a given disease, it is called 'case-finding'. A number of expert panels have suggested the application of specific criteria for deciding whether or not a given disease is amenable to secondary prevention.[8,9] The criteria required by the US Preventive Services Task Force include the following:

- The target condition (disease being screened for) must cause a significant burden of suffering: it must be relatively common, in terms of prevalence and incidence, and it must be clinically significant in terms of morbidity and mortality.

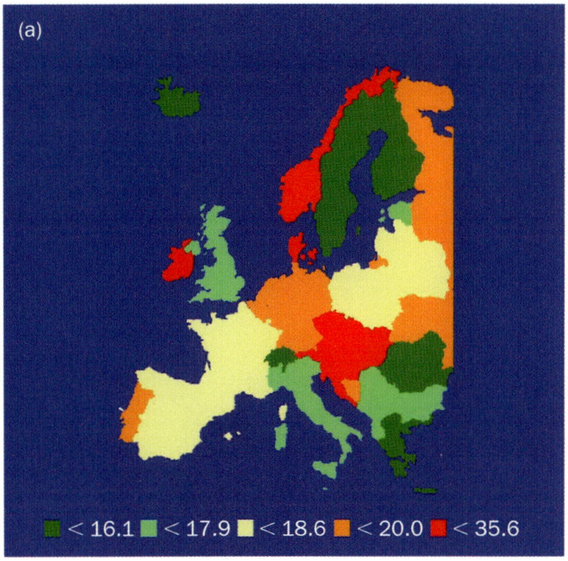

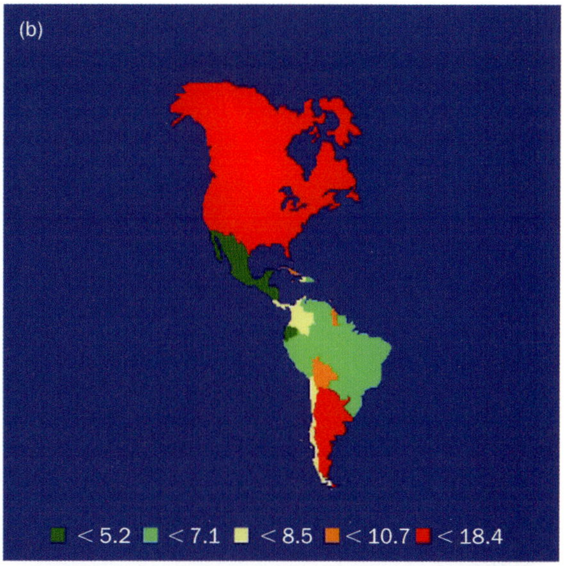

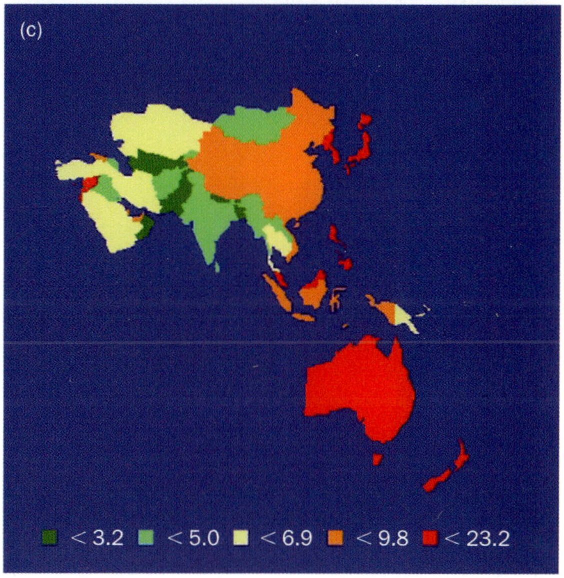

Figure 1.3 *Colorectal cancer mortality in males for 2002 in (a) Europe, (b) the Americas, and (c) Asia and Oceania, derived from GLOBOCAN 2002[1] and prepared by Ms S Bayua and Dr A Zauber, New York.*

- The screening test must be able to detect the target condition earlier than without screening, and with sufficient accuracy to avoid producing large numbers of false-positive and false-negative results.
- Screening for and treating persons with early disease should improve the likelihood of favorable health outcomes, such as decreased disease-specific morbidity or mortality, compared with treating patients when they present with symptoms and signs of the disease.[8]

False-negative test results can lead to false reassurance and a missed opportunity for early detection and treatment of the disease. *False-positive test* results usually lead to additional diagnostic tests and their associated expense and potential risk, as well as to psychologic anxiety in the patient who thinks he or she might have the disease. Test *sensitivity* is the probability that the test will be abnormal in a patient who has the disease of interest. The lower the test false-negative rate, the higher is its sensitivity. Test *specificity* is the probability that the test will be normal in a patient who does not have the disease

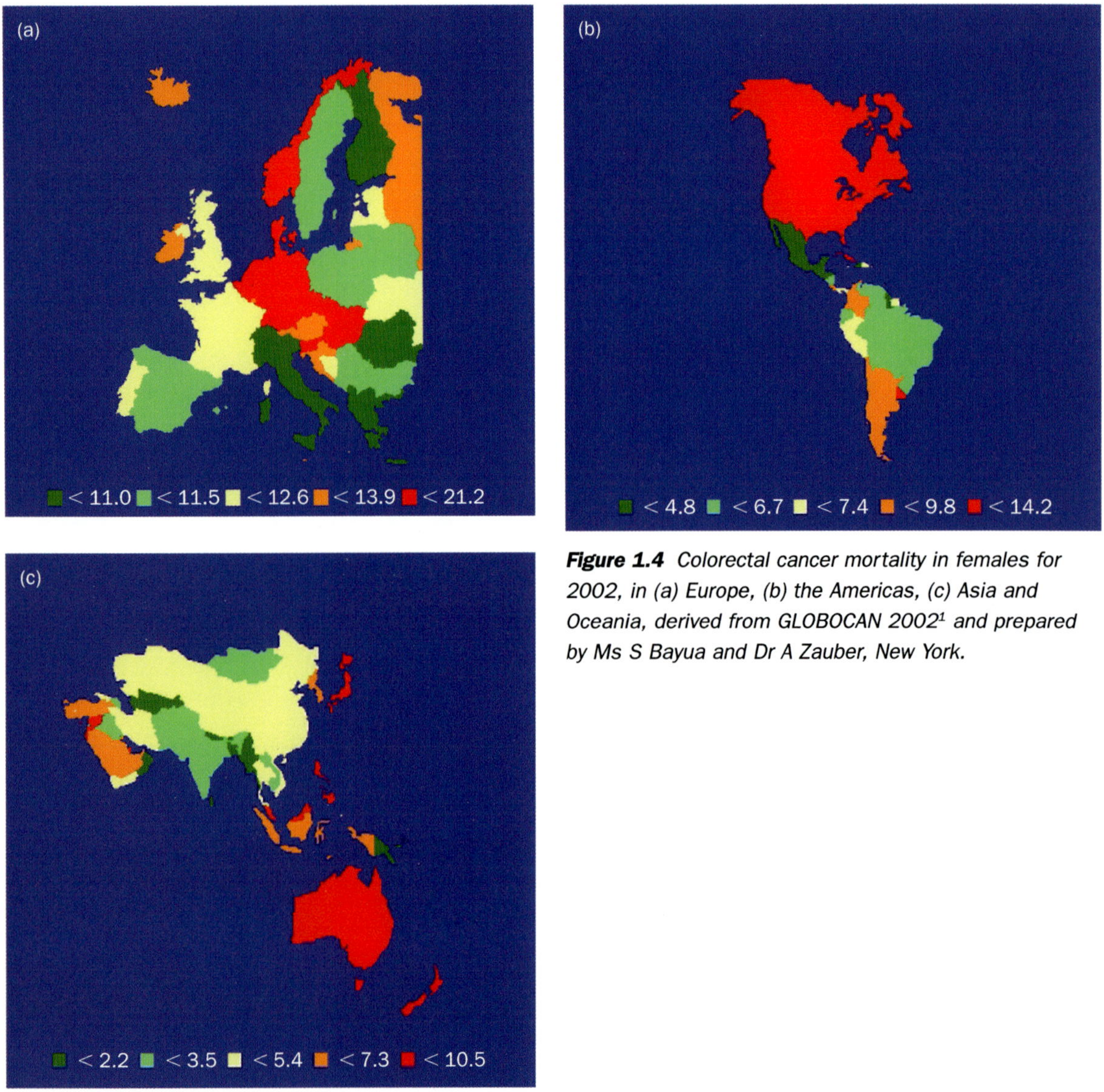

Figure 1.4 *Colorectal cancer mortality in females for 2002, in (a) Europe, (b) the Americas, (c) Asia and Oceania, derived from GLOBOCAN 2002*[1] *and prepared by Ms S Bayua and Dr A Zauber, New York.*

of interest. The lower the test false-positive rate, the higher is its specificity.

Clinicians are also interested in the predictive values of test results. *Positive predictive value* is the probability that a patient with a positive test does, in fact, have the disease of interest. *Negative predictive* value is the probability that a patient with a negative test is, in fact, free of the disease of interest (Table 1.4). Positive predictive value is directly proportional to test specificity: the higher the specificity of a test, the higher its positive predictive value. Negative predictive value is directly proportional to test sensitivity: the higher the sensitivity of a test, the higher its negative predictive value. Positive predictive value is directly proportional to the prevalence of the disease in the population tested: when screening a population at average risk for a given cancer, the positive predictive value will be low, since the prevalence rate will be low, by definition. Negative predictive value is indirectly proportional to the prevalence of disease in the population tested: in the average-risk screening situation, the negative predictive

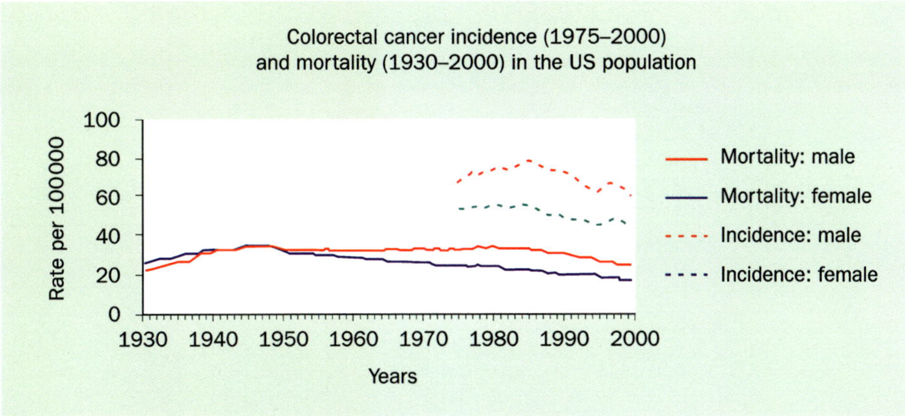

Figure 1.5 *Colorectal cancer incidence (1975–2000) and mortality (1930–2000) in the US population. There has been a recent fall in incidence in both sexes, and a reduction in mortality in females, especially in white women. Source: American Cancer Society: Cancer Statistics 2004. Available at http://www.cancer.org/docroot//stt//stt_0.asp*

value will be high. In other words, quite often a positive screening test of low specificity will be falsely positive, and the overwhelming majority of negative screening tests will be truly negative.

It can be challenging to establish that a screening test really leads to improved health outcomes; this is especially true for cancer screening tests. For most types of cancer, 5-year survival is higher for individuals identified with early-stage disease. It is tempting to conclude that early detection is effective because death appears to be delayed as a result of screening and early treatment. However, survival data may be influenced by *lead-time* bias: survival may appear to be lengthened when in fact screening has only advanced the time of diagnosis, lengthening the period of time between diagnosis and death without any true prolongation of life (Figure 1.7). Length bias can also cause unduly optimistic estimates of the effectiveness of screening for cancer: screening tests have a tendency to detect slow-growing tumors, as fast-growing tumors become symptomatic quicker. Patients found by screening may do better than unscreened patients even if the screening itself doesn't really affect the outcome. To determine whether or not a cancer-screening test is truly efficacious, it is best to conduct a randomized clinical trial, in which the experimental group receives the screening intervention of interest, and the control group does not. Both groups are then followed over time, and disease-specific mortality for that cancer is compared between the two groups. A randomized clinical trial showing decreased disease-specific mortality in the screening intervention group provides the most robust evidence of screening efficacy.[8,9] This enthusiasm is tempered by the observation that reducing the mortality

Table 1.4 *Definitions of terms which describe screening tests and their interpretation*

Term	Definition
True-negative	Non-diseased patient has a negative (normal) test
True-positive	Diseased patient has a positive (abnormal) test
False-negative	Diseased patient has a negative (normal) test
False-positive	Non-diseased patient has a positive (abnormal) test
Sensitivity (true-positive rate)	Probability that a diseased patient will have a positive (abnormal) test
Specificity (true-negative rate)	Probability that a non-diseased patient will have a negative (normal) test
Positive predictive value	Probability that a patient with a positive (abnormal) test does have the disease
Negative predictive value	Probability that a patient with a negative (normal) test does not have the disease

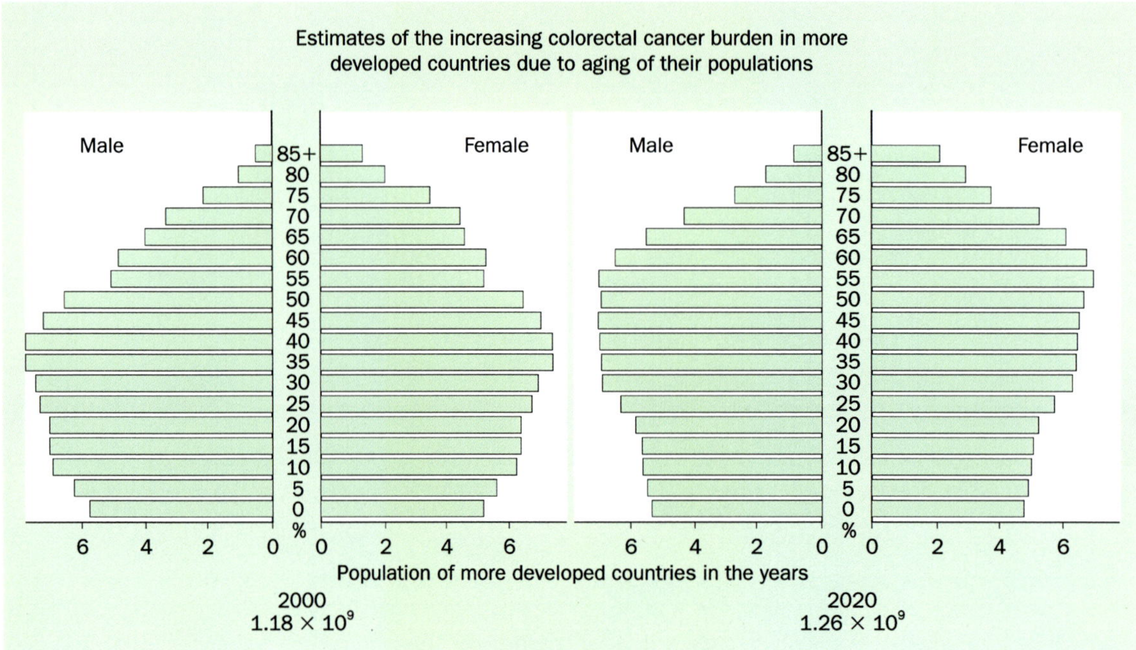

Figure 1.6 *Estimation of the future colorectal cancer prevalence in developed countries (including Europe, Northern America, Japan, Australia, and New Zealand), due to aging of their populations. Prepared from GLOBOCAN 2000, IARC Press, Lyon, 2001.*

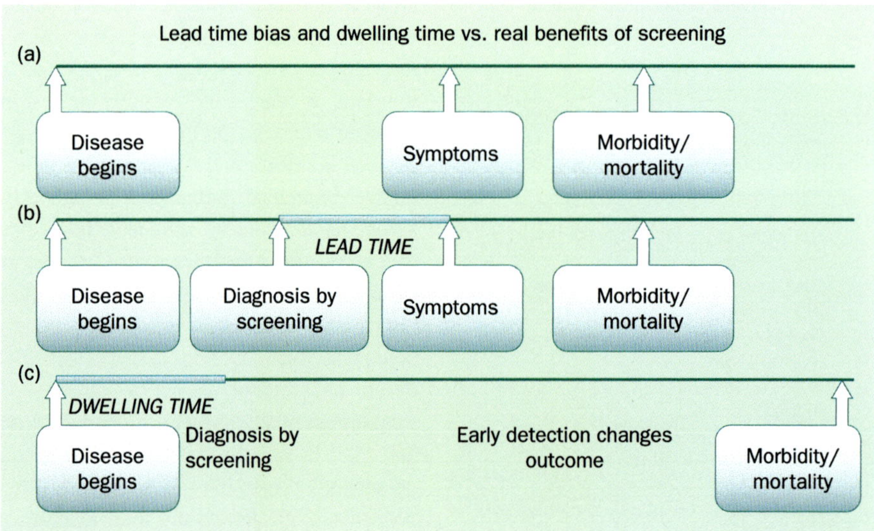

Figure 1.7 *Line (a) depicts the natural history of a disease in the absence of a screening test. Line (b) depicts the lead-time bias. Although the diagnosis of disease is made earlier with the screening test because of the lead time, the ultimate outcome of disease (morbidity/mortality) has not changed. Line (c) depicts the benefits of a good screening test. Timely early detection through screening changes the outcome by preventing or postponing morbidity/mortality from that disease.*

from one cause may not change overall mortality and prolong quality of life, as mortality is merely moved to another commonly occurring medical problem such as cardiovascular disease (see Chapter 10).

The best example of an accepted and promoted cancer-screening program is that of using mammography for breast cancer. This is actively promoted in many Western countries and has become the 'gold standard' when evaluating cost-effectiveness of other proposed cancer screening programs such as prostate or colorectal neoplasia screening. Colorectal cancer screening has an even better cost–benefit ratio than breast cancer screening (see Chapter 8).

Screening studies for colorectal cancer

See Chapter 8 for details on screening methodologies.

Fecal occult blood testing

Fecal occult blood testing (FOBT) meets the criteria for being an effective screening test for colorectal cancer. Four randomized trials have shown that FOBT is both efficacious and effective in lowering colorectal cancer mortality in individuals who undergo screening.[10–16]

Mandel and colleagues studied 46 551 participants aged 50–80 years old from the US state of Minnesota who agreed to be randomized to annual, biennial, or no screening for colorectal cancer with FOBT, using guaiac-impregnated paper slides with two smears from each of three consecutive stools. Eighty-three percent of slides were rehydrated. Participants with a positive test were evaluated with colonoscopy. The 13-year cumulative mortality per 1000 from colorectal cancer was 5.88 in the annually screened group, 8.33 in the biennially screened group, and 8.83 in the control group. Annual FOBT screening reduced the 13-year cumulative colorectal mortality by 33%. The number needed to screen annually, to prevent one death from colorectal cancer during the 13-year follow-up period, was 339 individuals.[10] After 18 years of follow-up, the annually screened group had a total of 417 colorectal cancers diagnosed, the biennially screened group 435, and the control group 507 colorectal cancers diagnosed. The cumulative incidence ratio for colorectal cancer was 0.80 in the annually screened group, and 0.83 in the biennially screened group, in comparison with the control group. These findings also support the hypothesis that screening leading to early identification and removal of neoplastic polyps decreases the incidence of, and ultimately mortality from, colorectal cancer.[11]

Kronborg and colleagues[12] randomized a population of 137 485 people aged 45–75 years old living in Funen, Denmark to (1) an invitation to biennial FOBT screening during a 10-year period (30 967), (2) no invitation to screening (30 966), or (3) non-enrollment in the study (75 552). After five rounds of screening (10 years) 481 people in the screened group had a diagnosis of colorectal cancer, compared with 483 in the unscreened control group. There were only 205 deaths attributable to colorectal cancer in the screened group, compared with 249 deaths in the control group, with a significant reduction in mortality of 18%. The number needed to screen biennially to prevent one death from colorectal cancer during the 10-year follow-up period was 704 individuals. After 9 rounds of screening the risk of dying from colorectal cancer was 11% lower in screened subjects compared with controls.[13] The reduction in effect size was attributed to some attrition in screening participation in the latter rounds of the study.

Hardcastle et al,[14] over a 10-year period, randomized a population of 152 850 individuals 45–74 years old living in the Nottingham area of the UK to biennial FOBT screening (76 466) or control (76 384). Median follow-up was 7.8 years. A total of 360 individuals died from colorectal cancer in the screened group, compared with 420 in the control group, with a significant 15% reduction in cumulative colorectal cancer mortality in the screened group. The number needed to screen biennially to prevent one death from colorectal cancer during the follow-up period in this study was 1275 individuals. A subsequent report after a median follow-up of 11 years found a 27% reduction in colorectal cancer mortality in the intervention group accepting screening.[15]

Faivre and colleagues,[16] in a French population-based, controlled study of biennial FOBT screening for colorectal cancer, allocated small-sized geographic areas, around Dijon, including 91 199 individuals aged 45–74 years old to invitation to screening, or no screening. The entire population was followed for 11 years. Six screening rounds were performed. Acceptability of the FOBT test was 52.8% in round one of screening, and ranged between 53.8% and 58.3% in subsequent rounds: 254 individuals died from colorectal cancer in the screened group, compared with 304 in the control group, with a

16% reduction in colorectal cancer mortality in the screened population.

The different effect sizes of these studies undoubtedly relate to the different screening methods used: unhydrated or rehydrated FOBT, test intervals, and different lengths of follow-up. The Minnesota study, with the greatest effect size (and smallest number needed to screen), had the shortest screening interval. The Funen study, with the smallest effect size (and largest number needed to screen), had the longer screening interval, and the longest follow-up period (Table 1.5).

Although the above-mentioned studies confirm the efficacy of FOBT colorectal cancer screening under study conditions, a recent demonstration pilot of FOBT screening in the UK (England and Scotland) supports the feasibility and effectiveness of population-based screening in a 'real world' setting. For the first round of screening, 478 250 residents of the pilot areas were invited to participate in the screening program, with 56.8% completing the FOBT screen. The overall rate of positive tests was 1.9% and the rate of detecting cancer was 1.62 per 1000 people screened. The positive predictive value was 10.9% for cancer and 35.0% for adenoma. Of 552 cancers detected by screening, 92 (16.6%) were polyp cancers; 48% of all screen detected cancers were Dukes' stage A, and only 1% had metastasized at the time of diagnosis.[17]

Screening sigmoidoscopy

The data on screening sigmoidoscopy are not quite as robust. There is one small randomized trial of this procedure. Thiis-Evensen and colleagues randomized 799 men and women aged 50–59 years old from the population registry of Telemark, Norway to an offer of a one-time screen with flexible sigmoidoscopy (400) or none (399): 81% of those invited accepted the screen. Individuals in whom polyps were identified underwent full colonoscopy and polypectomy, as well as surveillance colonoscopy 2 and 6 years later. All participants (intervention and control) received colonoscopy 13 years after initial randomization.[18] Two individuals in the intervention group and 10 individuals in the control group had developed colorectal cancer during the 13-year follow-up; 1 individual in the intervention group (who never had the sigmoidoscopy) and 3 in the control group died of colorectal cancer (number needed to screen to prevent one colorectal cancer death during 13 years = 200). Colonoscopy also demonstrated a preventive effect on the development of high-risk adenomas in the intervened group.[18]

Three case-control studies also provide evidence that screening sigmoidoscopy can reduce mortality from colorectal cancer. Selby and colleagues compared the screening history of individuals who died from colorectal cancer with that of matched controls. Rigid sigmoidoscopy was associated with a 59% reduction in risk of death from colorectal cancer located in a part of the colon reachable by the sigmoidoscope.[19] Newcomb and colleagues found an 80% reduction in the risk of death from rectosigmoid cancer in patients who had undergone one or more sigmoidoscopies, compared with those who had never done so.[20] Muller and Sonnenberg evaluated 4411 US veterans who died of colorectal cancer and matched controls, finding that proctosigmoidoscopy reduced mortality from colorectal cancer in the area examined by approximately 60%.[21] These studies suggest that sigmoidoscopy is efficacious in reducing colorectal cancer mortality risk.

The combination of FOBT and sigmoidoscopy, compared with sigmoidoscopy alone as a colorectal cancer screening strategy, was evaluated in one controlled trial. Patients

Table 1.5 *Summary of randomized controlled trials of screening for colon cancer with fecal occult blood testing (FOBT): their performance and efficacy*

Study	FOBT rehydration	Screening interval	Years of follow-up	Percent reduction in colorectal cancer mortality	No. needed to screen/cancer diagnosed
Mandel et al[10]	Yes	Annual	13	33	339
Kronborg et al[13]	No	Biennial	17	11	9091
Hardcastle et al[14]	No	Biennial	7.8	15	1275
Faivre et al[16]	No	Biennial	11	16	[a]

[a] Data provided do not allow calculation of number needed to screen.

were assigned to one or the other screening intervention according to the date of screening. Colorectal cancer mortality was lower in the group receiving the combined screening procedure.[22]

Randomized population trials of sigmoidoscopy, with or without FOBT, are taking place in the US, the UK, and Norway. There are no data available yet on the effect on colorectal cancer mortality.[23,24]

Screening colonoscopy

There are no results available from randomized studies of screening colonoscopy to demonstrate a significant reduction in colorectal mortality in the average risk population. A case-control study at Veterans Affairs hospitals in the United States found that patients with a diagnosis of colorectal cancer were less likely to have previously had a colonoscopy examination. The odds ratio for death from colorectal cancer was lower for patients with previous colonoscopy (0.43).[21] Also, the clinical evidence supporting screening colonoscopy is strong.[6,25] This has led to its inclusion by Medicare as an alternative screening method, once in 10 years, similar to what is available in Poland and Germany.[24,26] The Italian National Health Authorities have also made 5-yearly screening colonoscopy available for the average-risk population.[24]

Summary

The above trials and studies have provided the evidence for many countries to initiate colorectal cancer screening and for establishing the screening recommendations of the US Preventive Services Task Force, the American Cancer Society, and the American Gastroenterological Association.[25,27,28] These have been adopted by Medicare (the universal health insurance provided to US citizens from the age of 65 years old) (Table 1.6).[26] Similar screening programs, or their variations, have been initiated or are in place in other countries such as Germany, Poland, Czech Republic, United Kingdom, France, Italy, Japan, Australia, and Israel (Table 1.7).[24]

Compliance

Despite the proven efficacy of these screening tests for colorectal cancer, most individuals living in countries in which they are routinely recommended and offered do not participate in screening. In the United States, an analysis of the 2001 Behavior Risk Surveillance System conducted by the Centers for Disease Control and Prevention documented some improvement in use of colorectal cancer screening tests in the United States but underscored the need for efforts to further increase screening: only 23.5% reported receiving an FOBT within the previous 12 months;

Table 1.6 *Colorectal cancer screening tests covered by the US Medicare insurance plan*[a]

Patient risk status	FOBT[b]	Flexible sigmoidoscopy	Colonoscopy	Barium enema
Average risk (age = 50 years old)	Once every 12 months	Once every 48 months	Once every 10 years	May substitute for flexible sigmoidoscopy if physician determines that it will be equally effective for that individual
High risk (positive family history, previous colorectal cancer or precursor neoplastic polyps, history of inflammatory bowel disease, presence of appropriate gene markers, or other predisposing factors)			Once every 24 months	May substitute for colonoscopy if physician determines that it will be equally effective for that individual

[a]Adapted from reference 26.
[b]Fecal occult blood testing.

Table 1.7 Colorectal cancer screening in selected countries[a]

Country	Public health program	Pilot study	Screening method available or used		
			FOBT[b]	FS[c]	Colonoscopy
Australia	Planned	Yes	Yes		Yes
Austria	Yes		Yes		Yes
Croatia		Yes	Yes		
Czech Republic	Yes		Yes		
Denmark		Yes	Yes		
Finland	Yes		Yes		
France	Yes		Yes		
Germany	Yes		Yes		Yes
Hong Kong/China		Yes	Yes		Yes
Hungary		Yes	Yes		
Israel	Yes		Yes	Yes	Yes
Italy	Yes		Yes	Yes	Yes
Japan	Yes		Yes		Yes
Norway		Yes	Yes	Yes	
Poland	Yes				Yes
Slovakia	Yes		Yes		
Sweden		Yes	Yes		
Uruguay	Yes		Yes		
UK	Planned	Yes	Yes	Yes	

[a] Adapted from reference 24.
[b] *FOBT* = fecal occult blood test.
[c] *FS* = flexible sigmoidoscopy.

38.7% had received lower endoscopy within the past 5 years and 43.4% within the past 10 years; and 53.1% had received FOBT within the previous 12 months and/or lower endoscopy within 10 years.[29] Lieberman[30] has estimated that a 50% population compliance rate with an FOBT screening program would result in a 24% reduction in mortality from colorectal cancer. The issues of compliance for screening tests and implementation of screening by the treating physician are addressed in Chapter 10.

Symptoms and signs of colorectal cancer

Ideally, the majority of patients with colorectal cancer would be identified through screening, in an early, asymptomatic stage, with a high probability of cure. Regrettably, many patients today are still diagnosed because of symptoms of established disease, and only 37% of patients in the United States are found to have a localized stage of colorectal cancer at diagnosis.[7] Nonetheless, clinicians must remain alert for symptoms and signs that suggest the possibility of colorectal cancer, and be prepared to conduct the appropriate evaluation to rule out this disease.

Clinical presentation and evaluation

The clinical presentation of large-bowel cancer is dependent on its location within the colon and rectum, as well as the extent of spread. Right-sided lesions may present with abdominal pain, weakness (due to anemia), melena, and an abdominal mass. Left-sided lesions may also present with abdominal pain and melena, or bright red rectal bleeding, but constipation is also fairly common. Rectosigmoid and rectal lesions often present with bright red rectal bleeding, constipation, and tenesmus. Narrowing of the stool diameter is also common. The absence of constipation in the presence of right-sided lesions is due to the presence of liquid contents in the right side of the colon and the larger luminal capacity compared with the narrower lumen of the rectosigmoid and rectum.

The work-up of a patient with a suspected colorectal cancer includes a complete history, physical examination, and selected laboratory and radiologic tests. The history includes the patient's symptoms, prior removal of an adenoma or cancer, previous inflammatory bowel disease, and a family history of colorectal neoplasia or one of the inherited colorectal cancer syndromes. Physical examination may reveal evidence of Peutz–Jeghers or Gardner's syndrome or may suggest spread to the liver, peritoneal cavity, or lymph nodes. A digital rectal examination is necessary to determine the presence of a distal rectal cancer or of pelvic spread. In women, a thorough pelvic examination is required.

Laboratory tests may reveal liver enzyme abnormalities or iron deficiency anemia. In selected patients, a CEA (carcinoembryonic antigen) determination may be appropriate (see postoperative surveillance in Chapter 9).

Colonoscopy is the preferred approach for evaluating the patient with suspected large-bowel cancer. If this is not available or technically an incomplete examination, then computed tomography (CT) colonography will be useful to exclude significantly sized (>0.5–1 cm) mass lesions (see Figure 8.9). Another approach is to use flexible sigmoidoscopy followed by double-contrast barium enema. Colonoscopy is also indicated for examining patients in whom an abnormality has been detected on barium enema; in addition, the presence of synchronous cancers and adenomas can also be determined.

CT of the abdomen and pelvis may aid in determining the extent of spread. A chest radiograph will help to evaluate the possibility of lung metastasis. Endoscopic ultrasonography is being used more frequently to help in the staging of rectal cancers and depth of invasion can often be determined with accuracy (see Chapter 9).

The predictive value of common symptoms and signs

The frequency of presenting symptoms and signs varies by study and by location of the tumor in the bowel[31–34] (Tables 1.8 and 1.9). Of course, not all patients who present with these types of symptoms and signs have colorectal cancer: their positive predictive value for this disease is only moderate, and depends on the patient population. Studies evaluating patients with symptomatic rectal bleeding in general practice have shown positive predictive values for colon cancer ranging between 3.3% and 15.5%, and positive predictive values for adenomatous polyps ranging between 2.2% and 25%[35–37] (Table 1.10).

Rex[38] reviewed the literature on the diagnostic yield of colonoscopies performed on patients with various findings and symptoms suggestive of colorectal cancer. In 12 studies with a combined 1655 patients, reporting on colonoscopy results in patients with non-emergent rectal bleeding, the average prevalence of colorectal cancer was 11% (range 4–29%), and the average prevalence of adenomatous polyps was 22% (range 13–42%). In 4 studies with a combined 641 patients reporting on colonoscopy results in patients with symptoms of abdominal pain and/or change in bowel habits without rectal bleeding, the average prevalence of colon cancer was 2.8% (range 0–5%), and the average risk of adenomatous polyps was 16% (range 6–31%). Neugut and colleagues,[39] evaluated the diagnostic yield of colonoscopy for patients with abdominal pain, change in bowel habits, and rectal bleeding, referred to three colonoscopy practices in New York City between 1986 and 1989. Patients with rectal bleeding were again found to have a higher prevalence of colorectal cancer and adenomatous polyps than patients with other presenting symptoms (Table 1.11). Thus, it would appear that rectal bleeding is a more ominous symptom than are abdominal pain and/or change in bowel habits without rectal bleeding.

What is the appropriate work-up of a symptomatic patient?

There are three methods of imaging the entire colon: colonoscopy, flexible sigmoidoscopy plus double-contrast barium enema, or CT colonography. Colonoscopy is better for the detection of small adenomas, and provides opportunity for biopsy and polypectomy. Flexible sigmoidoscopy plus double-contrast barium enema has a sensitivity comparable to colonoscopy for detection of cancers and large polyps, and may be less expensive than colonoscopy in some settings. Irvine and colleagues[40] compared double-contrast barium enema plus flexible sigmoidoscopy vs colonoscopy in the evaluation of 71 patients with overt rectal bleeding. Patients were evaluated with all tests, and the results of the combination of tests were used as the gold standard. Colonoscopy was found to be 82% sensitive for diagnosing adenoma or carcinoma, compared with

Table 1.8 Frequency (%) of presenting symptoms and signs in patients diagnosed with colorectal cancer in different published series

Study	Rectal bleeding	Abdominal pain	Change in bowel habits	Anemia	Positive FOBT[a]
Majumdar et al[31]	58	52	51	57	77
Kyle et al[32]	44	41	56		
Speights et al[33]	34	22			

[a] FOBT, fecal occult blood test.

Table 1.9 Frequency (%) of presenting symptoms and signs of colorectal cancer, according to tumor location, in different series

Study	Tumor location	Abdominal pain	Rectal bleeding	Fatigue/ weakness	Weight loss	Change in bowel habits	Abnormal stools	Anemia	Abdominal mass	Abdominal tenderness	Rectal mass	Obstruction
Majumdar et al[31]	Proximal		73	31	46			70				
	Distal		70		34	30	30	47				
Lanier et al[34]	Proximal	62		38		30			37	28	23	
	Distal	42	68			68				12	61	18

a sensitivity of 73% for double-contrast barium enema plus flexible sigmoidoscopy. The positive predictive value of colonoscopy was 87%, compared to 91% for barium enema plus sigmoidoscopy. Jensen and colleagues[41] reported on the diagnostic accuracy of combined double-contrast barium enema plus rectosigmoidoscopy in the evaluation of 530 FOBT-positive patients identified through a randomized trial of colorectal cancer screening of the individuals aged 60–64 years old living in Funen County, Sweden. Patients with negative work-ups had repeat FOB testing, and positives underwent colonoscopy. Patients were followed longitudinally using local cancer and death registries. The combined test strategy was found to have a sensitivity of 90% for colorectal cancers, and a sensitivity of 96% for adenomas at least 1 cm in diameter. Rex and colleagues[42] randomized 380 patients with non-emergent rectal bleeding, aged 40 years old and over, to evaluation with flexible sigmoidoscopy plus air-contrast barium enema vs colonoscopy. Initial colonoscopy detected more polyps less than 9 mm in size, adenomas, and arteriovenous malformations, but fewer cases of diverticulosis. No significant difference was found between strategies in the number of patients found with cancers or polyps greater than 9 mm. Cancers were more common in subjects ≥55 years old (8%), than in younger subjects (1%). The authors conclude that flexible sigmoidoscopy plus air-contrast barium enema may be more cost-effective in evaluating patients <55 years old with rectal bleeding, but colonoscopy may be the more cost-effective strategy in older patients. In a subsequent study of similar design involving 156 patients with colorectal cancer symptoms without rectal bleeding, Rex and colleagues[43] found more adenomas in the initial colonoscopy group, but more diverticulosis in the sigmoidoscopy plus barium enema group. The overall prevalence of cancer (0.6%) and significant adenomas (4.6%) was low. The authors suggest that for this group of patients with symptoms other than rectal bleeding, sigmoidoscopy

Table 1.10 *The predictive value of rectal bleeding in the general practice setting*

Study	Study location	No. of patients	Patient ages (years)	Percent with cancer	Percent with polyps
Fijten et al[35]	Netherlands	269	18–75	3.3	2.2
Metcalf et al[36]	United Kingdom	99	>40	8	25
Norrelund and Norrelund[37]	Denmark	208	⩾40	15.5	7.7
Norrelund and Norrelund[37]	Denmark	156	⩾40	14.1	11.5

Table 1.11 *Diagnostic outcomes of colonscopies performed on referred patients with common symptoms of colorectal cancer*[a]

Symptom	No. of patients	Percent with colorectal cancer	Percent with adenomatous polyps
Rectal bleeding	861	8.6	25
Abdominal pain	113	4.4	17.7
Change in bowel habits	154	5.8	21.4
Abdominal pain and change in bowel habits	44	6.8	15.9

[a]Adapted from reference 39.

plus barium enema may be the more cost-effective evaluation strategy, especially for individuals under 55 years old.

Although colonoscopy is clearly the most sensitive test for evaluating patients with symptoms and signs suggestive of colorectal cancer, it may not always be readily available, or affordable. When this is the case, flexible sigmoidoscopy plus double-contrast barium enema may be an acceptable alternative diagnostic strategy. Because this testing strategy is less sensitive, every effort should be made to obtain a colonoscopy in symptomatic patients at highest risk of colorectal cancer: individuals ≥50 years old who present with rectal bleeding or anemia and follow-up after polypectomy.[44]

The third option, CT colonography is not yet widely available. Results published from dedicated specialist imaging units have been very favorable and equivalent to colonoscopy in identifying lesions greater than 0.5–1 cm.[45] An added advantage is the CT examination itself. It can identify extracolonic lesions that might benefit from treatment. The costs are anticipated to be lower than colonoscopy. The disadvantages, currently, are the limited experience with the methodology and the availability of quality performance. Clearly, the most important limitation is the inability to biopsy mass lesions and remove treatable polyps. There is no accepted policy of CT colonography as a screening test.

Conclusions

Colorectal cancer constitutes an important and increasing cause of morbidity and mortality worldwide. Efficacious and effective screening tests are available that improve disease outcomes. And yet, current compliance with screening recommendations is suboptimal, and needs to be improved. Clinicians must remain alert for symptoms and signs of established disease, as well. Patients displaying such findings should undergo complete visualization of the large intestine, preferably by colonoscopy.

References (*Reviews and general articles)

1. *Ferlay J, Bray F, Pisani P et al, GLOBOCAN 2002: Cancer Incidence, Mortality and Prevalence Worldwide, Version 2.0. IARC Cancer Base No. 5. Lyon: IARC Press, 2004. www.dep.iarc.fr/globocan/globoref.htm.
2. American Cancer Society, Cancer facts and figures 2004. http://www.cancer.org/downloads/STT/CAFF_finalPWSecured.pdf
3. Centers for Disease Control, Preventing chronic diseases: investing wisely in health. Screening to prevent cancer deaths. http://www.cdc.gov/nccdphp/pe_factsheets/pefs_cancer.pdf
4. Ries LAG, Eisner MP, Kosary CL et al (eds), SEER Cancer Statistics Review, 1975–2001, Bethesda, MD: National Cancer Institute, 2004. http://seer.cancer.gov//csr/1975_2001/.
5. Bonithon-Kopp C, Benhamiche AM, Are there several colorectal cancers? Epidemiological data. Eur J Cancer Prev 1999; 8: S3–S12.
6. *Winawer SJ, Zauber AG, Ho MN et al, Prevention of colorectal cancer by colonoscopic polypectomy. The National Polyp Study Workgroup. N Engl J Med 1993; 329: 1977–81.
7. Jemal A, Clegg LX, Ries LA et al, Annual report to the nation on the status of cancer, 1975–2001, with a special feature regarding survival. Cancer 2004; 101: 3–27.
8. *US Preventive Services Task Force, Screening for colorectal cancer. In: Guide to Clinical Preventive Services. Baltimore: Williams & Wilkins, 1996; 89–103.
9. The Canadian Task Force on the Periodic Health Examination. Screening for colorectal cancer. In: The Canadian Guide to Clinical Preventive Health Care (Solomon M, McLeod R, eds). Ottawa: Canada Communication Group—Publishing, 1994: 797–807.
10. Mandel JS, Bond JH, Church TR et al, Reducing mortality from colorectal cancer by screening for fecal occult blood. N Engl J Med 1993; 328: 1365–71.
11. *Mandel JS, Church TR, Bond JH et al, The effect of fecal occult-blood screening on the incidence of colorectal cancer. N Engl J Med 2000; 343: 1603–7.
12. Kronborg O, Fenger C, Olsen J et al, Randomised study of screening for colorectal cancer with faecal-occult-blood test. Lancet 1996; 348: 1467–71.
13. Kronborg O, Jorgensen OD, Fenger C et al, Randomized study of biennial screening with a faecal occult blood test: results after nine screening rounds. Scand J Gastroenterol 2004; 39: 846–51.
14. Hardcastle JD, Chamberlain JO, Robinson MHE et al, Randomised controlled trial of faecal-occult-blood screening for colorectal cancer. Lancet 1996; 348: 1472–7.
15. Scholefield JH, Moss S, Sufi F et al, Effect of faecal occult blood screening on mortality from colorectal cancer: results from a randomised controlled trial. Gut 2002; 50: 840–4.
16. Faivre J, Dancourt V, Lejeune C et al, Reduction in colorectal cancer mortality by fecal occult blood screening in a French controlled study. Gastroenterology 2004; 126: 1674–80.
17. UK Colorectal Cancer Screening Pilot Group. Results of the first round of a demonstration pilot of screening for colorectal cancer in the United Kingdom. BMJ 2004; 329: 133. doi:10.1136/bmj.38153.491887.7C (published 5 July 2004).
18. Thiis-Evensen E, Hoff GS, Sauar J et al, The effect of attending a flexible sigmoidoscopic screening program on the prevalence of colorectal adenomas at 13-year follow-up. Am J Gastroenterol 2001; 96: 1901–7.
19. Selby JV, Friedman GD, Quesenberry CP Jr et al, A case-control study of screening sigmoidoscopy and mortality from colorectal cancer. N Engl J Med 1992; 326: 653–7.
20. Newcomb PA, Norfleet RG, Storer BE et al, Screening sigmoidoscopy and colorectal cancer mortality. J Natl Cancer Inst 1992; 84: 1572–5.
21. Muller AD, Sonnenberg A, Prevention of colorectal cancer by flexible endoscopy and polypectomy. A case-control study of 32,702 veterans. Ann Intern Med 1995; 123: 904–10.
22. Winawer SJ, Flehinger BJ, Schottenfeld D et al, Screening for colorectal cancer with fecal occult blood testing and sigmoidoscopy. J Natl Cancer Inst 1993; 85: 1311–18.
23. *Rozen P, Cancer of the gastrointestinal tract: early detection or early prevention? Eur J Cancer Prev 2004; 13: 71–5.
24. Rozen P, Winawer SJ, Report of the OMED Colorectal Cancer Screening Committee Meeting, New Orleans, 2004—in collaboration with the IDCA. Eur J Cancer Prev 2004; 13: 461–4.
25. *Winawer S, Fletcher R, Rex D et al, Colorectal cancer screening and surveillance: clinical guidelines and rationale—update based on new evidence. Gastroenterology 2003; 124: 544–60.
26. Colorectal cancer screening, Medicare, http://www.cms.hhs.gov/media/press/release.asp?Counter=272
27. *US Preventive Services Task Force. Screening for colorectal cancer: recommendation and rationale. Ann Intern Med 2002; 137: 129–31.
28. *Smith RA, Cokkinides V, von Eschenbach AC et al, American Cancer Society guidelines for the early detection of cancer. CA Cancer J Clin 2002; 52: 8–22.
29. Centers for Disease Control and Prevention, Colorectal cancer test use among persons aged ≥50 years—United States, 2001. MMWR 2003; 52: 193–6.
30. Lieberman D, Mass screening: North American perspective. In: Prevention and Early Detection of Colorectal Cancer (Young GP, Rozen P, Levin B, eds). London: WB Saunders, 1996: 289–300.

31. Majumdar SR, Fletcher RH, Evans AT, How does colorectal cancer present? Symptoms, duration, and clues to location. Am J Gastroenterol 1999; 94: 3039–45.
32. Kyle SM, Isbister WH, Yeong ML, Presentation, duration of symptoms and staging of colorectal carcinoma. Aust N Z J Surg 1991; 61: 137–40.
33. Speights VO, Johnson MW, Stoltenberg PH et al, Colorectal cancer: current trends in initial clinical manifestations. South Med J 1991; 84: 575–8.
34. Lanier AP, Wychulis AR, Dockerty MB et al, Colorectal cancer in Rochester, Minnesota 1940–1969. Cancer 1973; 31: 606–15.
35. Fijten GH, Starmans R, Muris JWM et al, Predictive value of signs and symptoms for colorectal cancer in patients with rectal bleeding in general practice. Fam Pract 1995; 12: 279–86.
36. Metcalf JV, Smith J, Jones R et al, Incidence and causes of rectal bleeding in general practice as detected by colonoscopy. Br J Gen Pract 1996; 46: 161–4.
37. Norrelund N, Norrelund H, Colorectal cancer and polyps in patients aged 40 years and over who consult a GP with rectal bleeding. Fam Pract 1996; 13: 160–5.
38. Rex DK, Colonoscopy: a review of its yield for cancers and adenomas by indication. Am J Gastroenterol 1995; 90: 353–65.
39. Neugut AI, Garbowski GC, Waye JD et al, Diagnostic yield of colorectal neoplasia with colonoscopy for abdominal pain, change in bowel habits, and rectal bleeding. Am J Gastroenterol 1993; 88: 1179–83.
40. Irvine EJ, O'Connor J, Frost RA et al, Prospective comparison of double contrast barium enema plus flexible sigmoidoscopy v colonoscopy in rectal bleeding: barium enema v colonoscopy in rectal bleeding. Gut 1988; 29: 1188–93.
41. Jensen J, Kewenter J, Asztely M et al, Double contrast barium enema and flexible rectosigmoidoscopy: a reliable diagnostic combination for detection of colorectal neoplasm, Br J Surg 1990; 77: 270–2.
42. Rex DK, Weddle RA, Lehman GA et al, Flexible sigmoidoscopy plus air contrast barium enema versus colonoscopy for suspected lower gastrointestinal bleeding. Gastroenterology 1990; 98: 855–61.
43. Rex DK, Mark D, Clarke B et al, Flexible sigmoidoscopy plus air-contrast barium enema versus colonoscopy for evaluation of symptomatic patients without evidence of bleeding. Gastrointest Endosc 1995; 42: 132–8.
44. Winawer SJ, Stewart ET, Zauber AG et al, A comparison of colonoscopy and double-contrast barium enema for surveillance after polypectomy. National Polyp Study Work Group. N Engl J Med 2000; 342: 1766–72.
45. Pickhardt PJ, Choi R, Hwang I et al, Computed tomographic virtual colonoscopy to screen for colorectal neoplasia in asymptomatic adults. N Engl J Med 2003; 349: 2191–200.

2 What are the risk factors associated with colorectal cancer? An overview

Paul Rozen, Stephen J Spann, Graeme P Young, Bernard Levin

Introduction

In Chapter 1, colorectal cancer has been identified as a worldwide major medical problem in the established industrialized countries and also in those countries undergoing industrialization and adopting a Western lifestyle (Figure 2.1).[1,2] For some decades, the United States, which is a high incidence area, has recognized its public health importance. There, the incidence has recently shown a downturn, possibly because of the change in lifestyle and dietary habits that have also reduced the incidence of cardiovascular disease. Mortality has also declined, mainly in the US white population, and this reflects both its earlier diagnosis and improved therapy in the United States and in some of Western Europe (Figure 2.2; see also Figure 1.5).[3,4] This high incidence is also found in those ethnically diverse and non-Western countries such as Japan, Singapore, Hong Kong, and Israel and occurs within one or two generations in immigrants moving from low-incidence colorectal cancer countries to host countries of high incidence. From this, epidemiologists quickly concluded that acquired environmental and lifestyle factors must be the major etiologic causes.[5]

The main environmental culprit was identified as being the Western lifestyle and diet; however, in addition, it was clear that irrespective of diet certain families were at risk for colorectal cancer. These two major etiologies of colorectal cancer, acquired and inherited, are discussed more fully in Chapters 4 and 6 of this book and their references. This chapter will therefore be a synopsis of recognized risk factors and their relative contributions to the overall occurrence of colorectal cancer (Table 2.1). For simplicity, in this chapter, colon and rectum, cancer and adenomatous polyps, are considered as one entity, although there are slight differences in epidemiology for each of them.

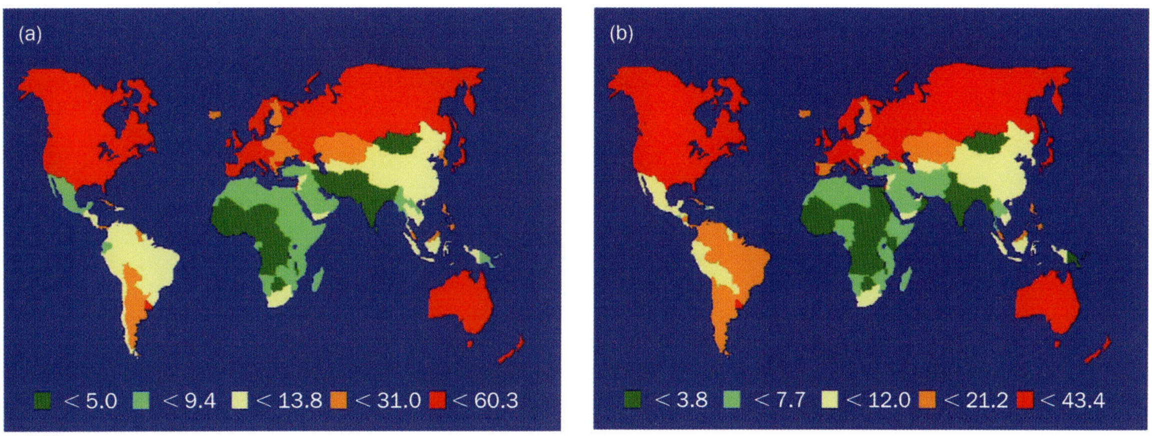

Figure 2.1 *Colorectal cancer incidence in (a) males and (b) females worldwide in 2002, derived from GLOBOCAN 2002[1] and prepared by Ms S Bayua and Dr A Zauber, New York.*

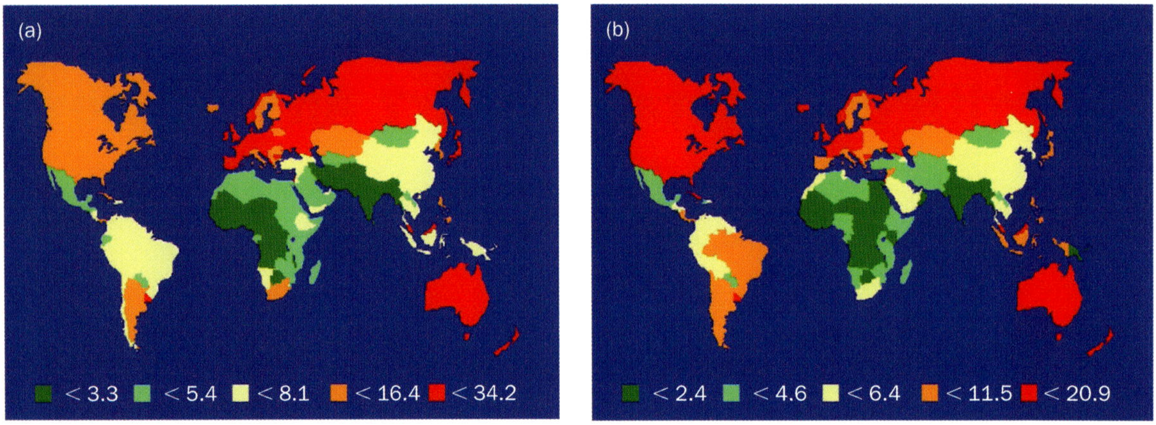

Figure 2.2 *Colorectal cancer mortality in (a) males and (b) females worldwide in 2002, derived from GLOBOCAN 2002[1] and prepared by Ms S Bayua and Dr A Zauber, New York.*

Table 2.1 *Genetic, dietary, lifestyle, personal and past history risk factors and an estimation of their relative contributions to the overall occurrence of colorectal neoplasia in industrialized countries*

Risk factor	Minimal	Minor	Moderate	Major
Inherited, dominant			+	
Inherited, recessive or low-penetrant			+	
Aging				+
Gender male		+		
Occupation	+			
Diet				+
Frequent meals	+			
Obesity, body build		+		
Physical activity, decreased			+	
Tobacco smoking		+		
Alcohol intake, chronic		+		
Laxative abuse, chronic	+			
Iron supplements, chronic	+			
Past colorectal cancer		+		
Past adenomatous polyp			+	
Inflammatory bowel disease, chronic and extensive		+		
Diabetes mellitus		+		
Cholecystectomy	+			
Acromegaly	+			
Breast, ovarian cancer, radiation therapy	+			

It is clear that there is no one major environmental factor that explains all the risk for colorectal cancer, and extensive evidence points to the etiology of large-bowel neoplasia as being multifactorial in origin. It may be easier to visualize the relationships of these etiologic factors if we think of the 'stepwise' progression to cancer as follows: factors initiating the expression of epithelial dysplasia, factors promoting adenomatous polyp growth, factors promoting progressive dysplasia, and factors allowing cancer to occur (Figure 2.3).

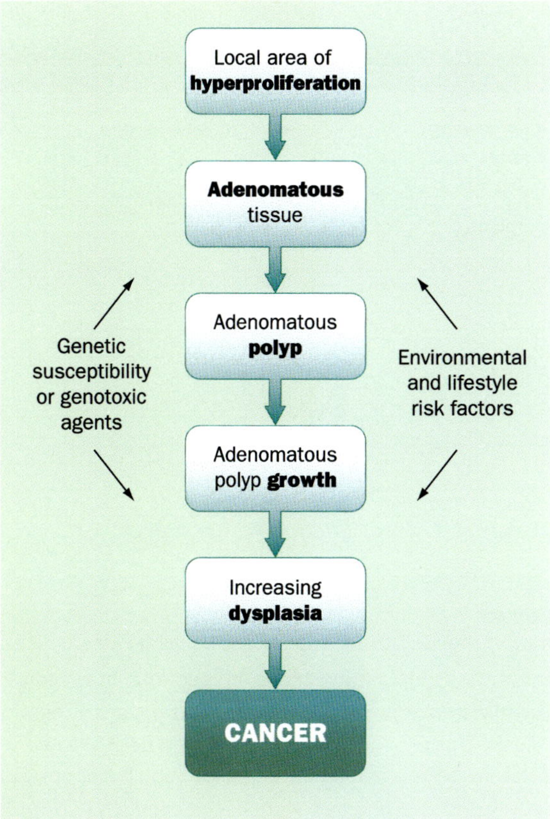

Figure 2.3 *Schematic representation of the stepwise progression with time to adenoma, to increasing dysplasia, and finally to cancer.*

Major risk factors

Diet

A consistently high caloric intake leading to obesity, especially if associated with low physical activity, are both factors associated with risk for colorectal cancer. The evidence is tenuous that eating frequent meals and therefore continuously promoting the flow of potentially carcinogenic bile salts is associated with a higher risk for large bowel cancer.[5] Specific dietary risk factors include a *high* intake of animal fat and beef and eating it fried or charred. On the other hand, risk is also associated with a *low* intake of grains, fruits, and vegetables, which contain protective dietary fiber, minerals, vitamins, and bioactive compounds. Minerals such as calcium, found mainly in dairy products, are also protective, as is also an adequate fluid intake. For more details, see Chapter 4 and its references.

The World Cancer Research Fund estimates that of the almost 1 000 000 cases occurring annually, 70% is preventable by following the ideal diet and exercise lifestyle.[6]

Inherited risk factors

Inherited risk factors include the defined genetic syndromes such as the Lynch syndrome (hereditary non-polyposis colorectal cancer), familial adenomatous polyposis, familial juvenile polyposis, and the Peutz–Jeghers syndromes. More common, but so far less well understood, is the familial clustering of colorectal and, or, other neoplasia, or the added risk of even having just a single first-degree relative with large-bowel cancer or adenomatous polyps. This is obviously a common occurrence, and probably points to the presence of a large pool of inherited genetic susceptibility factors in the general population.[5]

About 3–5% of all colorectal cancer is due to the defined syndromes. How much is due to weaker inherited factors is very unclear, but probably at least 10%. These conditions are discussed in detail in Chapter 6.

Genetic–environmental interaction

It has been hypothesized that exposure to environmental risk factors, especially in the diet, can facilitate the clinical expression of recessive or low-penetrance inherited genetic etiologies of colorectal cancer, or influence the age at which it appears. This might explain why some cases of colorectal cancer occur within the generation of persons who migrated from low-incidence countries such as Southern Greece or Italy to high-incidence areas such as Australia or the United States.[5] Commonly inherited systemic (germline) genetic variations (polymorphisms) can influence the rates of detoxification or activation of environmental carcinogens (Table 2.2) such as those that are created during the process of cooking, or from tobacco smoke, or alcohol metabolites. Also, there may be a concomitant lack of adequate amounts of dietary anticarcinogens, in the presence of an inability to metabolize these carcinogens.[5,7] This is an attractive explanation, but it is still uncertain that these genetic polymorphisms, i.e. minor variations in gene structure that do not lead to genetic disorders, represent a major contribution to the etiology of large-bowel neoplasia.

Table 2.2 *Examples of interactions between environmental factors and metabolic phenotype in the etiology of colorectal neoplasia*[a]

Risk factor	Inadequate or disordered metabolic pathway	Result of perturbation
Red meat and high-temperature cooking	Acetylation of heterocyclic amines	Tumor induction
Folate/methionine deficiency, chronic alcoholism	Methylation, thymidine synthesis	DNA damage and uncorrected mutations
Tobacco smoke	Glutathione conjugation, cytochrome enzyme AHH	DNA damage
Iron in meat, excessive intake	Hemochromatosis mutation	Excess free radicals

[a]Adapted from references 5 and 7.

How much risk do these major factors contribute to colorectal neoplasia?

At present, we can deduce that the etiology of more than 30% of large-bowel neoplasia is related directly to the environment, namely diet and lifestyle of industrialized (westernized) populations. Because of the family history of colorectal neoplasia, it is estimated that the etiology of more than 15% is inherited and the remainder are a result of an interaction between these etiologies (Figure 2.4).[5,7]

Other known risk factors

In this section we consider other risk factors for colorectal neoplasia. Even so, their quantitative contributions to the total cancer burden are relatively small compared with diet and genetic factors (see Table 2.1).

Demographic characteristics

Occupation

The only clear association of occupation with colorectal cancer is that of brewery workers who were given free access to their products.[5,8] There have been reports that asbestos workers were at slightly increased risk for colorectal neoplasia, but the overall evidence was not strong.[9] Today, because of public health measures preventing exposure to asbestos, this is not of clinical relevance.

Gender

On a country-to-country basis, the incidence of colorectal cancer is almost always higher in men than in women.[1–3] This difference is even greater for rectal cancer than for colonic cancer. These differences may be explained by different dietary and lifestyle habits, body build, physical activity, tobacco and alcohol use, consumption of NSAIDs (non-steroidal anti-inflammatory drugs), and body stores of iron. There is also a protective effect associated with

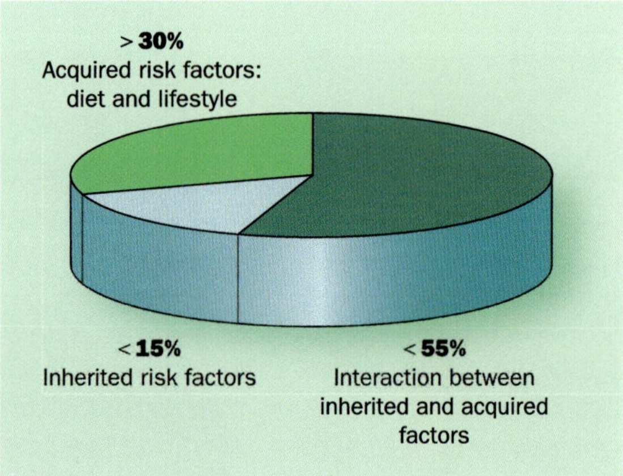

Figure 2.4 *Schematic representation of the relative contributions of acquired and inherited factors in the etiology of colorectal cancer and the interaction between them.*

the female premenopausal hormones and, at least temporarily, by the use of hormone replacement therapy (see Chapter 5).[5]

Age

The cumulative causes of colorectal neoplastic changes (see Figure 2.3) manifest themselves clinically as cancer in the later half of life (see Chapter 3). The incidence of colorectal cancer rises almost exponentially from the age of 50 years, and continues to rise dramatically for the duration of the population's lifespan (Figure 2.5).[10] About half will be diagnosed after the age of 65 years. Mortality rates increase in parallel at about 50% of the incidence in most Western countries, but more so in Eastern Europe, and show the same dramatic rise with aging. For those reasons, early detection programs are initiated at the age of 50 years and must be continued intensively throughout the life of the healthy aging, who are also at risk for a second primary colorectal cancer.[11]

Body build

Cancer risk and even the response to therapy (see Chapter 4) are associated with excess weight. In addition, the body mass index (BMI), which takes into account both height and weight (weight/height^2), and reflects the influence of growth factors, is also a risk factor for colorectal neoplasia when elevated.[5,12]

Lifestyle habits and medications

Physical activity

Industrialization and westernization has led to a marked decrease in physical activity for both work and even daily needs. This has been replaced, or at least supplemented, by engaging in recreational physical activity. Such activities have been shown to reduce the risks for colorectal cancer, even in older adults, and should be promoted, optimally from youth, and maintained throughout adult life.[13]

Tobacco smoking

The association is strongest for an increased prevalence of adenomas and less strong for risk of large-bowel cancer.[14] Even so, adenomas are potential precursors of cancers, and so tobacco smoking should also be considered in the etiology of colorectal cancer.

Alcohol

There is a weak association between alcohol consumption and risk for colon cancer.[8] The association is more consistent with rectal cancer, especially from beer drinking in most countries, but also for sake in Japan.[8] It is postulated that in the colon, the acetaldehyde metabolite of alcohol causes damage to the DNA and to the DNA protective dietary folic acid (see Chapter 4). There are individuals who cannot detoxify this metabolite and are therefore genetically susceptible.[15]

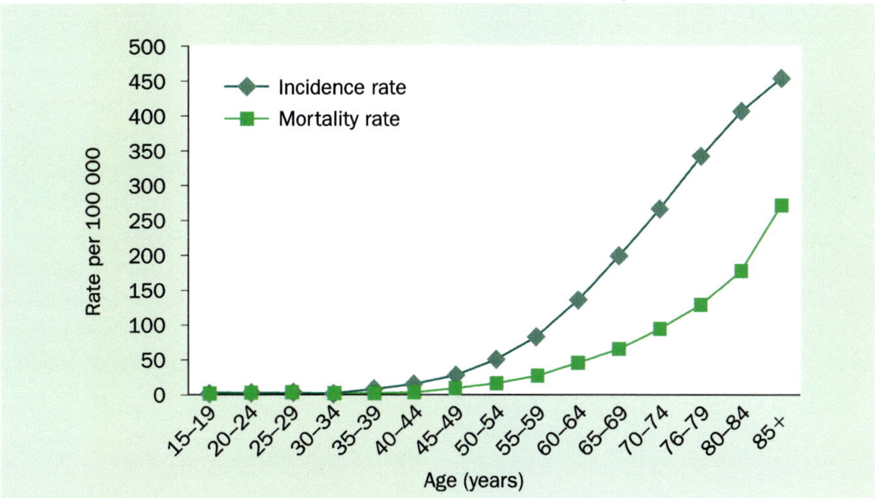

Figure 2.5 *Age-specific colorectal cancer incidence and mortality in the US general population, 1997–2001, age adjusted to the year 2000 US population. Note the sharp rise in incidence and mortality, with increasing age, after the age 50 years. Prepared by Ms S Bayuga and Dr A Zauber and derived from reference 10.*

Laxative usage

Chronic constipation had not been regarded as a risk factor for colon neoplasia, although there are now some studies to indicate this possibility.[16] In addition, there are also some reports that have identified the chronic ingestion of phenolphthalein, and especially senna-containing laxatives, as being a minor risk factor for large-bowel epithelial hyperproliferation and even being associated with a risk for cancer.[17]

Iron supplements and hemochromatosis

To date, physicians have believed that for optimal health the body stores of iron should be maintained full. There is some experimental and epidemiologic evidence that chronic iron supplementation is a minor risk factor for cancer of various sites, including the large bowel.[18,19] One suggested mechanism is that unabsorbed dietary iron produces free radicals, which can cause mucosal damage.[19] A similar increased risk has also been noted to occur in persons found to be heterozygous for hereditary hemochromatosis, but who do not manifest the disease, a condition that is estimated to occur in 15% of the American population.[20]

Personal history of disease

Inflammatory bowel disease

Chronic and extensive inflammatory bowel disease (IBD), which therefore leads to an increased turnover of epithelial cells, is associated with an increased risk for bowel cancer.[21] The risk is greater for ulcerative colitis than for Crohn's colitis. The longer the duration of disease, more than 8 years, and the more extensive the area of inflammation, more than the rectosigmoid, the greater the risk for cancer. However, with intensive and systematic medical therapy and earlier surgery, the cancer risk and mortality from colorectal cancer have decreased.[21] This is discussed more fully in Chapter 7.

Acromegaly

Acromegaly is an uncommon disorder that results from the pituitary gland secreting an excessive amount of growth hormone. This condition has been found to be associated with a significant risk for both colorectal adenomas and cancer.[22]

Diabetes mellitus

Meta-analyses of morbidity and mortality in diabetes mellitus patients showed that they had a slightly increased risk for colorectal cancer.[23] A prospective follow-up of HbA1c levels, which reflects average blood glucose levels over the preceding 3 months, in 10 000 individuals, demonstrated a significant correlation with risk for colorectal cancer.[24] Both the growth factor effect of hyperinsulinemia and systemic effects of hyperglycemia have been proposed to explain this.

Cholecystectomy

Several large population studies of women post-cholecystectomy confirmed that they are at slightly increased risk for right-sided colon cancer, 15 or more years after surgery.[25] It has been suggested that this was due to the constant free entry of bile into that site.

Breast and ovarian cancer, radiation therapy

Women who survive a breast or ovarian malignancy are at a slightly increased risk, about 1.5–2 times that expected, of developing a large-bowel malignancy.[26,27] The risk is probably related to unrecognized inherited risk factors and, or, common etiologic dietary and lifestyle causes.[28] A similar, slightly increased risk for colorectal cancer can also be found in first-degree relatives of breast cancer patients.[26] In the case of cervical or ovarian cancer, radiation therapy might have contributed to the appearance of rectal cancer.[27,29]

Past colorectal cancer or adenomatous polyp

Metachronous large-bowel cancer can appear in persons after successful surgery for a colorectal cancer. This is a lifetime risk and has been calculated as being 0.35% per year.[30] Similarly, persons who have had an adenomatous polyp are at risk for further polyps. This risk is least in persons having had a single small tubular adenoma without high-grade dysplasia, whereas there is an increased risk if the adenomatous polyps were large, sessile, multiple, villous, or showed high-grade dysplasia, and if there was a family history of colorectal neoplasia.[31] The magnitude of risk conferred varies from no increase to eight-fold, depending on the type of adenoma (see Chapter 7 for more details).

Human polyomavirus–JC virus

Infection with the polyomavirus is ubiquitous. There is some evidence for its oncogenic potential, and JCV gene sequences have been detected in colon cancer tissue.[32] The role of this virus, if any, in colon carcinogenesis, remains to be defined.

Conclusions

From the above review, it can be seen that some conditions are associated with a sizable increase in risk, whereas many conditions are associated with a slightly increased risk for colorectal cancer (see Table 2.1). However, the individual overall contributions to the total cancer burden, of the latter, are small. One must not lose sight that of the two most important etiologies that we know about, one is acquired (diet and lifestyle), and the other is inherited (susceptibility), and that they appear to interact. Prevention, therefore, is aimed at recognizing this susceptibility, correcting acquired risk habits, and detecting treatable neoplasia as early as possible.

References (*Reviews and general articles)

1. Ferlay J, Bray F, Pisani P et al, GLOBOCAN 2002: Cancer Incidence, Mortality and Prevalence Worldwide, Version 2.0. IARC Cancer Base No. 5. Lyon: IARC Press, 2004: www.dep.iarc.fr/globocan/globoref.htm.
2. Sant M, Capocaccia R, Coleman MP et al, Cancer survival increases in Europe, but international differences remain wide. Eur J Cancer 2001; 37: 1659–67.
3. Jemal A, Thomas A, Murray T et al, Cancer statistics, 2002. CA Cancer J Clin 2002; 52: 23–47.
4. Gatta G, Ciccolallo L, Capocaccia R et al, Differences in colorectal cancer survival between European and US populations: the importance of sub-site and morphology. Eur J Cancer 2003; 39: 2214–22.
5. *Potter JD, Epidemiologic, environmental and lifestyle issues in colorectal cancer. In: Prevention and Early Detection of Colorectal Cancer (Young GP, Rozen P, Levin B, eds). London: WB Saunders, 1996: 23–43.
6. *Food, Nutrition and the Prevention of Cancer: A global perspective. World Cancer Research Fund/American Institute for Cancer Research, Washington, DC: Banta Books, 1997.
7. *Gertig DN, Hunter DJ, Genes and environment in the etiology of colorectal cancer. Semin Cancer Biol 1998; 8: 285–98.
8. *Kune GA, Vitetta L, Alcohol consumption and the etiology of colorectal cancer: a review of the scientific evidence from 1957 to 1991. Nutr Cancer 1992; 18: 97–111.
9. Gamble JF, Asbestos and colon cancer: a weight-of-the-evidence review. Environ Health Perspect 1994; 102: 1038–50.
10. Surveillance, Epidemiology and End Results (SEER) Program, Database released April 2004, 1973–2001. Bethesda, MD: National Cancer Institute, http://seer.cancer.gov.
11. Shureqi I, Cooksley CD, Morris J et al, Effect of age on risk of second primary colorectal cancer. J Natl Cancer Inst 2001; 93: 1264–6.
12. *MacInnis RJ, English DR, Hopper JL et al, Body size and composition and colon cancer risk in men. Cancer Epidemiol Biomarkers Prev 2004; 13: 553–9.
13. Chao A, Connell CJ, Jacobs EJ et al., Amount, type, and timing of recreational physical activity in relation to colon and rectal cancer in older adults: the Cancer Prevention Study II nutrition cohort. Cancer Epidemiol Biomarkers Prev 2004; 3: 2187–95.
14. *Terry MB, Neugut AI, Cigarette smoking and the colorectal adenoma-carcinoma sequence: a hypothesis to explain the paradox. Am J Epidemiol 1998; 147: 903–10.
15. Murato M, Tagawa M, Watanabe S et al, Genotype difference of aldehyde dehydrogenase 2 gene in alcohol drinkers influences the incidence of Japanese colorectal cancer patients. Jpn J Cancer Res 1999; 90: 711–19.
16. Roberts MC, Millikan RC, Galanko JA et al, Constipation, laxative use, and colon cancer in a North Carolina population. Am J Gastroenterol 2003; 98: 857–64.
17. *van Gorkom BAAP, de Vries EGE, Karrenbeldd A et al, Anthranoid laxatives and their potential carcinogenic effects. Aliment Pharmacol Ther 1999; 13: 443–52.
18. *Stevens RG, Jones Y, Micozzi MS et al, Body iron stores and the risk of cancer. N Engl J Med 1988; 319: 1047–52.
19. Lund EK, Wharf SG, Fairweather-Tait SJ et al, Oral ferrous sulfate supplements increase the free radical-generating capacity of feces from healthy volunteers. Am J Clin Nutr 1999; 69: 250–5.
20. Nelson RL, Davis FG, Persky V et al, Risk of neoplastic and other diseases among people with heterozygosity for hereditary hemochromatosis. Cancer 1995; 76: 875–79.
21. *Munkholm P, Review article: the incidence and prevalence of colorectal cancer in inflammatory bowel disease. Aliment Pharmacol Ther 2003; 18(Suppl. 2): 1–5.
22. Ron E, Gridley G, Hrubec Z et al, Acromegaly and gastrointestinal cancer. Cancer 1991; 68: 1673–77.
23. *Chang CK, Ulrich CM, Hyperinsulinaemia and hyperglycaemia: possible risk factors of colorectal cancer among diabetic patients, Diabetologia 2003; 46: 595–607.
24. Khaw KT, Wareham N, Bingham S et al, Preliminary communication: glycated hemoglobin, diabetes, and incident colorectal cancer in men and women: a prospective analysis from the European prospective investigation into cancer—Norfolk Study. Cancer Epidemiol Biomarkers Prev 2004; 13: 915–19.

25. *Ekbom A, Yuen J, Adami H-O et al, Cholecystectomy and colorectal cancer. Gastroenterology 1993; 105: 142–7.
26. Howell MA, The association between colorectal cancer and breast cancer. J Chron Dis 1976; 29: 243–61.
27. Travis LB, Curtis RE, Boice JD Jr et al, Second malignant neoplasms among long-term survivors of ovarian cancer. Cancer Res 1996; 56: 1564–70.
28. Meijers-Heijboer H, Wijnen J, Vasen H et al, The *CHEK2* 1100delC mutation identifies families with an hereditary breast and colorectal cancer phenotype. Am J Hum Genet 2003; 72: 1308–14. Epub 2003 Apr 10.
29. Boice JD Jr, Day NE, Andersen A et al, Second cancers following radiation treatment for cervical cancer. An international collaboration among cancer registries. J Natl Cancer Inst 1985; 74: 955–75.
30. Cali RL, Pitsch PM, Thorson AAG et al, Cumulative incidence of metachronous colorectal cancer. Dis Colon Rectum 1993; 36: 388–93.
31. *Bochud M, Burnand B, Froehlich F et al, Appropriateness of colonoscopy: surveillance after polypectomy. Endoscopy 1999; 31: 654–63.
32. Niv Y, Goel A, Boland R, JC virus and colorectal cancer—a possible trigger in the chromosomal instability pathway. Curr Opin Gastroenterol 2004; 21: 85–9.

3 How does colorectal cancer develop?

Graeme P Young, Paul Rozen, Bernard Levin

Introduction

Colorectal cancer results from a series of genomic alterations that result in transformation of a normal epithelial cell into an adenocarcinoma. The process of development of colorectal cancer is characterized by a progressively disordered genome and perturbed biology. This process is subject to regulation, however, and involves interactions between the epithelial cell and its environment; these interactions are shown conceptually in Figure 3.1.[1] Both inherent genetic and externally determined environmental factors are important in colorectal oncogenesis (the process of development of a tumor) (see Chapter 2).[1,2] The colonic luminal environment is complex and subject to great variability, largely due to diet. It is not surprising therefore, that dietary lifestyle is important.[2] Variations in dietary lifestyle account for the characteristic international epidemiology of this disease, where colorectal cancer is more common in countries that follow, or are moving towards, a Western dietary lifestyle.[2]

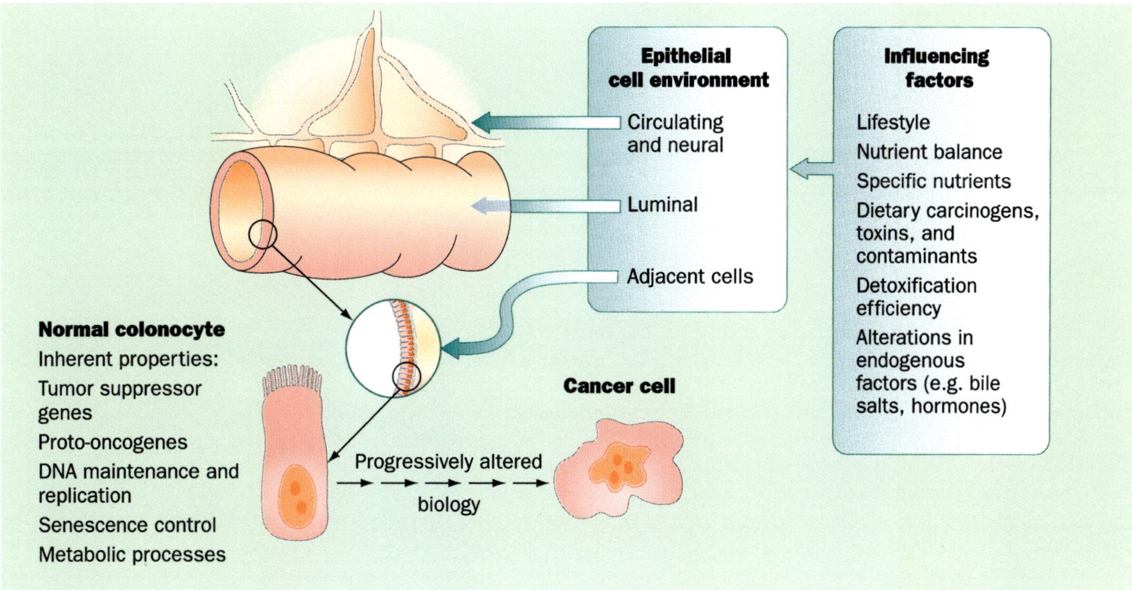

Figure 3.1 *Conceptual representation of interactions between the colonic epithelial cell and its environment. Influencing agents may be endogenous or exogenous in origin, with endogenous agents being affected by exogenous influences (e.g. bile salts by dietary fats). The epithelial environment is complex, with many variables and influencing agents acting via the lumen. The cell is not a passive target, and contains inherent protective processes that become disordered or overwhelmed as the progressively altered biology of oncogenesis is set in motion.*

The biology of gastrointestinal neoplasia is complex and involves concepts such as tumor genetics, multistage carcinogenesis, genomic alterations, oncogene activation, tumor suppressor gene inactivation, expansion of clones of neoplastic cells, homeostatic control of cell growth, and cell invasion. The purpose of this chapter is to provide a simplified presentation of these concepts to aid understanding of their relevance to primary prevention, early detection, and the clinical approach to management. The applied clinical genetics is presented in subsequent chapters, as is the approach to dietary prevention.

The biology of the colorectal cancer cell

In simple terms, four key biologic processes, as conceptualized in Figure 3.2a,b and c, are critical to normal behavior of a cell:[3]

1. Cell proliferation, regulated by checkpoints in the cell cycle.
2. Cell mortality, regulated by an inherent cellular process called programmed cell death or apoptosis.
3. Cell relationships with the immediate environment, i.e. cell-to-cell and intracellular signaling pathways.
4. Cell position, i.e. its anchorage to basement membrane in a normal cellular architecture.

In a cancer cell, proliferation and apoptosis (collectively often referred to simply as 'growth') plus relationship to environment and cell locale, are likely to be disturbed (Figure 3.2b).[4]

Proliferation—cell cycle checkpoints

The cycle of cell replication consists of five phases, which are critical to cancer development (Figure 3.2c).[4] The total

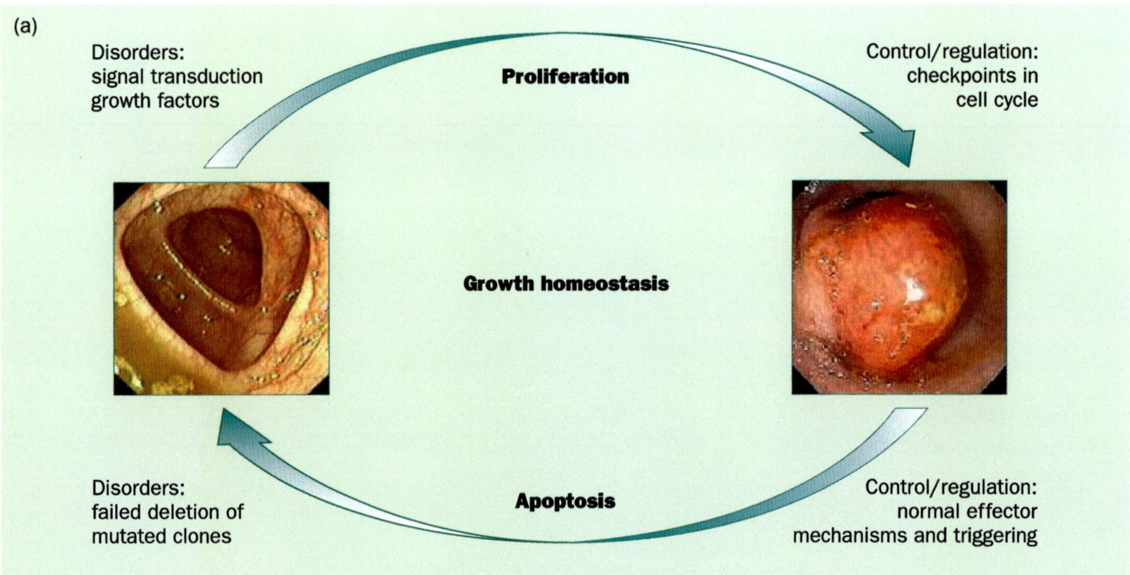

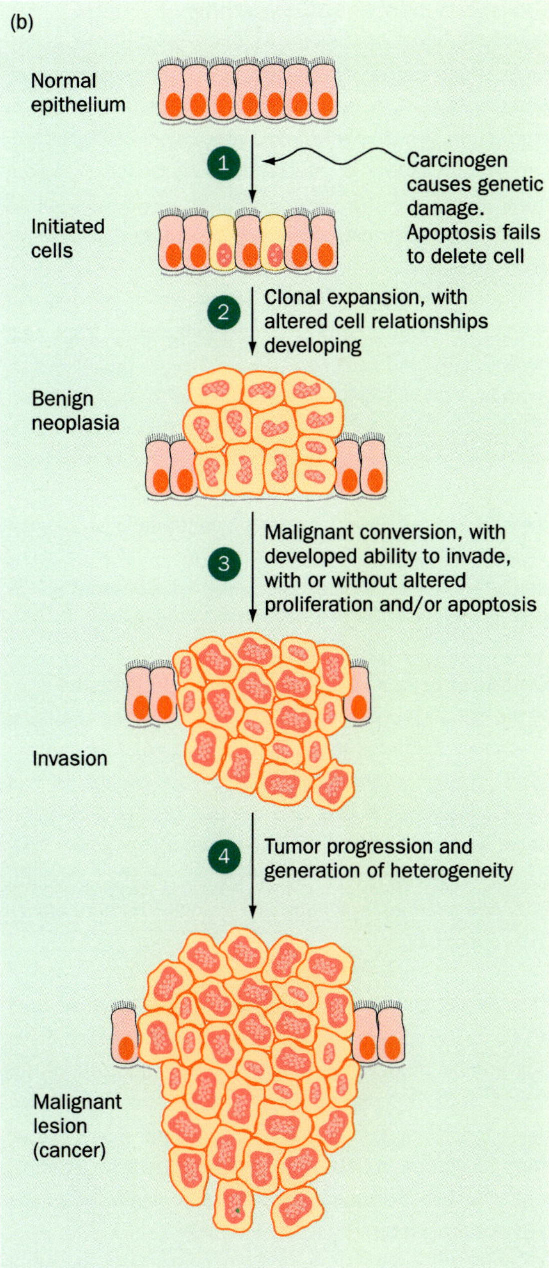

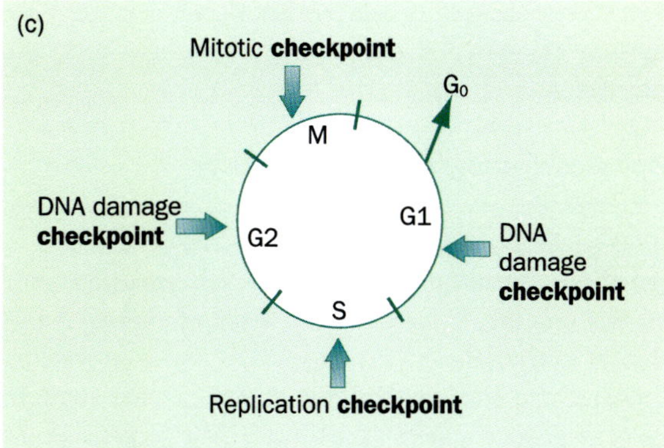

Figure 3.2 *Main biological processes inherent in control of cellular normality. (a) Conceptualization of growth control by regulated proliferation and apoptosis. (b) Conceptualization of morphologic progression through oncogenesis, incorporating altered cell relationships and invasion through basement membrane. Adapted from reference 3, with permission of publishers Lippincott, Williams, and Wilkins. (c) Diagrammatic representation of the cell cycle with its phases and the key checkpoints that control genomic stability: M, mitosis, S, synthesis; G_0, terminal differentiation; G_1 resting; G_2, preparation for mitosis.*

duration varies from 12 to 48 hours, depending on conditions causing changes in duration of G_1 (the resting phase). In the colonic crypt, 10–20% of cells are capable of DNA synthesis and chromosomal duplication (the S phase), at any one time. They then move into G_2, which is the preparation for cell division, and then mitosis, or the M phase. Following this, cells return to G_1. A controlled proportion of cells exit the cycle at G_1 for G_0, where they undergo terminal differentiation and eventual apoptosis (cell death). Various cell cycle checkpoint proteins regulate this ordered process.

In cancer cells, it is becoming increasingly apparent

that these checkpoints become disordered, with the result that proliferation and apoptosis are no longer controlled processes.

Apoptosis—programmed cell death

Programmed cell death, or apoptosis, is a physiologic process inherent in normal tissue turnover, deletion of genetically damaged cells, and embryonic development.[5] By this process, a cell dies as a result of internal activation of nucleus-destroying enzymes. It is an irreversible process, and ensures that cells do not become immortal or pass genetic abnormalities on to their progeny. In the colon, apoptosis controls the rate of growth and prevents undue expansion of the proliferative compartment towards the surface from the base of the crypt (Figure 3.3). In cancers, the mechanisms controlling apoptosis, which are dependent in part on proteins coded by the *APC* and the *bcl-2* gene family, become disordered and uncontrolled.[6] As a consequence, genetically damaged cells may be able to survive and replicate. Overexpression of cyclooxygenase-2 (COX-2) confers resistance to normal apoptotic homeostasis.

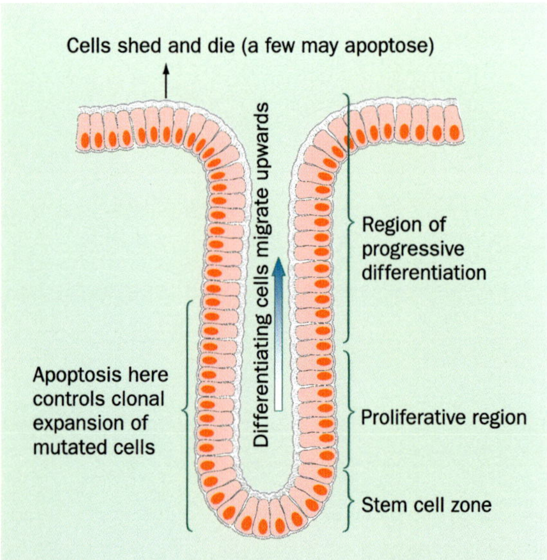

Figure 3.3 *Epithelial compartments of the normal colonic crypt, demonstrating the proliferative and differentiative compartments and showing how apoptosis may prevent expansion of mutated cells.*

Cell relationships and signaling

Gastrointestinal epithelium requires neighboring cells to form a tight barrier. Normal complexing between the APC protein, E-cadherin, and β-catenin ensures normal cell–cell interaction, growth control, and maturity of cell function. In cancers, a variety of molecular disturbances, including mutation of the *APC* and *b-catenin* genes, disrupt this complexing, with resultant disturbances in growth control and function.[7]

Interaction between epithelial and other mucosal cells is also important. Growth factors originating from neighboring cells bind to a receptor on the epithelial cell and modulate growth characteristics. Binding activates intracellular signaling pathways. In cancer, this process of signal transduction becomes disordered in a variety of ways.[3] In some instances, e.g. mutation of the *K-ras* oncogene, the signaling pathway becomes continually and uncontrollably activated, and growth is no longer effectively regulated. Other similar disorders occur such as with transforming growth factor β_1 (TGF-β_1) receptor.

Cell anchorage to the basement membrane

In the colon, the essential difference between the benign precancer epithelial lesion (i.e. dysplasia) and cancer is local invasion, where anchorage of the cell to its basement membrane is lost and the cell passes through the basement membrane.[3] Loss of normal basement membrane anchorage and secretion of invasion-mediating enzymes such as urokinase are biologic characteristics of the cancer cell.

The genetic nature of the colorectal cancer cell

A neoplastic colonic epithelial cell is characterized by various combinations of the above biologic aberrations (see Figure 3.2). For such biologic processes to become deranged, changes in the cell genome must occur.[8,9] These might be in DNA bases themselves (i.e. genetic) or else in the surrounding chromatin such that gene expression is altered (i.e. epigenetic).

Colorectal cancer results from progressive accumulation of genetic and epigenetic alterations that lead to transformation of the normal cell to a cancer cell.[4] There are four key elements of the molecular genesis:

- Cancer arises from a multistep process at the genetic, biologic and morphologic levels.

- The genetic and epigenetic (i.e. genomic) alterations underlying it provide a growth advantage to a clone of cells that displaces less-affected cells.
- Genomic instability is a key characteristic of cancer formation.
- Most of the genetic defects that drive colorectal oncogenesis are acquired. Where inherited (i.e. germline) factors are responsible, these frequently correspond to the acquired (i.e. somatic) defects.

Several forms of genomic instability are generally observed in cancer:[10]

1. subtle DNA base sequence changes such as the various types of mutations or microsatellite instability (termed MSI)
2. alterations in chromosome number, termed aneuploidy or chromosomal instability (CIN)
3. chromosomal translocation
4. gene amplification.

Virtually all colorectal cancers display either MSI or CIN, and these represent the two main genetic types or pathways of colorectal oncogenesis. These two types of genomic instability are exclusive and inversely related; they drive the oncogenic process and are progressively disordered during oncogenesis.

Approximately one-third of genes in the human genome encode for proteins that regulate DNA fidelity (i.e. maintain genomic stability). Some of these are characteristically affected early in colorectal cancer development (oncogenesis). The specific implications of these changes are best understood from a more detailed consideration of colorectal oncogenesis.

Models of colorectal cancer development

It is apparent that cancer is a genetic disease. Although in a minority, the familial etiology is the dominant cause, most of the genetic changes are acquired, resulting from exposure over many years to inherent errors or breakdowns in normal cellular homeostasis, to environmental carcinogens or to other factors.[9]

The initiation–promotion model of colorectal oncogenesis

Colorectal oncogenesis was initially described in terms of the classic 'initiation–promotion model'.[1,3] In this model, the first step involves direct damage to DNA, which results in mutations, i.e. 'initiation'. Surviving mutated cells proliferate and, if the mutations are biologically significant, then this eventually progresses through to cancer, driven to completion by promotional factors that in themselves do not necessarily damage DNA but modify biologic responsiveness. The initiation and promotion processes were conceived of as being strictly sequential.

The multistep model of colorectal oncogenesis

A new model, termed 'multistep carcinogenesis', appears to better explain the process.[1,3] The process is largely driven by genetic alterations, randomly occurring at different points in time, at multiple sites on DNA. It could be thought of as multiple, superimposed, initiation–promotion models, but such a description would not adequately allow for the biologic complexity or widespread genomic instability characteristic of oncogenesis in the colon.[1]

Inherent in the multistep model of oncogenesis are several important molecular genetic concepts:

1. The genome of the cell becomes progressively unstable over a prolonged period of time.
2. Abnormalities occur in specific genes which are critical to maintaining the non-neoplastic phenotype.
3. The broad pattern of genomic instability is usually one of two main types—CIN or MSI.

Genomic stability is maintained by what may be termed caretaker genes.[8] Abnormalities in these genes increase the likelihood that further, more profound and pathogenetically important, genetic abnormalities will occur. If, by chance, an abnormality arises in a gene with a fundamentally important biologic role, then a function important for the neoplastic phenotype may be acquired. These latter genes are termed *gatekeepers*.[8] How specific genes play a role is outlined below.

No single genetic abnormality is so critical to the process that it alone will result in cancer, although certain inherited or acquired mutations, especially in caretaker genes, may accelerate the process. Early in the process, genomic instability gives rise to spontaneous genetic abnormalities that further drive the process.[4]

Cells developing genetic abnormalities that provide a growth and/or survival advantage may displace the neighboring normal cells through successive waves of cellular clonal expansion and selection. With time, a subclone may acquire the full malignant phenotype (see Figure 3.2). Eventually, further biologic changes may occur that confer metastatic capacities.

The likelihood of accumulating such events increases with time such that colorectal cancer incidence rises as an exponential function of age.

Precancer events in colorectal oncogenesis

Cell phenotype progressively changes during oncogenesis. The evidence suggests a broad 'field' change throughout the colon characterized by cellular hyperproliferation, followed by development of focal change. The earliest focal change is the formation of cellular dysplasia within single crypts, with gradual enlargement and evolution through to carcinoma, i.e. the adenoma–carcinoma sequence (Figure 3.4).

The adenoma–carcinoma sequence

The concept of cancer development via benign neoplasms characterized as adenomatous polyps has progressively gained creditability over almost three decades.[11] Although sometimes called the polyp–cancer sequence, this description is technically incorrect in that 'polyp' simply describes a shape and need not refer to an early neoplasm.[12] The key morphologic hallmark of the precancer lesion is dysplasia.[13] Dysplasia is characterized by progressive cytologic and architectural abnormalities, but the cells are not invasive. Adenoma is the term applied to

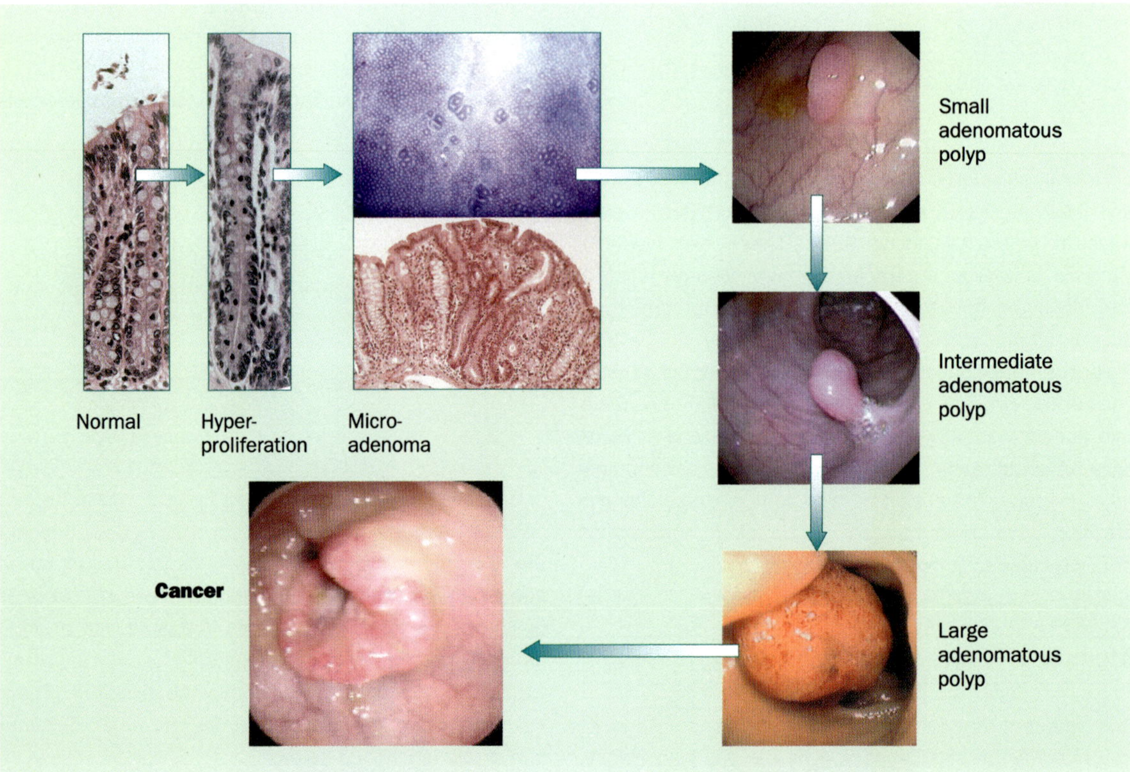

Figure 3.4 *Phenotypic stages in the adenoma–carcinoma sequence. Note that the hallmark of the adenoma is dysplasia, which represents the premalignant lesion. Dysplastic tissue may not take on the form of a polyp (i.e. it may remain a flat adenoma).*

localized dysplasia. Adenomatous tissue does not always take on the shape of a polyp and it might be flat or very diffuse—hence a more correct term is the 'dysplasia–carcinoma' sequence.

Although most colorectal carcinomas arise one way or another from dysplastic epithelium, it is also clear that most adenomas do not develop into carcinomas.[14] The exact frequency and time course of this neoplastic progression is not clearly defined, because (for ethical reasons) polyps once identified are usually removed, but predictions can be made based on observational studies. The peak age at which adenomas develop is 50 years, and precedes the peak age of development of carcinomas by about 7 years.[15] This suggests that adenomas progress over a period of 5–10 years before becoming cancers, although this rule applies to cancers developing by the CIN pathway (Figure 3.5). MSI pathway tumors may develop more rapidly.

Evidence for the adenoma–carcinoma sequence

The evidence for the adenoma–carcinoma sequence is derived from epidemiologic, morphologic, biologic, anecdotal clinical, and therapeutic data. There is a close association between adenomas and carcinomas.[1] For instance, 30% of patients with colorectal cancer have at least one synchronous adenoma, and in patients with two or more synchronous cancers, 50–85% have a synchronous adenoma.

Although it is ethically difficult to leave adenomas untreated, the available evidence suggests that progression to cancer does occur. Cancers have been found to develop at the site of adenomas left untreated because of patient non-compliance or technical difficulties in their removal. Additional evidence comes from studies involving detection and removal of adenomatous polyps. For instance, in a large study, the frequency of carcinomas occurring in the 7–14 years subsequent to polypectomy was about a third of the expected rate in an untreated population.[16]

The term 'de novo' or 'in situ' cancer development has emerged to address the possibility that a cancer did not develop from a macroscopically obvious adenomatous polyp.[17] The possibility that a dysplastic lesion does not precede the invasive cancer phenotype, however, seems unlikely. Small colorectal carcinomas normally arise in adenomas, whereas small carcinomas not associated

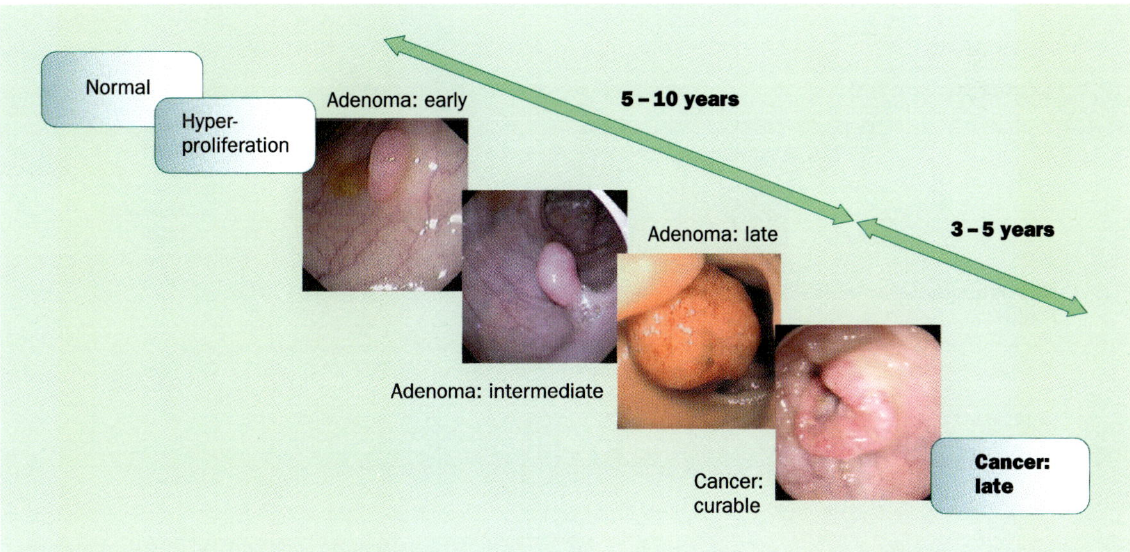

Figure 3.5 *Time course of sporadic colorectal cancer development in the human colon. Subsequent figures show the alternative pathways for the dominantly inherited cancer syndromes. Progression of oncogenesis may be characterized by (all or some of) increasing polyp size, amount of villous histology, degree of dysplasia, and increasing number of polyps.*

with adenomas are relatively rare in Western countries. Whether or not we can always recognize the precancer state, it clearly exists.

Genetic events occurring during oncogenesis

With progression of adenomas to carcinomas there is a progressive accumulation of genomic changes consistent with the multistep model.[10] The biologic significance of some of these is discussed in a subsequent section, but the following is a brief synopsis of the timing of genetic abnormalities occurring in the various pathways of colorectal oncogenesis. A simplified presentation of current conceptualization of these events is presented for the CIN and MSI pathways in Figure 3.6. Events and their timing are better understood for the CIN pathway.

CIN pathway

In the CIN pathway, aneuploidy is a key characteristic, with high rates of chromosomal loss or gain. The timing of events is fairly well conceptualized. Up to 85% of colorectal cancers develop by this pathway.

The most prevalent molecular genetic abnormality in the earliest focal neoplastic pathology identifiable—termed aberrant crypt foci or microadenomas (i.e. dysplastic crypts)—is that of mutations in the *K-ras* proto-oncogene or *APC* tumor suppressor gene.[18,19] Such mutations are passed to subsequent expanding clones, as about half of larger adenomas and cancers have been found to have such mutations. Mutations in the *APC* gene, found on chromosome 5, may be inherited and cause FAP (familial adenomatous polyposis).[19]

More random genomic instability becomes increasingly apparent in the early adenoma stage, and mutations in cell cycle checkpoint genes that control CIN (e.g. the *BUB*

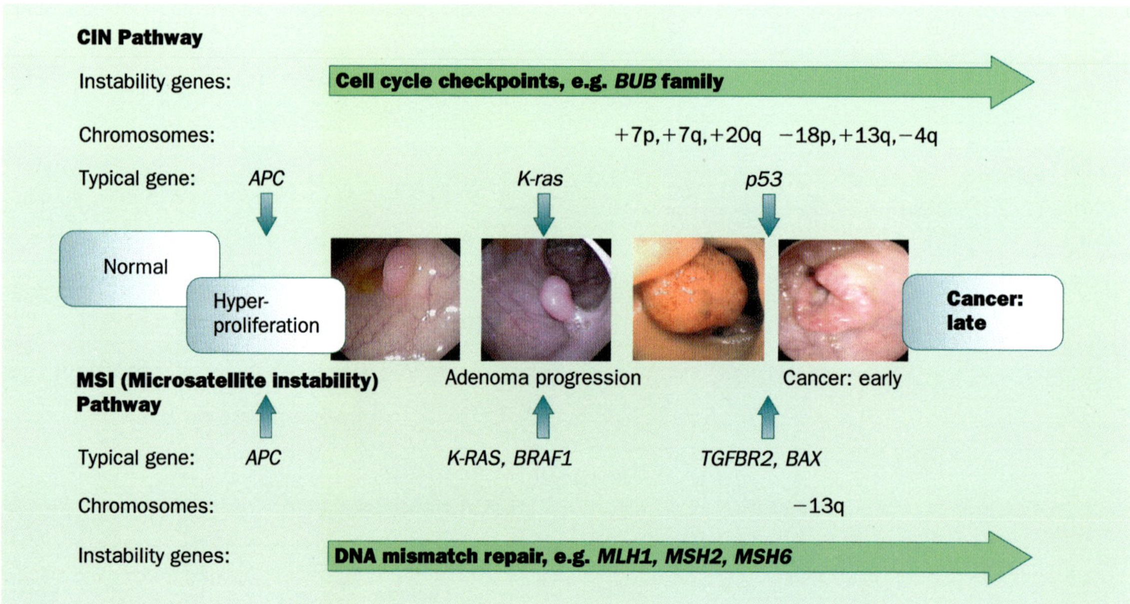

Figure 3.6 *Main molecular events occurring in each of the two main pathways of development of colorectal cancer. Not all cancers developing in each pathway possess each of these events, as abnormalities in other genes with similar function can lead to the same type of biologic progression. The stage during progression at which a typical gene might be affected is shown by the vertical arrows. Typical chromosomal changes and their timing are indicated by chromosome number and arm (p or q), with plus or minus for gain or loss. 'Instability genes' refers to the genes responsible for the genomic instability in the relevant pathway.*

gene family) can be observed at this stage.[4] Colonic adenomas harbor, on average, 11 000 genomic alterations![20]

Loss of chromosomal alleles and allelic imbalance is observed in larger adenomas. Allelic losses of chromosome 5 (a mechanism for APC changes in sporadic cancers) and/or of chromosome 18 (site of the DCC gene), are progressively common in larger adenomas and cancers.[21]

A pivotal event associated with transition from dysplasia to the cancer phenotype is loss of function of the p53 protein, whose gene is found on chromosome 17.[22]

MSI pathway

In the MSI pathway, cancers are diploid and do not show abnormal chromosome loss or gain. The timing of events is much less well understood and the spectrum of gene changes is characteristically different, although there are some common points. This pathway results specifically from dysfunction of a DNA mismatch-repair (MMR) gene (see below). These mutations may be inherited, and cause the Lynch syndrome (hereditary non-polyposis colorectal cancer, HNPCC), or may occur as an acquired epigenetic event. Up to 15% of sporadic colorectal cancers develop by this pathway.

In focal dysplastic lesions, mutations in K-RAS or APC are seen at the same time as in the CIN pathway but at a lower frequency.

The characteristic microsatellite mutator genotype, detected by assaying for alterations in microsatellite loci throughout the genome, becomes more frequently observed in adenomas but at rates not yet known with confidence.

Specific genes more vulnerable to mutation in this pathway include the TGF-β receptor type II (at the time of adenoma–cancer transition), *BAX* (a gene important for apoptosis), *IGFR2* (a gene important in growth/differentiation homeostasis), and a range of other biologically important genes.[4]

Mechanisms causing genomic instability

Gene dysfunction is the driving force behind oncogenesis.[1,3,4] Genomic alterations are either inherited or acquired. Those that are acquired may affect specific points in certain genes and be due to chance mutations occurring as part of the normal cellular life span, or to dietary lifestyle, or they may be less targeted and due to progressive genomic instability (Table 3.1).

Inherited mutations

Inherited mutations may be direct and powerful, such as mutations of the *APC* gene, responsible for familial adenomatous polyposis (FAP), or of the DNA mismatch-repair genes (see below), responsible for HNPCC (Lynch syndrome). They may be indirect and less powerful, such as the genes which control metabolism of dietary procarcinogens present in cooked meats (see Chapter 4). These are represented schematically in Figures 3.7 and 3.8. Further details on the inherited syndromes are presented in Chapter 6.

Table 3.1 Examples of genetic abnormalities relevant to colorectal cancer and the possible reasons as to why they might occur

Nature of abnormality	Genes involved
Inherited	Tumor suppressor genes: *APC* DNA mismatch-repair genes: *MLH1*, *MSH2*, etc. Carcinogen-metabolizing genes: *NAT1*, *NAT2*, etc.
Acquired	
Spontaneous due to base instability: e.g. point mutations	*APC, p53, K-ras*
Induced by carcinogens: e.g. point mutations	*K-ras, myc, myb*
DNA rearrangement or deletions: e.g. unstable genome	*APC, p53, p16, DCC*
Epigenetic events: e.g. promoter methylation	*MLH1*
Failure of DNA repair:	
e.g. MMR gene mutation	*TGFβ-R2, BAX*
e.g. mitotic checkpoint failure	*BUB* family
e.g. DNA checkpoint failure	*p53*

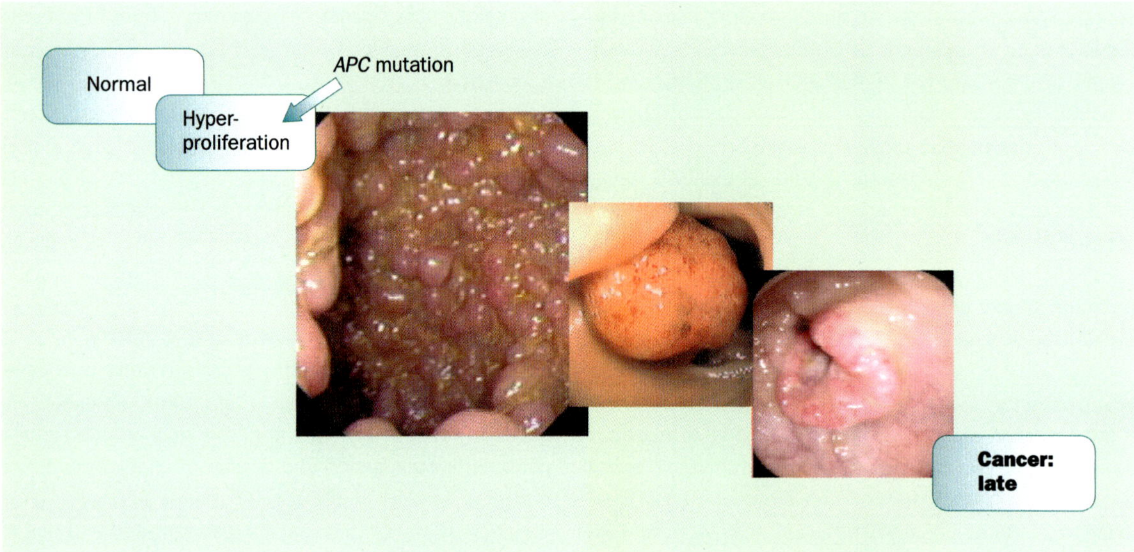

Figure 3.7 *Schematic representation of oncogenesis in familial adenomatous polyposis (FAP). The early development of massive numbers of adenomatous polyps is the key biologic change.*

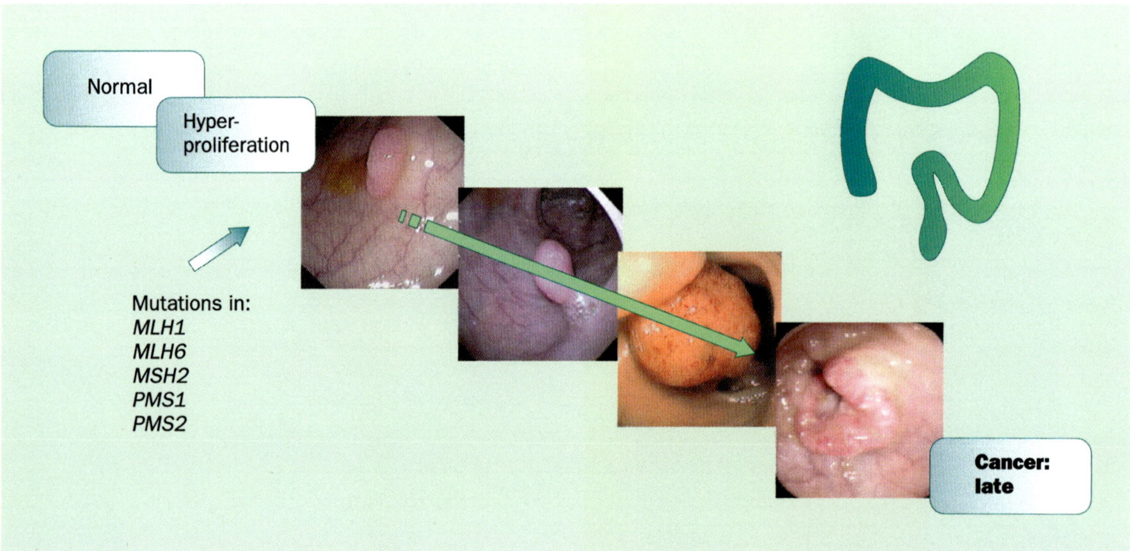

Figure 3.8 *Schematic representation of oncogenesis in hereditary non-polyposis colorectal cancer (HNPCC). The rapid progression through the adenoma/dysplasia phase occurs because of already existing genetic perturbations and results in predominantly right-sided lesions.*

Acquired abnormalities

Several environmental factors predictably induce damage to DNA, including viral infections, chemical carcinogens, and radiation (ionizing radiation such as X-rays and γ-rays, and particle radiation such as electrons, α-particles, and heavy ions). With colorectal cancer, viral infections (see Chapter 2, JC virus) and radiation are rare causes, but dietary chemical carcinogens are important because of the direct exposure of the gut.

Chemical carcinogenesis

Chemical carcinogens are ubiquitous in the human diet, and studies have demonstrated increased mutagenic activity in the stools of patients at risk for colorectal neoplasia.[23] Typically, carcinogens occur in foods in a form needing to be activated (i.e. procarcinogens), and are modified by metabolic processes in the liver and colonic mucosa to either activate or deactivate them. The microbial flora of the gastrointestinal tract and certain phytochemicals (bioactive components of plants) are also important in their activation and deactivation.[24]

Carcinogen metabolism

There are large individual differences in cancer susceptibility. In colorectal cancer, evidence points to an increased risk in those who are rapid acetylators.[25] Heterocyclic amines are formed by high-temperature cooking of meat (red or white) and fish, especially when exposed to direct flame. These heterocyclic amines may undergo oxidation and/or acetylation and eventually be converted into carcinogens that are known to induce colorectal cancer in rodents and alter DNA bases, thus inducing mutations. Oxidation, in the liver, and acetylation are under control of genetically determined enzymes. Cooking methodologies may well be critically important to the risk status in fast acetylators (see Chapter 4).[26]

Mechanisms by which gene dysfunction may occur[3]

There are many ways in which gene function may be affected: in broad terms, these changes can be small, such as a mutation, or gross such as a chromosomal loss. For the purposes of this review, we will present a simplified approach to the subject. Note that gene abnormalities can interact and perpetuate each other. Genomic instability by its nature is self-perpetuating.

Point mutation

Point mutation, i.e. a change in a single base pair, affects a range of genes important in human colorectal oncogenesis. These include *K-ras*, *APC*, and *p53*. Carcinogens and inflammation act to cause mutations in this way. Inflammation gives rise to reactive oxygen species, which create several forms of DNA damage, including point mutations and strand breaks in DNA.

Inactivation of DNA repair

Damage can occur to normal cellular genes through a variety of spontaneous and induced mechanisms. Mutations may be spontaneous, due to the instability of the purine and pyrimidine bases themselves. If these are not corrected by the inherent surveillance and repair systems (DNA checkpoint genes, MMR genes) they are perpetuated during the next round of replication as a mutation.[4,10] When DNA is damaged, e.g. by carcinogens, it is repaired by specific proteins that excise the damaged DNA and repair the defect by matching it against the complementary DNA strand.[10]

Of significance in the gastrointestinal tract is inactivation of the MMR system for DNA, as it is responsible for ensuring accurate copying of DNA during cell replication (Figure 3.9). Germline mutations in *MSH2*, *MLH1*, and *MSH6*—genes that encode the MMR proteins—have been identified and shown to be the major causes of HNPCC (see Chapter 6). Somatic inactivation of the *MLH1* gene through epigenetic silencing by hypermethylation of the gene promoter region has also been identified in sporadic tumors that show MSI. Defective MMR means that point mutations may more easily transmit during cell replication.

Genomic instability in colorectal cancer

The critical caretaker function lost in colorectal oncogenesis is the destabilization of DNA fidelity, resulting in genomic instability.[1,3] This accelerates the accumulation of genetic abnormalities throughout the genome. Even though many will not be relevant to the neoplastic process, an occasional rare event will occur that alters its biology, allowing a cell and its progeny to overgrow its neighbors. As described above, there are two types of genomic instability: chromosomal instability or CIN and microsatellite instability or MSI.

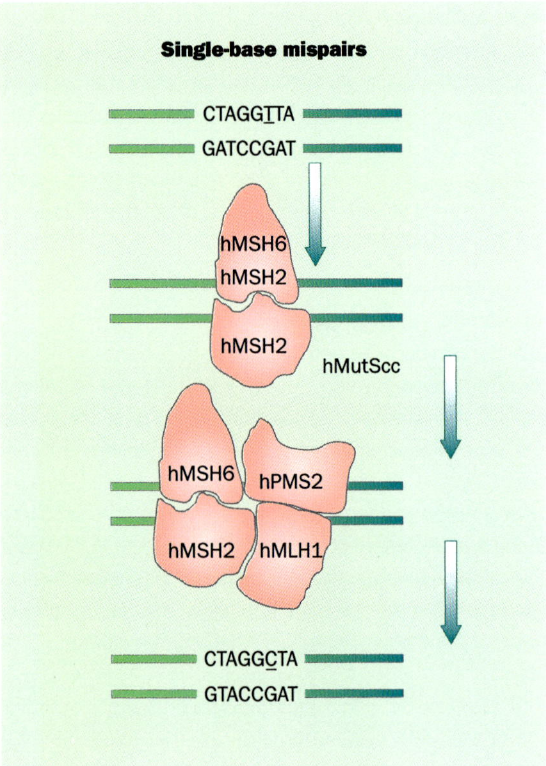

Figure 3.9 *Example of DNA mismatch repair. Mismatch-repair proteins identify mistakes after DNA replication and arrange for the repair. The repair proteins form a complex around the error, the mistake is excised, and correct bases are inserted. In this example, the incorrect base thymidine (T) is replaced by the correct base cytosine (C). Adapted from Carethers & Boland[3] with permission from publishers Lippincott, Williams and Wilkins.*

Chromosomal instability

This type of genomic instability is found in most colorectal cancers and results from asymmetric division of chromosomes during mitosis such that one progeny gets both copies of a gene while the other gets neither. This problem is characterized by aneuploidy, i.e. an abnormal complement of DNA, and loss of heterozygosity (LOH), i.e. loss of the two copies of a gene. By chance, LOH may result in the loss of copies of tumor suppressor genes.

The underlying cause of genomic instability in the CIN pathway is much more complex than MSI, as many more genes cause CIN.[4] It is beyond the scope of this review to address this rapidly evolving area, but 'checkpoint' genes that control mitotic spindle function, telomere formation, and DNA fidelity are being increasingly recognized as important in the early events. CIN causes the chromosomal losses and gains characteristic of aneuploidy. Thousands of genetic events of consequence may result but, interestingly, certain chromosomal regions are more likely to be affected as part of this process (see Figure 3.6). This, in turn, can result in frequent dysfunction of certain key genes. Deletion affects genes such as *p53* or *APC*.

Gene expression can also be modified by gross rearrangement of chromosomes and DNA sequences. Chronic myelogenous leukemia is the classic example. With progression during oncogenesis in the colon, chromosomal breaks and rearrangements become progressively frequent due to genomic instability and so change the function of genes that maintain normal cell behavior.

Microsatellite instability

This pathway for colorectal oncogenesis has emerged during the search for the genetic disorder responsible for HNPCC (Lynch syndrome). Repetitive segments of DNA between coding areas called microsatellites were found to be highly susceptible to mutation in HNPCC tumors: mutations in these are termed microsatellite instability (MSI). Mutation in one of the genes causing HNPCC confers a mutator phenotype which puts certain key oncogenic genes at risk of mutation and therefore dysfunction. MSI reflects sensitivity to mutation resulting from defects in repair of DNA. Neoplasms with MSI do not demonstrate the chaotic nuclear disorganization produced by LOH, and are more likely to be diploid rather than aneuploid. Although characteristic of HNPCC, microsatellite instability is also found in about 15% of sporadic, nonfamilial colorectal cancers, particularly those in the proximal colon. This is discussed below.

Biologic importance of genetics events

Key genes, their function, and their mechanism of alteration are listed in Table 3.2.

Important specific genes

APC, *a caretaker gene*

The *APC* (adenomatous polyposis coli) gene is considered to be a gatekeeper for colorectal oncogenesis. Its function is frequently affected in sporadic and inherited colorectal cancer.

Table 3.2 Examples of major genes that may be abnormal in colorectal cancer, and their function

Gene	Chromosomal location	Function
Tumor suppressor genes:		
p53	17p	Initiates apoptosis in response to DNA damage
APC	5q	Regulates binding of β-catenin
p16	9p	Inhibits CDK4 and CDK6 and so controls cell cycle
SMAD4	18q	TGF-β signal transduction
DCC	18q	Netrin-1 receptor
Oncogenes:		
K-ras		Membrane-associated ATPase
myc		DNA-binding protein and hence transcription regulation
myb		DNA-binding protein and hence transcription regulation
DNA fidelity genes:		
MSH2	2p	DNA mismatch repair
MLH1	3p	DNA mismatch repair
MLH6	2p	DNA mismatch repair
BUB family		Mitotic checkpoint gene
ATM		DNA damage checkpoint

FAP is due to an inherited mutation in the tumor suppressor gene *APC*, the gatekeeper for adenoma formation in FAP.[7] Nonsense mutations of the *APC* gene lead to a shortened (truncated) and dysfunctional protein with resultant defective regulation of cell death due to loss of its function.

Mutant *APC* leads to overactivation of the Wnt signaling pathway and permits tolerance to development of aneuploidy and genomic instability.[4]

K-ras *gene mutations*

For a small adenoma to progress, additional changes must occur. In adenomas, mutations have been identified in the *K-ras* proto-oncogene.[18] Mutations at certain critical positions in the gene alter the Ras protein such that extracellular signaling of proliferation is constitutively activated, thus causing a gain in function even when the other allele is normal. Such mutations are seen in many colorectal neoplasms.

The p53 *gene, gatekeeper for progression to cancer*

Advanced adenomas remain benign while they have not invaded the muscularis mucosae. A gene often associated with malignant conversion is the *p53* gene, which is affected by the two-hit mechanism characteristic of tumor suppressor genes.[22] A mutation in one allele must be associated with loss of the other allele for function to be compromised. *p53* is a transcription factor important in maintaining genomic stability. To facilitate DNA repair, it blocks cell cycle progression and activates apoptotic deletion of damaged cells. Inactivation of the gene permits mutated DNA to be passed on to cell progeny. Mutations in *p53* are usually missense in that they lead to a stable and overexpressed but non-functional p53 protein.

MLH1*, an example of epigenetic regulation*

As with the *APC* gene, this gene is also relevant to both sporadic and familial colorectal cancer. Inherited mutations have been discussed above. In addition, epigenetic regulation of MLH1 function through silencing of the promoter region by hypermethylation also leads to oncogenesis via the MSI pathway.[27] This accounts for the majority of MSI-positive tumors, and these tumors are sporadic, not familial.

Other genetic alterations in colorectal cancer

There are many other genetic abnormalities that occur in colorectal neoplasia and may participate in multistep carcinogenesis. Some substitute for others: for example, amplification of the *myc* oncogene, hypomethylation of DNA, and activation of the cellular proto-oncogene *src*. Other oncogenes are mutated or otherwise abnormally regulated in colorectal cancer, but their roles in carcinogenesis remain to be elucidated. COX-2 is often overexpressed in colorectal cancers—this is associated with disordered apoptosis and resistance to chemotherapeutic drugs.

Pathways of colorectal oncogenesis

The two main pathways are shown in Figure 3.6.

CIN Pathway

The CIN pathway is the most common and reflects the most common genetic abnormalities associated with many colorectal cancers, especially sporadic (sometimes called 'common') colorectal cancer. A range of observations suggest that the adenoma phase is about 5–10 years, whereas the cancer phase is up to 5 years in duration if untreated (see Figure 3.5).[15,16]

Other pathways may exist which vary in biologic and/or genetic sequence and speed of progression (Table 3.3).

In FAP, the CIN pathway is followed, but the ubiquitous presence of APC mutations in all colonic epithelial cells leads to a much earlier formation of massive numbers of adenomas.

In colorectal carcinoma complicating long-standing ulcerative colitis, there is no precursor polyp, and the cancer develops from a dysplastic focus that may assume a raised plaque-like appearance. The molecular pathway is not well defined but *p53* mutations occur early in dysplasia and MSI can be observed. Thus, it probably represents a variant of the MSI pathway.

MSI pathway

In HNPCC (Lynch syndrome), the process is quite different and follows the MSI pathway. Carcinomas arise rapidly through small precursor polypoid and flat adenomas due to an accumulation of oncogene mutations or suppressor gene deletions. Tumor pathology also differs: more mucinous tumors at a more proximal location and a more prominent lymphoid reaction. MSI due to defective DNA mismatch repair is the hallmark feature of this pathway and serves to facilitate diagnosis (see Chapter 6).

Methylation and serrated adenoma pathways

Gene expression is also subject to epigenetic regulation. Evidence is now emerging for several oncogenic pathways where altered methylation of regulatory regions in certain genes is responsible for progression to cancer.

One pathway involves *MLH1*, which is silenced by hypermethylation of its promoter region. This leads to oncogenesis via the MSI pathway and accounts for most (three-quarters) of cancers developing by this pathway—such cancers are not familial, in contrast to those due to HNPCC.

Another pathway is the serrated adenoma pathway. In this pathway, dysplasia develops in hyperplastic polyps. It accounts for about 1% of colorectal cancer.[28] Although still controversial, it appears that the genetic characteristics of this pathway are sufficiently different to justify designation of a separate pathway.[29] The main genetic characteristics include absence of MSI, as seen in HNPCC tumors; aberrant and widespread methylation of CpG islands, which

Table 3.3 *Alternative pathways for colorectal cancer development and their contribution to the overall burden of colorectal cancer*

Setting	Pathway (burden)	Characteristics			
		Relative speed of progression	Adenomas	Age for cancer appearance	Colon cancer site
Sporadic	CIN (up to 85%)	Slow	Few, typical	>50 years	Distal
	MSI (10–15%)	Uncertain	Few	>30 years	Proximal or distal
FAP	CIN (<1%)	Moderate	Polyposis	>15 years	Distal
HNPCC	MSI (<5%)	Rapid	Frequent as polyps or flat dysplasia	>30 years	Proximal
Ulcerative colitis	MSI (<1%)	Uncertain	Flat dysplasia	Varies	Distal
Serrated adenoma	CpG methylation[a] (1%)	Uncertain	Serrated	>50 years	Proximal
'De novo'	Uncertain	Uncertain	Flat dysplasia	Varies	Uncertain

[a]As yet, there is no commonly accepted label for this pathway. Low rates of MSI are observed and some label it 'MSI-low'.

increases with histologic progression; early methylation of *SLC5A8*; and additional methylation of several other genes, including *p16* and *MGMT*.[29]

Other pathways

At present, the possibility of even another molecular pathway for the 'de novo' cancers, observed especially in Japan but increasingly identified in Western countries, remains to be explored.[17]

External regulation of colorectal oncogenesis

The wide variation in international incidences of colorectal cancer suggests the importance of external regulatory factors in terms of their induction of genomic changes and/or the regulation of the biologic consequences.[2] Ethnic groups migrating from low-risk into high-risk regions quite rapidly experience an increase in the incidence of colorectal cancer, underscoring the importance of environment. Epidemiologic studies looking for environmental associations with such phenomena have found that a large proportion of this variance is related to the dietary lifestyle itself (see Chapters 1, 2 and 4). As is apparent from the discussion above on the process of oncogenesis and the mechanisms of genomic change that lead to cancers, many of these genomic events must be acquired. However, dietary factors do more than influence changes in DNA; they also, and perhaps at least as importantly, regulate the biologic consequences of altered DNA.

The following discussion sets out to establish some principles and examples of how this might occur. More clinical advice is provided in Chapters 2 and 4. First we will discuss the common aspects by which diet might regulate oncogenesis and then outline the mechanisms possibly operative for certain nutrients.

General themes explaining dietary regulation

Many possible general themes account for external regulation of oncogenesis (Table 3.4). The luminal environment within the colon seems likely to play a major role, as it is subject to great variation related to diet, but systemic and epithelial factors are also of relevance.[30]

Luminal factors

The luminal environment is complex and subject to great variation. Apart from unabsorbed dietary factors, whether

Table 3.4 *Dietary factors that may regulate colorectal oncogenesis, classified by site of action*

Site of action	Examples of factor and effect on risk[a]
Luminal	Probiotics (↓) Transit rate (↓) Bulk and dilution (↓) Bile salt type and modification (↓↑) pH (↓) Short-chain fatty acids (↓) Long-chain fatty acids (↓↑) Calcium (↓) Carcinogens (↑) Dietary fiber (↓)
Epithelial	Rate of proliferation (↓↑) Procarcinogen activation (↑) Phytochemicals (↓) Apoptosis threshold (↑)
Systemic	Fish oil (↓) BMI[b] >30 (↑) Physical inactivity (↑)

[a]↓, reduced; ↑, increased.
[b]BMI, body mass index.

modified by digestion or not, the influence of luminal bacteria and their metabolic activity seem likely to be important.

Simple physical factors are important. Diet (including fluid intake) influences transit rates and determines fecal bulk. Hastened transit may serve to reduce exposure times to dietary carcinogens and increased bulk may dilute them. Dietary fiber has been shown to bind and inactivate luminal carcinogens as well.[1]

Antioxidants may reduce DNA damage and inactivate carcinogens. To date, there is no direct proof that this occurs. Some dietary phytochemicals have the potential to inactivate carcinogens, but direct proof of such an effect is still lacking.[2]

Products of ingested foods are important. Luminal bacteria ferment unabsorbed carbohydrate (non-starch polysaccharides and starch resistant to digestion) to produce the short-chain fatty acids acetate, propionate, and butyrate. This acidifies the luminal environment, and an acid environment seems associated with a lower risk for colorectal cancer. Butyrate has a broad range of biologic actions of relevance to suppression of oncogenesis, including an ability to promote cell maturity and facilitate apoptosis.[31] In the test tube, it directly regulates certain genes of importance in tumor development. Activation of apoptosis, and hence deletion of genetically damaged cells by butyrate, represents a mechanism by which a dietary factor restores genomic stability. Butyrate also inhibits histone deacetylase, and this can lead to epigenetic regulation of gene expression of relevance to prevention.

There is increasing evidence, although yet incomplete, that different bacterial species (probiotics) are associated with a healthier luminal environment. Whether we eventually confirm that probiotics, commonly taken as yoghurt, are beneficial, remains to be proven. Although there is increasing laboratory basis to support how probiotics might act, there is as yet no proof in humans. The observations that bacteria can also activate or inactivate carcinogens, modify bile salts to more toxic forms, and generate differential amounts of short-chain fatty acids suggests that they are beneficial.

Endogenous luminal factors may also play a role. Bile salt composition and amount are altered by changes in pH and dietary fats.[32] Different types of fatty diet are associated with different rates of oncogenesis. It has been suggested that secondary bile salts such as deoxycholic and lithocholic acid, produced by bacterial action in the colonic lumen, act as tumor promoters or indeed carcinogens. They are toxic to the epithelium and stimulate proliferation.

Epithelial factors

In skin, the rate of cell proliferation at the time of exposure to a carcinogen has a major impact on the process of carcinogenesis, because DNA is more sensitive to carcinogens during the S phase (time of DNA synthesis) of the cell cycle. Such an idea has been proposed for the colon, but has never been substantiated due to conflicting observations. It is well known that dietary fiber, especially when actively fermented in the colon, stimulates epithelial proliferation and maintains epithelial cell mass, thus preventing atrophy and maintaining the integrity of the epithelial barrier.[33] Overall, fiber is protective against colorectal oncogenesis. On the other hand, toxic bile salts seem to promote oncogenesis and certainly stimulate epithelial proliferation, which could be a step to carcinogenesis.

Certain procarcinogens require activation to become carcinogenic. The hydrocarbons generated by high-temperature cooking of animal protein, such as the heterocyclic amines PhIP and IQ, fall into this category and their activation depends on the genetic polymorphisms associated with acetylator status. Individuals who inherent a fast acetylator status may be more at risk of colorectal oncogenesis, especially if they eat large quantities of heavily cooked (charred) meat, red or otherwise, and also fish, because there is activation of these procarcinogens in epithelial mitochondria.[26] Whether there are other such examples remains to be determined.

Programmed cell death or apoptosis is an inherent defense mechanism and, as outlined above, becomes progressively disordered in colorectal oncogenesis due to defective function of the DNA checkpoint and apoptosis-controlling genes. Certain diet-derived agents or dietary components facilitate apoptosis by altering the cellular threshold for its activation.[31] These include curcumin in curry, omega-3 fatty acids in fish oil, and butyrate from fermentation of polysaccharides. The biologic concept is that activation of apoptosis leads to more efficient removal of cells with damaged DNA. Experimental studies suggest it to be of importance, but definitive proof is lacking to establish it as the fundamental way in which dietary factors regulate oncogenesis by directly influencing epithelial behavior.

Systemic factors

The relevance of diet-dependent systemic factors to colorectal oncogenesis is less obvious than the above mechanisms, but may still be important. For instance, dietary fish oil seems to be protective.[34] Fish oil has numerous effects, including suppression of mucosal prostaglandin production and changed membrane lipid composition (and hence signal transduction). Both are changed in the colon after absorption of the lipids in small intestine.

The link between obesity and colorectal cancer might be mediated by systemic factors such as insulin and insulin-like growth factor activity.

Although not of dietary origin, non-steroidal anti-inflammatory drugs (NSAIDs) have a systemic action on oncogenesis; they may achieve this by regulating apoptosis and hence stabilizing the genome.[35]

Specific dietary components and oncogenesis

A report from the World Cancer Research Fund has examined in depth the relationships between diet and colorectal cancer and discusses the possible mechanisms.[2] The following discussion touches on the mechanisms of a few of these relevant foods (Table 3.5).

Dietary fats

The mechanism by which a high-fat diet enhances oncogenesis relates in part to the effect of dietary fats on bile acids and the subsequent effect on colonic epithelial proliferation. Increasing animal fat intake increases total fecal bile acid and fatty acid excretion in humans. Experimental models show increased cellular proliferation and increased reactive oxygen radicals in the colon of animals on a high-fat diet.

Other oils, however, seem protective. Fish oils are rich in omega-3 polyunsaturated fatty acids, and geographic regions where people consume large amounts of fish tend to have lower incidences of colorectal cancer. Fish oils protect against colorectal cancer in animal models. The mechanism by which they protect remains uncertain, but reduction of mucosal prostaglandins in colorectal tumors may be part of the explanation.

Non-digestible polysaccharides, including dietary fiber

Dietary fiber consists of a heterogeneous mixture of non-starch polysaccharides, undigested starch (resistant starch), and other plant-derived products such as lignin. A number of mechanisms seem likely to explain their protective action against colorectal cancer. Fiber hastens luminal transit time and, together with water, increases fecal bulk as a result of fermentation, thus tending to dilute the concentration of other luminal constituents.[1] Both of these would minimize contact between carcinogens and colonic epithelium. Fiber polymers can bind toxic substances and render them unable to make contact with epithelium. As outlined above, it is also subject to fermentation by luminal anaerobic flora, which reduces fecal

Table 3.5 *Examples of dietary factors that regulate oncogenesis and how they might achieve this*

Food	Mechanism	Risk for cancer
Saturated fats, *n*-6 polyunsaturated fats	Increases bile salts, increase epithelial proliferation and oxygen free radicals	Increased
Fish oil	Decreases prostaglandins and epithelial proliferation	Decreased
Fiber and resistant starch	Increases fecal bulk, transit rate, and short-chain fatty acid concentrations Binds carcinogens, alters bacterial species, and decreases pH	Decreased
Meat (red)	Possibly undigested protein is fermented to form genotoxic compounds	Increased
Charred meats	Increased procarcinogens	Increased
Calcium	Precipitates free fatty acids and decreases damage	Decreased
Phytochemicals	Detoxify toxins, induce metabolizing enzymes, antioxidants	Decreased

pH and generates short-chain fatty acids: one of these, butyrate, is present in high concentrations in the colonic lumen and is an important energy source for colonic epithelium.[31] Different fiber sources vary in their capacities to alter these factors, but all mechanisms seem likely to be important to varying degrees. The strongest support for a protective role comes from early experiments using wheat bran.[36]

Dietary protein

There is an association between colorectal cancer and red meat consumption above 140 g per day.[37] The mechanism for this is unclear, and appears to be independent of fat content or charring of meat. Some suggest it is due to the heme or iron content (see Chapter 4). Colonic bacteria produce a range of toxic nitrogenous compounds while fermenting undigested protein; this process, together with the iron content and means of cooking, have all been suggested as being involved in the process of carcinogenesis.

Micronutrients

Micronutrients are specific chemicals in the diet that do not supply energy but are nutritionally relevant. Our understanding of how these interact with the process of oncogenesis is developing. What follows is a short summary of some of the relevant or topical issues from a mechanistic perspective. The reader is again directed to reference 2 for supporting detail.

Calcium Calcium tends to normalize the generalized disturbance in the regulation of cell proliferation seen in the colons of patients with adenomatous polyps or cancers. It has been suggested that the damaging and mitogenic effects of free fatty acids and bile acids could be reduced by luminal calcium precipitating free fatty acids as calcium soaps.

Selenium Low levels of selenium have been associated with an increased risk for colorectal cancer, and some clinicians view it as an antioxidant. It is a constituent of the enzyme glutathione peroxidase, which prevents damage to tissue by free radicals; it also minimizes toxicity caused by certain heavy metals. Recent experience with other cancers raises questions as to its value.

Vitamins A, C, and E Indirect studies show that these agents have promise as anticarcinogenic agents, especially because of their powerful antioxidant activities. Retinoids also function as differentiating agents and reduce epithelial proliferation. The benefit of these agents has not been obvious in interventional studies, which suggests that antioxidant activities are not sufficiently powerful to suppress oncogenesis in the colon. It seems that other substances in the food sources of these agents are also contributing to the protective actions.

Folate Folate status relates to risk for cancer. Folate-replete animals are less susceptible to oncogenesis as they are less at risk of DNA hypomethylation, a non-specific effect on DNA that can result in changes in gene regulation.

Other phytochemicals A range of other components in plant foods, especially those strongly associated with protection and found in fresh vegetables, are summarized in Chapters 4 and 5. Their mechanisms of action include inactivation of carcinogens, detoxification, and scavenging of free radicals. They include benzyl isothiocyanate, a naturally occurring constituent of cruciferous vegetables, organosulfur compounds from *Allium* species (i.e. the garlic and onion families), monoterpenes found in citrus fruits, polyphenols in teas, flavones, tannins, protease inhibitors, terpenes, curcumin, glycyrrhetinic acid, and glucarates. Many of these agents have been proposed as potential chemopreventive substances for human studies.

Carcinogens and procarcinogens in foods

From the perspective of colorectal cancer, there are no known naturally occurring colorectal carcinogens in food. However, carcinogens may be produced during cooking of meats, as described above, or may be derived from endogenous bile salts subjected to metabolic changes by colonic bacteria.

How do dietary regulators affect genomic instability and/or mutations?

If procarcinogens in the diet do drive colorectal oncogenesis, then dietary modification of these (by removal from the diet and consumption of inactivating agents) should be protective. There is no direct evidence yet that dietary carcinogens are of great importance but the mechanisms to study this are only now becoming available.

Factors might act to counteract the biologic consequences of genomic instability. Activation of apoptosis is one such obvious mechanism. Reduction in S phase and cell proliferation is another. Proving that these are the operative mechanisms is challenging.

Factors might also regulate expression of key genes, either directly or indirectly. Again, the evidence is suggestive for a few agents but has not been systematically explored, largely because the genetic factors driving oncogenesis are complex and any single genetic process does not drive oncogenesis.

Much more work needs to be done to show how the environment interacts with the genome and the disordered events characteristic of colorectal oncogenesis.

Conclusions

Colorectal cancer is a genetic disorder in which most of the genetic abnormalities are acquired but some are inherited. Colorectal cancer develops by a process termed 'multistep carcinogenesis', in which progressive genomic instability affects the function of genes that are important in oncogenesis. The whole process may take as long as 10–15 years but it can be accelerated in certain familial cancer syndromes. Benign dysplasia precedes invasive cancer, the former often taking the form of an adenomatous polyp. The principal genetic pathways of development are the CIN pathway, where aneuploidy is common and chromosomal defects frequent, and the MSI pathway, where cells remain diploid but pathogenetically important genes are affected. In the former, tumor suppressor genes and oncogenes are often involved. Specific events leading to genomic instability are well understood for the MSI pathway but not the CIN pathway. Some of these genetic disorders and the resultant biologic disturbances seem to be able to be regulated by dietary lifestyle. Observational studies support this, but very few studies have been undertaken to show how dietary factors regulate genomic instability or its consequences. There are a variety of ways in which these agents might be responsible for such regulation, and events in the colonic luminal environment might be critical as these are easily altered.

References (*Reviews and general articles)

1. *Boland CR, Malignant tumors of the colon. In: Textbook of Gastroenterology, 4th edn (Yamada T, Alpers DH, Kaplowitz N et al, eds). Philadelphia: Lippincott, Williams & Wilkins, 2003: 1940–89.
2. *World Cancer Research Fund and American Institute for Cancer Research, Food, Nutrition and the Prevention of Cancer; A Global Perspective. Washington, DC: American Institute for Cancer Research, 1997.
3. *Carethers JM, Boland CR, Neoplasia of the gastrointestinal tract. In: Textbook of Gastroenterology, 4th edn (Yamada T, Alpers DH, Kaplowitz N et al, eds). Philadelphia: Lippincott, Williams & Wilkins, 2003: 557–83.
4. *Grady WM, Genomic instability and colon cancer. Cancer Metast Rev 2004; 23: 11–27.
5. Carson DA, Ribeiro JM, Apoptosis and disease. Lancet 1993; 341: 1251–4.
6. Morin PJ, Vogelstein B, Kinzler KW, Apoptosis and *APC* in colorectal tumorigenesis. Proc Natl Acad Sci USA 1996; 93: 7950–4.
7. Aberle H, Schwartz H, Kemler R, Cadherin-catenin complex: protein interactions and their implications for cadherin function. J Cell Biochem 1996; 61: 514–23.
8. Kinzler K, Vogelstein B, Gatekeepers and caretakers. Nature 1997; 386: 761–3.
9. *Fearon ER, Vogelstein B, A genetic model for colorectal oncogenesis. Cell 1990; 61: 759–67.
10. Lengauer C, Kinzler KW, Vogelstein B, Genetic instability in colorectal cancers. Nature 1997; 386: 623–7.
11. *Morson BC, Evolution of cancer of colon and rectum. Cancer 1974; 34: 845–9.
12. *Young GP, Macrae FA, Neoplastic and non-neoplastic polyps of the colon and rectum. In: Textbook of Gastroenterology, 4th edn (Yamada T, Alpers D, Kaplowitz N et al, eds). Philadelphia: Lippincott, Williams & Wilkins, 2003: 1883–913.
13. Muto T, Bussey HJR, Morson BC, The evolution of cancer of the colon and rectum. Cancer 1975; 36: 2251–70.
14. *Atkin WS, Morson BC, Cuzick J, Long-term risk of colorectal cancer after excision of rectosigmoid adenomas. N Engl J Med 1992; 326: 658–62.
15. Kozuka S, Nogaki M, Ozeki T et al, Premalignancy of the mucosal polyp in the large intestine. II. Estimation of the periods required for malignant transformation of mucosal polyps. Dis Colon Rectum 1975; 18: 494–500.
16. *Winawer SJ, Zauber AG, Ho MN et al, Prevention of colorectal cancer by colonoscopic polypectomy. N Engl J Med 1993; 329: 1977–81.
17. Rozen P, Brazowski E, Flat colorectal neoplasia: identification, pathogenesis and clinical significance. Dig Liver Dis 2003; 35: 135–7.
18. Vogelstein B, Fearon ER, Hamilton SR et al, Genetic alterations during colorectal-tumor development. N Engl J Med 1988; 319: 525–32.
19. Powell SM, Zilz N, Beazer-Barclay Y et al, *APC* mutations occur early during colorectal oncogenesis. Nature 1992; 359: 235–7.
20. Stoler DL, Chen N, Basik M et al., The onset and extent of genomic instability in sporadic colorectal tumor progression. Proc Natl Acad Sci USA 1999; 96: 15121–6.
21. Law DJ, Olschwang S, Monpezat J-P et al, Concerted nonsyntenic allelic loss in human colorectal carcinoma. Science 1988; 241: 961–5.

22. Kikuchi-Yanoshita R, Konishi M, Ito S et al, Genetic changes of both *p53* alleles associated with the conversion from colorectal adenoma to early carcinoma in familial adenomatous polyposis and non-familial adenomatous polyposis patients, Cancer Res 1992; 52: 3965–71.
23. Lang NP, Butler MA, Massergill J et al, Rapid metabolic phenotypes for acetyltransferase and cytochrome p4501A2 and putative exposure to food-borne heterocyclic amines increase the risk for colorectal cancer or polyps. Cancer Epidemiol Biomarkers Prev 1994; 3: 675–82.
24. Miller EC, Miller JA, Searches for ultimate chemical carcinogens and their reactions with cellular macromolecules. Cancer 1981; 47: 2327–45.
25. Loeb LA, Mutator phenotype may be required for multistage carcinogenesis. Cancer Res 1991; 51: 3075–9.
26. Roberts-Thomson IC, Ryan P, Khoo KK et al, Diet, acetylator phenotype and risk of colorectal neoplasia. Lancet 1996; 347: 1372–4.
27. Kim HC, Kim CN, Yu CS et al, Methylation of the hMLH1 and hMSH2 promoter in early-onset sporadic colorectal cancers with microsatellite instability. Int J Colorect Dis 2003; 18: 196–202.
28. Jass J, Serrated adenoma and colorectal cancer. J Pathol 1999; 187: 499–502.
29. Dong SM, Lee EJ, Jeon ES et al, Progressive methylation during the serrated neoplasia pathway of the colorectum. Modern Pathol 2005; 18: 170–8.
30. *Cummings JH, Wiggins HS, Jenkins DJA et al, Influence of diets high and low in animal fat on bowel habit, gastrointestinal transit, fecal microflora, bile acid, and fat excretion. J Clin Invest 1978; 61: 953–63.
31. *Young GP, Gibson PR, Butyrate and the human cancer cell. In: Physiological and Clinical Aspects of Short Chain Fatty Acid Metabolism (Cummings J, Sakata T, Rombeau JL, eds). Cambridge: Cambridge University Press, 1994: 319–35.
32. Reddy BS, Dietary fat and its relationship to large bowel cancer. Cancer Res 1981; 41: 3700–5.
33. Cummings JH, Cellulose and the human gut. Gut 1984; 25: 805–10.
34. Anti M, Marra G, Armelao F et al, Effect of omega-3 fatty acids on rectal mucosal cell proliferation in subjects at risk for colon cancer. Gastroenterology 1992; 103: 883–91.
35. Piazza GA, Kulchak Rahm AL, Krutzsch M et al, Antineoplastic drugs sulindac sulfide and sulfone inhibit cell growth in inducing apoptosis. Cancer Res 1995; 55: 3110–16.
36. MacLennan R, Macrae F, Ward M et al, Randomized trial of intake of fat, fiber and betacarotene to prevent colorectal adenomas. J Natl Cancer Inst 1995; 87: 1760–6.
37. Giovannucci E, Rimm EB, Stampfer MJ et al, Intake of fat, meat, and fiber in relation to risk of colon cancer in men. Cancer Res 1994; 54: 2390–7.

4 Is diet important in preventing colorectal cancer?

Paul Rozen, Graeme P Young, Bernard Levin

Introduction

From studies of migrants moving from areas of low colorectal cancer incidence to westernized or industrialized countries having a high incidence, it became apparent that within one or two generations these immigrants developed cancer rates similar to those of the indigenous populations of the host countries. This pointed to the environment as providing the major risk factors for colorectal neoplasia, the conclusions being that diet and lifestyle are the main etiologies in at least 30% of cases. This does not negate the importance of genetic risk factors in dominant high-penetrance disorders such as familial adenomatous polyposis, Lynch syndrome, or chronic and extensive inflammatory bowel disease. However, altogether, these can only contribute to about 5% of colorectal cancer cases. The remainder, about 60%, is probably explained by the widespread presence of inherited low-penetrance genetic perturbations that interact with the dietary and lifestyle factors and lead to adenoma and/or cancer of the large bowel (Figure 4.1).[1–4] So, even though diet has a very important role in the etiology and prevention of large-bowel cancer, it must also take into consideration interaction with race, gender, genetic make-up, occupation, age, and lifestyle.[3] These are also discussed in Chapter 2.

What preventive dietary recommendations can we make?

What is the relevance of body weight?

A higher than recommended body weight is a preventable risk factor for important chronic disorders such as cardiovascular disease, and several common cancers such as the hormone-dependent malignancies and colorectal cancer or adenomas.[4–8] It has been well known from both experimental studies in animals and from human epidemiologic studies that the risk for colorectal neoplasia, adenomas or cancer, is related to the caloric intake and body mass index (BMI).[6,7] Measurement of body weight is scientifically less useful than the BMI, which takes into account both weight and height, the formula being weight in kilograms divided by height in meters squared (w/h^2).[6] A simplified classification of weight status and risk for colorectal cancer is given in Table 4.1. The importance of obesity is illustrated by the observation that it is easier to promote cancer in the overweight experimental animal than in the active, non-obese rodent.[9] In humans, the risk for neoplasia, including that of the large bowel, is statistically

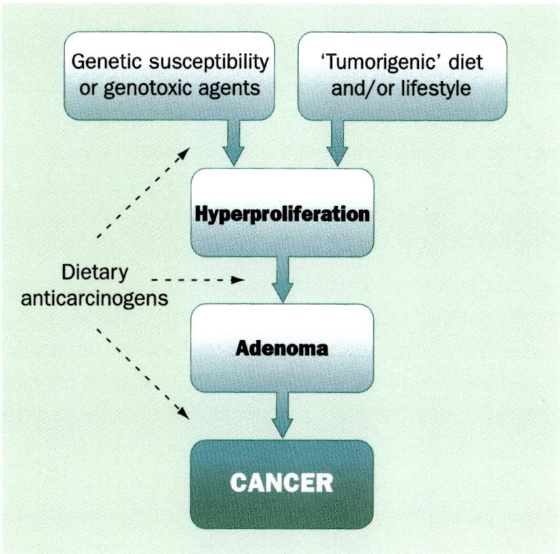

Figure 4.1 Schematic representation of the interactions between dietary and genetic tumor-promoting factors and preventive dietary factors.

Table 4.1 Body Mass Index (BMI)[a], approximate classification of weight status, and risk for colorectal and other cancers

BMI range	Weight status	Cancer risk[b]	
		Any	Colorectal
10–<18.5	Underweight		
18.5–<25	Ideal weight		
25–<30	Overweight		
30–<40	Obese	Yes	
40–70	Gross obesity		Yes

[a]BMI = weight in kilograms/height in meters squared.
[b]Derived from references 1, 4, and 6.

most significant in men, especially those having central (waist) obesity and those being extremely obese, for proximal colon cancer.[10] Obesity is not only related to the risk for neoplasia but is also associated with a poorer response to chemotherapy and less chance of sphincter preservation in men with rectal cancer.[11,12]

Calories

When evaluating diet, the first consideration is the *total amount of calories* that we eat. Clearly, the amount ingested should depend on what we need to replace our daily expenditure. In a westernized society, once we grow to adulthood and become physically less active, we tended to continue with previous dietary habits and not reduce our caloric intake in line with reduced needs (see Chapter 1). So, in general, being mildly to moderately overweight is a common phenomenon in men, and is even more of a problem in the economically disadvantaged of both sexes due to the easier availability of cheaper but high-caloric foods. Another recent phenomenon is the overfeeding of these same foods to infants, so now it is not uncommon to see overweight babies and children. Hormonal changes in these obese children are similar to those associated with cancer risk in obese adults.[13]

Maintaining close-to-ideal body weight is a lifetime habit and should be instilled from childhood by parents. Access of experimental animals to less calories leads to fewer cancers than in free-eating animals.[9] Similarly, food shortage in early life, due to war and poverty, has been associated with a lower incidence of colorectal cancer.[14]

Are there commonly consumed dietary additives or contaminants that have been identified as certain carcinogens?

Considerable public health efforts have and are being made to maintain the optimal quality of water and food products. This has included the identification and removal from consumption of those substances which are potentially carcinogenic, such as the breakdown products of fertilizers, preservatives, food colors and antibacterial or antifungal agents (none of which are known to cause colorectal neoplasia). In westernized countries, this goal has been achieved; known carcinogens are searched for and contaminated foods destroyed before marketing.[2,3,15] Chlorinated water has been extensively investigated and not proven to be a risk factor for colon cancer.[4] However, it was recently shown that long-term intake of groundwater heavily contaminated with nitrates (from fertilizers and manure), together with a low dietary intake of vitamin C, was associated with a risk for colorectal cancer.[16] Carcinogens produced by various methods of cooking are discussed below.

What should we eat so as to minimize the risk for colorectal cancer?

In contrast to the experimental animal, which is constantly fed a diet whose constituents have been artificially standardized, the free-living human eats a mixed diet. This diet varies from day to day, by seasons, changing tastes and habits, and with age. So, it is difficult to draw conclusions for humans from animal studies or from the epidemiologic studies of populations that are not uniform genetically, or by gender, or in their diet and lifestyle habits.[4,5]

Almost all the constituents of our usual diet have been identified both from experimental studies and by epidemiologists to have some measure of cancer-promoting or cancer-preventive value (Table 4.2). However, in general, these have only a mild to moderate influence on the process of carcinogenesis, especially when comparing the occasional intake of a specific food within a mixed diet to the constant habit of tobacco smoking. Even so, the following conclusions can be drawn regarding food constituents and specific foods. Their use as short-term cancer-preventive dietary supplements is also described in Chapter 5.

Table 4.2 Lifestyle and dietary factors and their estimated relative roles in colorectal carcinogenesis

Lifestyle/dietary factor	Relative role	Protective	Promoting
Physical activity	Moderate	+	
Total caloric intake	Moderate		+
Obesity	Minor		+
Alcohol	Minor		+
Tobacco	Minor		+
Chronic NSAID[a] use	Moderate	+	
Total fluid intake	Minor	+	
Tea	Minor	+	
Fried, charred, smoked foods	Moderate		+
Total fat intake	Moderate		+
Animal fat	Moderate		+
Fish oil	Minor	+	
Olive oil	Moderate	+	
Total fiber intake	Moderate	+	
Wheat bran	Moderate	+	
Cane sugar	Minor		+
Micronutrients	Moderate	+	
Calcium/vitamin D	Minor	+	
Iron	Minor		+
Folic acid	Minor	+	
Beef	Moderate		+
Poultry	Minor	+	
Vegetables	Minor	+	
Fruits	Minor	+	
Milk products (low fat)	Minor	+	

[a]Non-steroidal anti-inflammatory drugs.

Main food constituents (macronutrients)

Fats

The evidence of a strong relationship between the amount of fat ingested and the risk for large-bowel neoplasia is less clear in humans than from animal studies, where induction of tumors is easier when increasing their dietary intake of fat. In the US population, dietary fat of animal origin is regarded as an important risk factor for colorectal cancer, especially when taking into account the major contribution dietary fat makes to the total caloric intake, and as a means of cooking.[4,15,17] But, in some European and Mediterranean populations, the evidence is less conclusive, as there are countries, e.g. Greece, southern Italy, and Spain, where there is a relatively high intake of different types of fat and yet not a high incidence of large-bowel cancer.[4] These countries have a high intake of fish, whose oil contains omega-3 fatty acids, and of olive and canola oils containing monounsaturated fat, which seem neutral or protective, whereas the animal fats in the US diet may be more of a risk factor.[18–20]

There has been a strong recommendation in the United States to reduce total fat intake to 30–35% of total caloric intake, and this seems to have contributed to the marked reduction that recently occurred in the incidence of coronary artery disease. It is still not clear if this is also the reason for the slight reduction in the incidence of large-bowel cancer that has recently been noted, mostly in the American Caucasian female population (see Chapters 1 and 2).

Carbohydrates

Studies of animal models of carcinogenesis and some epidemiologic studies of large-bowel neoplasia have shown an inverse relationship between increased total carbohydrate intake and risk for colorectal adenomas.[4,7]

The strongest evidence for protection is from ingestion of the complex long-chain carbohydrates, rather than from the simple sugar sucrose. Actually, in both experimental and epidemiologic studies, a high intake of sucrose was found to potentiate the risk for colorectal cancer.[4] A consistently high intake of sucrose and easily digested and absorbed foods, mainly starches having a high 'glycemic index', is usually accompanied by a relatively low intake of other dietary constituents, including protective dietary factors. It has also been suggested that persistent hyperglycemia, and consequent insulin response, is a stimulus for colonic epithelial proliferation and risk for cancer.[8] The complex carbohydrate-containing foods should provide 45–60% of the total energy intake and refined sugar <10%.[4]

Fiber and fluid intake

The fermentation breakdown products of complex carbohydrates are important in maintaining healthy colonic epithelial cells and bowel function.[21] In addition, meta-analysis of epidemiologic studies evaluating fiber intake in preventing colorectal cancer indicates a low but protective role for fiber, especially from that of wheat origin.[4,7,15] The strongest evidence is from a multinational European study of fiber intake in over 500 000 persons, which demonstrated a significantly reduced risk for cancer in those having the highest intake. The effect was mainly on colonic and not rectal cancers and was independent of the source of fiber.[22] Similarly, in a large US screening study, dietary fiber, independent of source, was significantly associated with a reduced risk for colonic adenoma.[23] The beneficial effects of whole grain foods are also discussed below.

It was recently shown in epidemiologic studies of both colorectal cancer and adenoma patients that the protective effect provided by fiber was potentiated by the individual's total fluid intake, independent of type of fluid drunk.[7] The type of fiber ingested and types and amounts of other dietary constituents (e.g. fat, calcium, and fluid) are likely to influence the protective role that fiber has to play within the intracolonic environment.[7] The recommended daily intake of fiber is 25–35 g.[4]

Protein

As protein is derived from both vegetable and animal sources, it is difficult to evaluate its role in colorectal carcinogenesis separately from these food sources or from the means of food preparation. Protein intake is highest in those countries at highest risk for colorectal cancer and is probably in excess of physiologic needs. However, there is little evidence relating protein intake to neoplasia per se; the protein foods and the effects of their cooking are discussed below.[4]

Minor dietary constituents (micronutrients)

These are the vitamins and minerals that have been extensively investigated and, in the main, are protective against colorectal cancer. Their anticarcinogenic roles seem to be minor, acting on the intraluminal contents and/or by strengthening the resistance of the large-bowel epithelium to carcinogens and by correcting genetic damage. The list of these nutrients is numerous and they have various functions; they include selenium, calcium, vitamins A (carotenoids), C, D, and E, and folic acid.[4,20,24] Their beneficial or deleterious pharmacologic use as chemopreventive agents is discussed in Chapter 5. Vitamin supplements are not needed when eating the recommended five portions per day of fruits and salads.

There has been considerable interest in the colon cancer protective role of *calcium* and *vitamin D*. The strongest evidence for this is experimental, as shown by giving a 'Western-style' diet to mice and suppressing the resulting hyperproliferative response of the colonic epithelium by adding dietary calcium.[25] The epidemiologic evidence is not supportive for a strong anticarcinogenic role, but rather for a modulating, protective role within a 'carcinogenic' Western diet (see section on milk products). In adenoma patients, suppression of rectal epithelial proliferation by long-term calcium dietary supplements is greatest when their dietary intake is high in carbohydrate, fiber, and water and low in fat, with low tobacco use.[26] Long-term calcium supplements will slightly but significantly reduce the recurrence rate of large-bowel adenomatous polyps by 18%, especially when allied to an adequate intake of vitamin D.[27] The vitamin D plasma metabolite 25-hydroxyvitamin D levels were found to have been significantly lower in persons eventually developing distal colorectal cancer after long-term follow-up. This was notable in the older-aged study population and could also be related to their inadequate sun exposure as well as diet.[28]

What seems important about the calcium intake is not its source, but rather its total intake: up to 1500–2000 mg calcium ion/day. The dietary reference intake for calcium has been increased to 1200 mg/day for adults aged

50 years or older.[29] This discrepancy in dosage probably reflects the difference between desirable minimal amounts for physiologic needs and pharmacologic effects. Very few adults have even this minimal intake when eating their Western diet. A higher intake of calcium can be obtained by providing a diet rich in calcium, such as calcium-containing low-fat milk products. This diet has been shown to be practical in volunteers and suppresses their large-bowel epithelial proliferation.[30] However, it has not been proven to prevent neoplasia, nor are its long-term effects known. Other, non-dairy sources of dietary calcium are listed in Table 4.3.

There is now some epidemiologic and experimental evidence to link a high intake of *iron* and having high body stores of iron, especially when due to supplements or genetic reasons for iron overload, with an increased risk for colorectal cancer. High dietary or supplemental sources of iron lead to increasing concentrations of intraluminal free radicals, which have been associated with risk for cancer.[4,31] If confirmed, these observations may have an important implication on the clinical practice of maintaining full body stores of ion.

A low intake of *folic acid* has been associated with risk for colorectal cancer. These patients have a lower intake and blood levels of folic acid. This is exacerbated in chronic alcoholism and in persons having a specific genetic polymorphism that interferes with folic acid metabolism.[32,33] The importance of folic acid on overall health led the Health Authorities in the United States and Canada to require all flour and uncooked cereals be fortified with folic acid.[33]

Table 4.3 Dietary sources and their relative calcium content

Food	Calcium content
Cheese	Highest
Kelp	
Sardines	Moderate
Vegetable greens	
Nuts	Lower
Beans	
Tofu	
Whole milk	
Spinach	
Sesame	

The above foods have a calcium content ranging from about 1000 mg/100 g in the highest calcium-containing food to 100–200 mg/100 g in the lowest calcium-containing food.

The overall impression is that an adequate dietary intake of *all* these micronutrients is important in the defense against carcinogenesis (see also Chapter 5).

Bioactive compounds

Bioactive compounds is a general term that includes numerous chemicals found in fruits, vegetables, spices, condiments, herbs, etc., that in some cases have been proven to have anticarcinogenic properties. Some of the best known and studied are those found in green tea, tomatoes, onions, carrots, lemons, curry, and garlic. A partial list is given in Table 4.4. Even though their effects have been demonstrated experimentally, it is not clear how important is their occasional ingestion within the mixed Western diet. However, there are some national groups or individuals where their consistent intake may have a significant contribution as anticarcinogens, e.g. green tea, curry, etc.[20,34–36] The consistent ingestion of isoflavonoids and lignans found in soya beans and rye cereal have been associated with a lower risk of cancer, especially breast cancer, in Asia and Scandinavia.[37,38] Their effect in preventing colorectal cancer is less well documented.[38]

Specific food sources

Most evidence for or against an anticarcinogenic property of specific food groups or foods is based on epidemiologic and experimental studies. However, foods vary in their composition from season to season, from one geographic area to another, and between food product manufacturers. So, it is not always possible to extrapolate from one study to another. In addition, and most important, we eat a mixed and varied diet, and national and personal habits change from time to time.

Cereals

In the main, countries having national habits of a high intake of complex carbohydrates, whole grain cereals such as whole grain wheat, rye, and pasta, have a lower incidence of colorectal or other cancers.[4,5,20,22,35,39] This is probably also by displacing fats as an energy source (Figure 4.2). The recommendations for an adult are 600–800 g/day.[4]

Table 4.4 Classification and sources of phytochemicals (examples)[a]

Class	Sources	Action
Allium	Garlic	Induce enzymes, detoxify
Dithiolthiones	Cruciferous vegetables	Induce enzymes, detoxify
Isothiocyanates	Spices, vegetables	Induce enzymes
d-Limonene	Citrus fruits	Induce glutathione S-transferase
Phytoestrogens	Cereals, pulses	Alter steroid hormone metabolism
Flavonoids	Tea, fruit, vegetables	Antioxidants
Polyphenols	Tea, fruit, vegetables	Detoxify, inhibit *N*-nitrosation

[a] Adapted from reference 4.

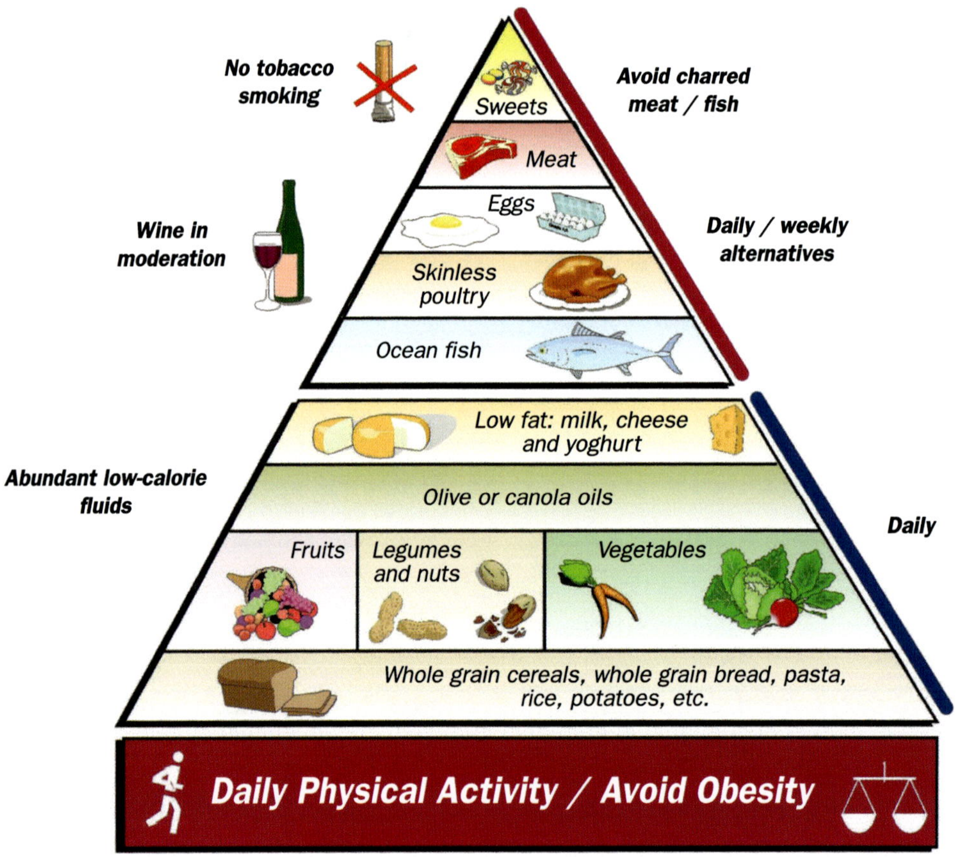

Figure 4.2 *Schematic representation of the amounts and types of food groups recommended daily or weekly to promote health. Adapted from information in references 4, 20, 56, 58, and 64.*

Vegetables and fruits

An extensive meta-analysis has confirmed the significantly reduced risk for colorectal cancer with high consumption of fruits and vegetables.[40] The fruits and vegetables contain vitamins, minerals, and some poorly digestible fiber, which clearly may all play protective roles. Considerable efforts have been made to identify other protective bioactive constituents, some of which have been discussed above.[20,35,36] These natural anticarcinogens act together at different stages of carcinogenesis and are most effective in correcting the deleterious effects of their inadequate consumption, rather than having a pharmacologic effect.[41]

Legumes, a food group that includes beans and nuts, are often consumed in small amounts in the mixed diet, but are staple elements of vegetarians' diets and they have significantly increased life expectancy.[42] This food family also includes soybean, which is consumed frequently in Asia. Epidemiologic studies have demonstrated a lower risk for cancer in consumers of soybean; however, this effect is less prominent in preventing large-bowel cancer than for hormone-dependent malignancies.[37,38] It has not been conclusively proven that their beneficial effect is just from the contents of phytoestrogens (lignans and isoflavonoids); it could also be from other nutrients in these foods.

Surprisingly, a recently published prospective study of mortality in vegetarians did not demonstrate a reduction in their cancer mortality compared with non- vegetarians, but they do have a significantly longer survival.[42,43] The recommendations for fruits and vegetables are 400–800 g/day, about five or more servings.[4]

Meat

Beef and lamb ('red' meat) and poultry and pork need to be considered separately.

Red meat

The epidemiologic studies tend to indicate a risk for colorectal cancer in persons having a high dietary intake of beef (greater than 80–140 g/day) and processed meat.[4,15,44] However, it is also necessary to take into account the meat's content of fat, iron (also from the blood), and means of cooking, e.g. fried or charred—all of which increase the risk for cancer (see below).[4] It has been demonstrated that the meat heme molecule can be cytotoxic and cause a hyperproliferative colonic mucosa, more so than just mineral ion added to the diet of experimental animals.[45] This has been extended to metabolic studies in volunteers and showed that increasing the ingested heme, by increasing red meat intake (not poultry) to more than 60 g/day, resulted in markedly elevated amounts of carcinogenic fecal nitroso compounds.[46] So, the daily consumption of red meat, one adult size serving, should be less than 80 g/day. However, it has been calculated that decreasing the red meat consumption to only 70 g/week would reduce the colorectal cancer risk in men by 18% in Australia and 12% in North America.[44]

Poultry and pork

Here, the epidemiologic evidence is that the intake of low-fat meat of poultry and pork origin is of less risk for large-bowel neoplasia.[4,44,46] However, this assumes that the poultry skin is removed after roasting. Carcinogenic heterocyclic amines are formed there due to the high temperature causing an interaction between the skin protein and fat content (see below).[47,48]

Fish

Fish from the cold-water oceans are rich in omega-3 oils that are believed to be protective for both cardiovascular disease and colorectal neoplasia. Residents of Mediterranean and other countries having a low dietary intake of meat but a high consumption of ocean fish have less risk for large-bowel cancer.[4,5,18–20] This is not necessarily true if the consumption is of pond-bred fish, as the biochemical constitution of the fish's body fat depends on its source of artificial food. Again, heterocyclic amines can be produced on the fish surface if cooked at high temperature, and this surface layer should be removed.[48]

Eggs

Eggs are obviously a rich source for fat, especially cholesterol. In the large bowel, intraluminal metabolites of cholesterol promote carcinogenesis. Eggs are probably a risk factor not only for cardiovascular disease but also for colorectal cancer, especially in men.[4]

Milk products

These need to be considered as low- or high-fat milk products and whether they contain vitamin D or calcium supplements. Low-fat dairy products can provide calcium and vitamin D, which have a large-bowel cancer preventive role—as shown by short-term intervention studies in humans and experimental studies in animals.[25,30] However, the inconsistent epidemiologic evidence for a protective role for milk products might have been related to the fat content of the milk and its products.[4,26,35] This has now been addressed by a meta-analysis of 10 studies, from 5 countries, including over 500 000 individuals followed up for 6–16 years.[49] There was a significant reduction of colorectal cancer occurrence (mainly distal cancers) in those having the highest intake of calcium. Interestingly, the threshold for the protective calcium effect was calculated to be 1000 mg/day, which is less than the amount used in intervention studies.[49]

Food preparation

The relationship of food preparation to carcinogenesis has been extensively evaluated. High-temperature cooking by grilling, frying, and charring of meat produces heterocyclic amines, which are carcinogenic.[15,48] Epidemiologic studies of persons consistently eating such prepared foods show that they have an increased risk for colorectal neoplasia.[4,5,50] There is evidence that this risk is greatest in persons of a specific genetic phenotype—fast acetylators—who have a reduced capability to metabolize these carcinogenic products.[51] This is further complicated by the biochemical interactions that occur during cooking between proteins and other constituents such as fats and sugars, to produce compounds that are also carcinogenic.[52]

Processing meat, by smoking or curing has been associated with the production of carcinogenic nitrosamines from nitrites. Consistent intake of such products has been associated with an increased risk for large-bowel neoplasia.[4,15,44]

Hypothesis for colorectal carcinogenesis

Fat ingestion causes an increased flow of intestinal bile, and some of this fat and bile reaches the colon, where bacteria degrade them to fatty and bile acids. These damage the large-bowel epithelium, and thereby stimulate proliferation, which leaves the epithelium susceptible to carcinogenesis. The usual by-products of bile metabolism and food preparation may themselves act as carcinogens, especially if there is genetic susceptibility. In addition to these effects of foods on the intraluminal contents and bowel wall, the products of digestion are absorbed and release local peptides and hormones such as gastrin and insulin, which are also factors promoting epithelial hyperproliferation.

Dietary fiber, by its bulk and fluids, dilutes the colonic contents and shortens transit time, permitting less contact time of the contents with the bowel wall. The bacterial fermentation of cereal fibers produces short-chain fatty acids, which are important for the metabolism and health of the colonic epithelium, and help maintain its integrity. The resultant intraluminal acidic pH inhibits bile acid dehydroxylation and dehydrogenation, events that can lead to the production of carcinogenic by-products. Micronutrients and bioactive compounds protect through several mechanisms: systemically they promote cell differentiation and apoptosis and help maintain epithelial integrity, whereas intraluminally, they help detoxify carcinogenic dietary and metabolic by-products (see Figure 4.1).

See also Chapter 3 for a discussion of biologic mechanisms.

Risk and protective diets

There are apparently dietary lifestyle patterns that have been associated with greater or less risk for colorectal cancer.[5,17,20,53] Different risk factors have been associated with colon and not rectal cancer.[6,17,20,22,40,53–55] This has been attributed in part to ethnic habits and to gender.[56,57] The Mediterranean diet is not ethnic-specific, but geographic, and its variations are found in many non-European countries, i.e. in the Mediterranean basin, Middle East, and Asia.[20,35] However, with westernization of these areas and subsequent lifestyle change, colorectal cancer and other diseases have become prevalent.[56,58]

Aging and the risk for colorectal cancer

Caloric excess, obesity from childhood, is associated with metabolic changes seen in adults at risk for colorectal cancer.[13,14] In addition, in westernized populations, dietary intake of vitamins and minerals is less than recommended.[29] In Western countries, adults frequently have a fruit and vegetable intake below the recommended amounts, and this is more apparent in men than in women due to their lack of knowledge on nutrition.[57] Aging, itself, has been associated with global hypomethylation of genomic DNA, which potentates tumorigenesis in general.[59] Nutrition advice can modulate these processes by promoting caloric restriction, increased fruits and vegetables intake, and, if necessary, chemoprevention with phytoestrogens, folic acid, and other vitamin and mineral supplements.[60]

Intervention trials

A number of clinical trials have added food items, or food groups, or even modified dietary habits.[4,20,33,61,62] Some of the results have been inconclusive or negative, possibly as the duration of intervention had been too short and the process of carcinogenesis too well established so as to be influenced by dietary intervention (see Chapter 5). Important trials are the American Women's Health Initiative, which is a very large, multifactorial trial, and the Polyp Prevention Trial, whose results will tell us not only about the recommended relative proportions and amounts of its dietary constituents that are most health-promoting but also about their success in modifying the dietary habits of a large-sized healthy American population.[61,62]

Dietary recommendations

What conclusions about diet and colorectal cancer can be drawn? Well there is an *imbalance* between protective and deleterious dietary factors and lifestyle, interacting in some cases with a genetic susceptibility. There is no one individual food item or micronutrient that causes or prevents colorectal cancer, but it is the total long-term lifestyle and diet that is important (see Table 4.2). What has happened in Europe and also in some parts of the Asia-Pacific region and Latin America is that with increasing affluence there was not only an increased consumption of cereals, vegetables, fruits, and milk but also a disproportionate increased consumption of meat and added fats.[4]

The US National Academy of Sciences and the American Cancer Society felt that there was enough evidence to recommend a multipurpose 'health' regimen, good for preventing obesity, hyperlipemia, adult-type diabetes, cardiovascular disease, and some cancers.[63] This was published as the US Department of Agriculture's 'Food Pyramid', but was criticized for not placing sufficient emphasis on promoting physical activity, preventing obesity, promoting more consumption of whole-grain cereals and low-fat dairy products, less consumption of red meat, using olive and canola oils, and avoiding high-temperature cooking.[64] This has now undergone modification in line with the above recommendations (see Food and Nutrition in www.usda.gov/wps/portal/usdahome).

This regimen can be summarized (and modified slightly) as follows:

1. Be physically active, eat in moderation, and avoid obesity throughout life.
2. Use complex carbohydrates and high-fiber grains to displace fat as an energy source. Avoid a high intake of sucrose and refined 'white' flour products.
3. Reduce fat intake as a source of energy. Ideally, it should not contribute more than 25–30% of daily caloric intake. Use monounsaturated olive or canola oils for cooking and salad dressing.
4. Eat adequate amounts of fruits and fresh vegetables and have an adequate low-calorie fluid intake.
5. Substitute lean chicken, pork, fish, and low-fat dairy products for red meat.
6. Avoid high-temperature and direct-flame overcooking of meats and fish. Remove the charred portion.
7. Reduce alcohol consumption and cease or never begin tobacco smoking.

This diet and lifestyle is not only healthful but also palatable, economic, and multipurpose for the prevention of common diseases.

Based on these recommendations, the Western-style diet has been modified and is being tried by a large number of Americans (see above).[61,62] Another recommended diet and lifestyle modification is that of being vegetarian. In general, studies have shown vegetarians to have a longer life expectancy.[42,43] A third dietary pattern is that of Mediterranean countries, where a high intake of fruits, vegetables, cereals, fish, and olive oil have been associated with a lower incidence of cardiovascular disease and cancer.[4,5,20,35,56,58,64] This is illustrated in Figure 4.2, which is typical of the Mediterranean type of diet; a similar example is now shown on the US Department of Agriculture website (see above).

In conclusion, the choice of any one of the above long-term diets and lifestyles is individual. Based on the numerous data available, any one of them may provide a better dietary protection against colorectal cancer than the present Western diet.

References (*Reviews and general articles)

1. Lutz WK, Carcinogens in the diet vs. overnutrition. Individual dietary habits, malnutrition, and genetic susceptibility modify carcinogenic potency and cancer risk. Mutat Res 1999; 443: 251–8.
2. *Manson MM, Benford DJ, Factors influencing the carcinogenicity of food chemicals. Toxicology 1999; 134: 93–108.
3. Labadarios DL, Parke DV, Nutrition and diet in the prevention and treatment of cancer. J Clin Biochem Nutr 1999; 26: 135–53.
4. *World Cancer Research Fund and American Institute for Cancer Research, Food, Nutrition and the Prevention of Cancer: A Global Perspective. Washington, DC: Banta Books, 1997.
5. *Schatzkin A, Dietary prevention of colorectal cancer. In: Prevention and Early Detection of Colorectal Cancer (Young GP, Rozen P, Levin B, eds). London: WB Saunders, 1996. 103–13.
6. Ford ES, Body mass index and colon cancer in a national sample of adult US men and women. Am J Epidemiol 1999; 150: 390–8.
7. *Lubin F, Rozen P, Arieli B et al, Nutritional and lifestyle habits and water-fiber interaction in colorectal adenoma etiology. Cancer Epidemiol Biomarkers Prev 1997; 6: 79–85.
8. *Calle EE, Thun MJ, Obesity and cancer. Oncogene 2004; 23: 6365–78.
9. Weindruch R, Albanes D, Kritchevsky D, The role of calories and caloric restriction in carcinogenesis. Hematol Oncol Clin North Am 1991; 5: 79–89.
10. *Moore LL, Bradlee ML, Singer MR et al, BMI and waist circumference as predictors of lifetime colon cancer risk in Framingham Study adults. Int J Obesity 2004; 28: 559–67.
11. Meyerhardt JA, Catalano PJ, Haller DG et al, Influence of body mass index on outcomes and treatment-related toxicity in patients with colon carcinoma. Cancer 2003; 98: 484–95.
12. Meyerhardt JA, Tepper JE, Niedzwiecki D et al, Impact of body mass index on outcomes and treatment-related toxicity in patients with stage II and III rectal cancer: findings from Intergroup Trial 0114. J Clin Oncol 2004; 22: 648–57.
13. Gascón F, Valle M, Martos R et al, Childhood obesity and hormonal abnormalities associated with cancer risk. Eur J Cancer Prev 2004; 13: 193–7.
14. Dirx MJM, van den Brandt PA, Goldbohm RA et al, Energy restriction early in life and colon carcinoma risk. Cancer 2003; 97: 46–55.
15. Ferguson LR, Natural and man-made mutagens and carcinogens in the human diet. Mutat Res 1999; 443: 1–10.
16. De Roos AJ, Ward MH, Lynch CF et al, Nitrate in public water supplies and the risk of colon and rectum cancers. Epidemiology 2003; 14: 640–9.
17. Satia-Abouta J, Galanko JA, Martin CF et al, Food groups and colon cancer risk in Africans-Americans and Caucasians. Int J Cancer 2004; 109: 728–36.
18. Rose DP, Connolly JM, Omega-3 fatty acids as cancer chemopreventive agents. Pharmacol Ther 1999; 83: 217–44.
19. *de Deckere EAM, Possible beneficial effect of fish and fish n-3 polyunsaturated fatty acids in breast and colorectal cancer. Eur J Cancer Prev 1999; 8: 213–21.
20. *Simopoulos AP, The traditional diet of Greece and cancer. Eur J Cancer Prev 2004; 13: 219–30.
21. *Slavin JL, Martini MC, Jacobs DR Jr et al, Plausible mechanisms for the protectiveness of whole grains. Am J Clin Nutr 1999; 70(Suppl): 459S–63S.
22. *Bingham SA, Day NE, Luben R et al, Dietary fibre in food and protection against colorectal cancer in the European Prospective Investigation into Cancer and Nutrition (EPIC): an observation study. Lancet 2003; 361: 1496–501.
23. Peters U, Sinha R, Chatterjee N et al, Dietary fibre and colorectal adenoma in a colorectal cancer early detection programme. Lancet 2003; 361: 1491–5.
24. *Weisburger JH, Nutritional approach to cancer prevention with emphasis on vitamins, antioxidants and carotenoids. Am J Clin Nutr 1991; 53: 226S–37S.
25. Richter F. Newmark HL, Richter A et al, Inhibition of Western-diet induced hyperproliferation and hyperplasia in mouse colon by two sources of calcium. Carcinogenesis 1995; 16: 2685–9.
26. Rozen P, Lubin F, Papo N et al, Calcium supplements interact significantly with long-term diet while suppressing rectal epithelial proliferation of adenoma patients. Cancer 2001; 91: 833–40.
27. *Grau MV, Baron JA, Sander RS et al, Vitamin D, calcium supplementation and colorectal adenomas: results of a randomized trial. J Natl Cancer Inst 1999; 340: 101–7.
28. Feskanich D, Ma J, Fuchs CS et al, Plasma vitamin D metabolites and risk of colorectal cancer in women. Cancer Epidemiol Biomarkers Prev 2004; 13: 1502–8.
29. Institute of Medicine, Dietary Reference Intakes for Calcium, Phosphorus, Magnesium, Vitamin D and Fluoride. Food and Nutrition Board, Washington, DC: National Academy Press, 1997.
30. Holt PR, Atillasoy EO, Gilman J et al, Modulation of abnormal colonic epithelial cell proliferation and differentiation by low-fat dairy foods. JAMA 1998; 280: 1074–9.
31. *Weinberg ED, The role of iron in cancer. Eur J Cancer Prev 1996; 5: 19–36.
32. Pufulete M, Al-Ghnaniem R, Leather AJM et al, Folate status, genomic DNA hypomethylation and risk of colorectal adenoma and cancer: a case control study. Gastroenterology 2003; 124: 1240–8.
33. *Kim Y-I, Role of folate in colon cancer development and

progression. J Nutr 2003; 133: 3731S–9S.
34. *Borrelli F, Capasso R, Russo A et al, Systematic review: green tea and gastrointestinal cancer risk. Aliment Pharmacol Ther 2004; 19; 497–510.
35. Gerber M, Biofactors in the Mediterranean diet. Clin Chem Lab Med 2003; 41: 999–1004.
36. *Giovannucci E, Tomatoes, tomato-based products, lycopene, and cancer: review of the epidemiologic literature. J Natl Cancer Inst 1999; 91: 317–31.
37. Thiagarajan DG, Bennink MR, Bourquin, LD et al, Prevention of precancerous colonic lesions in rats by soy flakes, soy flour, genistein, and calcium. Am J Clin Nutr 1998; 68: 1394S–9S.
38. *Adlercreutz H, Epidemiology of phytoestrogens. Baillière's Clin Endocrinol Metab 1998; 12: 605–23.
39. *Nestle M, Animal v. plant foods in human diets and health: is the historical record unequivocal? Proc Nutr Soc 1999; 58: 211–18.
40. *Riboli E, Norat T, Epidemiologic evidence of the protective effect of fruit and vegetables on cancer risk. Am J Clin Nutr 2003; 78(Suppl): 559S–69S.
41. *Temple NJ, Gladwin KK, Fruit, vegetables and prevention of cancer: research challenges. Nutrition 2003; 19: 467–70.
42. Singh PN, Sabaté J, Fraser GE, Does low meat consumption increase life expectancy in humans? Am J Clin Nutr 2003; 78(Suppl): 526S–32S.
43. Key TJ, Fraser GE, Thorogood M et al, Mortality in vegetarians and nonvegetarians: detailed findings from a collaborative analysis of 5 prospective studies. Am J Clin Nutr 1999; 70(Suppl): 516S–24S.
44. *Norat T, Riboli E, Meat consumption and colorectal cancer: a review of epidemiologic evidence. Nutr Rev 2001; 59: 37–47.
45. Sesink ALA, Termont DSML, Keibeuker JH et al, Red meat and colon cancer: the cytotoxic and hyerproliferative effects of dietary heme. Cancer Res 1999; 59: 5704–9.
46. Cross AJ, Pollock JR, Bingham SA, Haem, not protein or inorganic iron, is responsible for endogenous intestinal N-nitrosation arising from red meat. Cancer Res 2003; 63: 2358–60.
47. Solyakov A, Skog K, Screening for heterocyclic amines in chicken cooked in various ways. Food Chem Toxicol 2002; 40: 1205–11.
48. *Sugimura T, Wakabayashi J, Nakagama H et al, Heterocyclic amines: mutagens/carcinogens produced during cooking of meat and fish. Cancer Sci 2004; 94: 290–9.
49. *Cho E, Smith-Warner SA, Spiegelman D et al, Dairy foods, calcium, and colorectal cancer: a pooled analysis of 10 cohort studies. J Natl Cancer Inst 2004; 96: 1015–22.
50. Sinha R, Chow WH, Kulldorff M et al, Well-done, grilled red meat increases the risk of colorectal adenomas. Cancer Res 1999; 59: 4320–4.
51. Roberts-Thomson IC, Butler WJ, Ryan P, Meat, metabolic genotypes and risk for colorectal cancer. Eur J Cancer Prev 1999; 8: 207–11.
52. *Corpet DE, Stamp D, Medline A et al, Promotion of caloric microadenoma growth in mice and rats fed cooked sugar or cooked casein and fat. Cancer Res 1990; 50: 6955–8.
53. Fung T, Hu FB, Fuchs C et al, Major dietary patterns and the risk of colorectal cancer in women. Arch Intern Med 2003; 163: 309–14.
54. Friedenreich CM, Orenstein MR, Physical activity and cancer prevention: etiologic evidence and biological mechanisms. J Nutr 2002; 132: 3456S–64S.
55. Wei EK, Giovannucci E, Wu K et al, Comparison of risk factors for colon and rectal cancer. Int J Cancer 2004; 108: 433–42.
56. Trichopoulou A, Costacou T, Bamia C et al, Adherence to a Mediterranean diet and survival in a Greek population. N Engl J Med 2003; 348: 2599–608.
57. Baker AH, Wardle J, Sex differences in fruit and vegetable intake in older adults. Appetite 2003; 40: 269–75.
58. Hu FB, The Mediterranean diet and mortality—olive oil and beyond. N Engl J Med 2003; 348: 2595–6.
59. Lui L, Wylie RC, Andrews LG et al, Aging, cancer and nutrition: the DNA methylation connection. Mech Ageing Dev 2003; 124: 989–98.
60. *Davis CD, Uthus EO, DNA methylation, cancer susceptibility and nutrient interactions. Exp Biol Med 2004; 229: 988–95.
61. *Anderson G, Cummings S, Freedman L et al, Design of the Women's Health Initiative: clinical trial and observational study. Controlled Clin Trials 1998; 19: 61–109.
62. Lanza E, Schatzkin A, Daston C et al, Implementation of a 4-y, high-fiber, high-fruit-and-vegetable, low-fat dietary intervention: results of dietary changes in the Polyp Prevention Trial. Am J Clin Nutr 2001; 74: 387–401.
63. *National Academy of Sciences, National Research Council (USA), Committee on Diet and Health. Diet and Health: Implication for Reducing Chronic Disease Risk. Washington, DC: National Academy Press, 1989.
64. Willet WC, Stampfer MJ, Rebuild the food pyramid. Sci Am 2003; 288: 64–71.

5 Can non-dietary and dietary agents prevent colorectal cancer?

Paul Rozen, Graeme P Young, Bernard Levin

Introduction

For more than two decades there has been a concerted effort made to identify and evaluate chemical compounds, termed chemopreventive agents, that could prevent, inhibit, or change the course of carcinogenesis. These studies were based on observations and beliefs that certain foods or additives, e.g. green tea or garlic, had beneficial anticarcinogenic properties. In addition, there were both astute epidemiologic correlations and clinical observations that pointed to the anticancer chemopreventive properties of non-steroidal anti-inflammatory drugs (NSAIDs) such as aspirin, and the use of other NSAIDs to cause the regression of polyps in familial adenomatous polyposis (FAP) patients.

These chemopreventive agents include medications (e.g. aspirin) that have non-chemopreventive attributes, chemicals derived from foods and believed to have anticarcinogenic properties (e.g. lycopene from tomatoes), and chemicals especially developed for their antineoplastic properties (e.g. nitric oxide–NSAIDs or NO–NSAIDs). However, it is not possible to completely address this topic without including chemicals that are natural constituents of foods (e.g. calcium, vitamins and minerals). These agents and their studies in animals and man are numerous and have been collected onto an extensive database.[1]

The sites of action and mechanisms of chemoprevention are numerous and vary from agent to agent. The characteristics needed for an effective agent, the steps needed for their evaluation, and their chemopreventive mechanisms are summarized in Tables 5.1, 5.2, and 5.3, respectively.

A review of mechanisms and sites of chemopreventive action, types of agents being evaluated, and results of tri-

Table 5.1 Characteristics needed for a chemopreventive agent

- **Safe**: proven by long-term experimental and clinical follow-up studies
- **Effective**: proven by long-term experimental and clinical follow-up studies
- **Cheap**: for mass use
- **Easy to take**: possibly as a dietary supplement

Table 5.2 Steps in evaluation of possible antineoplastic agents

1. A **clinical** impression of efficacy and/or a scientific hypothesis
2. **Animal** studies (given a carcinogen), looking for a reduction in adenomatous polyp and/or cancer occurrence
3. **Human** studies evaluating:
   - Epithelial proliferation
   - Adenomatous polyp occurrence or recurrence
   - Side-effects and dosage needed for therapeutic effect

Table 5.3 Outline of chemopreventive mechanisms

- Inhibition and/or deactivation of possible carcinogens
- Correction of genetic damage
- Inhibition of proliferation
- Promotion of terminal cell differentiation and/or programmed cell death (apoptosis)
- Antiangiogenesis

als are available elsewhere.[2] In brief, once an agent has been identified as potentially having anticancer properties, it is evaluated for its usefulness in an animal model, which is usually given a carcinogen. It is obvious that the genetic susceptibility for cancer, the gastrointestinal tract of the test animal, and the diet given are far different from those of humans, who are genetically dissimilar one to another, are eating a mixed and varied diet, and are certainly not subjected deliberately to a carcinogen. If promising results are obtained from the animal model, then short-term studies are performed in humans, looking at 'intermediate biomarkers' of response to the chemopreventive agent. These biomarkers include, for example, suppression of epithelial proliferation and/or promotion of terminal differentiation and apoptosis (cell death).[3] The next step might be a clinical trial in persons at high risk for developing adenomatous polyps, e.g. persons having had an ileorectal anastomosis for FAP. Randomized placebo-controlled trials in persons having sporadic adenomatous polyps are usually the last stage, as it would take too long and too large a study to evaluate each compound for its anticolorectal cancer effect (see Table 5.2).[1,4]

In this chapter, we will refer to some of the chemopreventive agents that have been or are being evaluated clinically and could reach clinical application.

Pharmaceutical drugs

Several drugs that have been investigated or specifically developed for their chemopreventive properties will now be considered.[1]

Non-steroidal anti-inflammatory drugs

Aspirin

The strongest epidemiologic evidence that medications prevent colorectal cancer is for the NSAIDs family in general and specifically for aspirin.[1,2] The clinical evidence is for a 50% reduction in incidence of large-bowel cancer. However, this evidence is indirect, as a by-product of epidemiologic and follow-up studies in chronic aspirin users and users of other non-specific cyclooxygenase (COX) inhibitors. The aspirin effect is greater in those having a high intake of vegetables and is influenced by having a specific polymorphism of the ornithine decarboxylase gene.[5,6] There is further supportive evidence for the significant efficacy of aspirin from intervention trials in adenoma patients followed up for adenoma recurrence.[1,2]

Most evidence for the daily dosage of aspirin needed to prevent recurrent colorectal adenomas is for one adult-size tablet, about 325 mg. However, it is not known for how many years it should be given and what is its long-term benefit.[7] In addition, what are the side effects (such as gastrointestinal bleeding or hemorrhagic stroke) that can be expected vs the benefit in reducing the likelihood of dying from cancer? This has been noted to be a concern in the elderly, who are often taking multiple medications for a variety of disorders.[8] The overall conclusions have been that routine colorectal screening saves more lives and at a lower cost than chemoprevention with aspirin.[9] For these above reasons, chronic aspirin use has not gained general acceptance for cancer prevention.

Cyclooxygenase

How does aspirin affect the gastric mucosa and also protect against colorectal neoplasia? Cyclooxygenase 1 (COX-1) is a naturally occurring and physiologically important enzyme involved in the synthesis of prostaglandins; it is found in the kidney, brain, and gastrointestinal mucosa, where it is cytoprotective. It is also expressed in the early phase of carcinogenesis in the large bowel.[10] COX-2 is induced during the inflammatory processes and during the process of cellular hyperproliferation and progression to neoplasia.[11] In order to reduce the production of prostaglandins, aspirin, and the other commonly used non-NSAIDs, while aiming at the COX-2 (which was induced by some inflammatory or neoplastic process), have a non-specific effect and inhibit both COX-1 and 2.[2,9] This non-specific inhibition can result in the loss of cytoprotection and allow damage to occur to the gastroduodenal mucosa.

Cyclooxygenase inhibition COX-2 inhibition studies have been performed with specific COX-2 inhibitors thought to act as promoters of apoptosis and inhibitors of invasion and angiogenesis, which may provide a better complication–benefit ratio than that obtained with aspirin.[11] New NSAIDs that are COX-1-sparing and are COX-2-specific inhibiting medications have been developed and marketed. These include the less-specific nimesulide (Mesulid, Helsinn Healthcare, Switzerland), which has been noted to cause the side effect of hepatotoxicity, and nabumetone (Relifex, SmithKline Beecham, UK). The highly specific COX-2 inhibitors include celecoxib (Celebrex), and valdecoxib (Bextra) Pfizer Inc., USA). So far, none of these have been approved for preventing sporadic colorectal neoplasia, but trials had been initiated.[1,2,4] Their dose-dependent side effects include edema, a slight reduction in renal function, and elevation of blood pressure. Bextra and Rofecoxib (Vioxx, Merck & Co., Inc., USA) have been withdrawn from the market because of an increased risk for cardiovascular and skin events. Celecoxib has been approved by the US Food and Drug Administration (FDA) as an adjunct therapy for FAP patients (see Chapter 6) as it has been demonstrated to significantly reduce their polyp sizes and numbers.[1,2,4] However, because of the increased risk for cardiovascular events occurring with COX-2 inhibitor drugs, it is not known if they will continue to be available for use even in young people with polyposis.

There is good clinical evidence that NSAIDs such as sulindac will inhibit the growth of adenomatous polyps in the retained rectum of FAP patients.[12] Sulindac and one of its metabolites, sulindac sulfide, also inhibit cellular proliferation and promote apoptosis. However, while reducing the number and size of adenomatous polyps in FAP patients, they inhibit both COX-1 and COX-2. Unfortunately, this is an incomplete therapeutic effect and adenomatous tissue is still present within the mucosa, and colorectal cancer can even occur while under treatment.[12] This is not unexpected, as experimental studies using a carcinogen demonstrated that the magnitude of therapeutic response depended on how early sulindac was administered in relationship to the carcinogen administration. So, in an ongoing genetic disorder such as FAP, it is very unlikely that NSAIDs can provide a complete therapeutic effect. COX-2 is also strongly expressed in other genetically driven familial neoplasia syndromes, so that COX-2 inhibitors might also have a role in their management (see Chapter 6).

Sulindac sulfone is the second metabolite of sulindac. It has no antiprostaglandin effect, but promotes apoptosis.[13] It, too, has an effect on the number of adenomatous polyps and their growth in the retained rectum of patients with FAP. But, clinically important dose-dependent hepatotoxicity has been reported to occur. This drug is still under investigation and is not yet marketed.

In conclusion, even though specific inhibition of COX-2 is beneficial in partially preventing colorectal neoplasia, COX-1 has a role to play in the early phases of carcinogenesis and later there are non-COX pathways also involved. In addition, the COX-2 specific inhibitors do not have the cardioprotective attributes of aspirin.

Other NSAIDs

There are studies with newer and safer aspirin preparations and other NSAIDs. These include *nitric oxide–aspirin* (NO-aspirin). Short-term human studies have demonstrated that, compared with aspirin, there is no gastric damage, and experimental studies have demonstrated inhibition of carcinogenesis. As yet, there are no published long-term human colorectal neoplasia prevention studies.[14,15]

5-aminosalicylic acid (5-ASA) preparations are used for treating inflammatory bowel disease (ulcerative colitis and Crohn's diseases). They are given in the acute state, but also chronically, to reduce the frequency of disease relapses. There is epidemiologic evidence of less colorectal neoplasia occurring in those persons who keep taking 5-ASA.[16] This has been attributed to the transient COX-2 inhibition that occurs while taking therapy.[17]

Ursodeoxycholic acid

Ursodeoxycholic acid is a synthesized bile acid, as it is found only in minute amounts in human bile. It has pharmaceutical properties that could make it useful as a chemopreventive agent. Its administration changes the usual constitution of hepatic bile by replacing and therefore reducing the amounts of deoxycholic acid produced and reaching the large-bowel epithelium. Deoxycholic acid and fatty acids in the colon are metabolized by bacteria to products that may be damaging to the colorectal epithelium and therefore cause cellular hyperproliferation, and they themselves also have a carcinogenic potential. Ursodeoxycholic acid prevents this and colorectal cancer from occurring in the experimental animal and reduces the risk for colorectal adenomas in patients with primary biliary cirrhosis. However, there are no supportive, published, long-term large clinical studies in humans.[1,2,4,18]

Eflornithine

Eflornithine or α-difluoromethylornithine (DFMO) is an inhibitor of the synthesis of polyamines, which are important in stimulating cell proliferation. This compound reduces the risk for colorectal and other cancers in animal experiments.[1,2,19] In humans, toxicity studies demonstrated a dose-dependent but reversible hearing impairment.[19] This drug is undergoing clinical trials in humans, with or without the addition of COX-2 inhibitors.[2,4]

Polyethylene glycol

Polyethylene glycol (PEG) is an inert laxative agent that is commonly used to prepare the bowel for colonoscopy; it significantly reduces the risk for colorectal neoplasia in experimental studies.[1,20] There are no published intervention studies in humans.

Postmenopausal hormones

The evidence for a protective effect of estrogen replacement therapy, with or without progesterone, is from meta-analyses of large follow-up studies in treated women.[21] This is consistent with the observation that large-bowel cancer is slightly less common in premenopausal women than in men, and that the rates rise in postmenopausal women. Even though the estrogen–progesterone combination significantly reduces the risk for postmenopausal colorectal cancer, the other side effects do not make it a useful preventive therapy.[21] Estrogens alone may have a protective effect.[2]

Naturally occurring agents

Fiber

In contrast to the overall conclusion that an adequate long-term intake of dietary fiber has a beneficial role to play in preventing colon neoplasia, the beneficial effect of short-term fiber supplements is not established (see also Chapters 3 and 4). This has been evaluated by studies looking at the effects of fiber supplements, from different sources, on large-bowel epithelial proliferation and/or adenoma recurrence. The effect, if preventive, was not prominent.[1,2,22]

Calcium

This mineral has been extensively investigated epidemiologically, experimentally, and clinically for its large-bowel anticancer properties. Its importance as a long-term dietary factor in colorectal cancer prevention is discussed in Chapter 4. Here, we will consider its usefulness as a pharmaceutical agent.

The strongest evidence for its use as a chemopreventive agent comes from a trial where calcium or placebo was given for 4 years to individuals with a prior history of adenomatous polyps. There was a small, but significantly reduced risk for adenomatous polyp recurrence in the intervened group, especially in those having an above-median serum level of vitamin D.[23] The daily dosage used, 3 g of calcium carbonate, added 1200 mg of calcium ion to the daily intake of dietary calcium.

Other studies used a slightly higher dose of calcium carbonate, so as to provide 1500 mg of calcium ion per day. The sources of calcium used, and whether they were insoluble or soluble salts did not seem to be important, and the different compounds gave similar results. Only a small proportion of ingested calcium, about 30–40%, is absorbed, and the remainder reaches the large bowel mixed with the intestinal contents, makes some contact with the mucosa, and finally is lost in the stools. So, there is evidence that 4–6 calcium carbonate tablets/day, each providing 300 mg of calcium ion, is a dosage proven to modestly suppress the risk for colorectal neoplasia in persons having had an adenomatous polyp and/or large-bowel epithelial proliferation in persons having had an adenoma or family history of colorectal cancer.[1,2,23,24] However, no such studies have been performed in the average-risk population.

Calcium supplementation

Because of the mounting evidence supporting the beneficial effect of calcium in preventing colorectal neoplasia and other more common disorders in high-risk persons, there is greater concerted public health action to supplement diets with more calcium.[25] The recommended intake of calcium ion for mature adults has now been increased to 1200 mg/day; however, very few people in the United States have this intake. A number of low-fat, high-calcium, dairy and breakfast-food products and juices are now being marketed and gaining popularity for the prevention of osteoporosis. Calcium should be given together with informative dietary counseling so as to provide a well-balanced diet (see also Chapter 4).[24] Contraindications to giving calcium supplements or for increasing the dietary calcium intake include hypercalcemia, nephrolithiasis, renal insufficiency, and gastrointestinal intolerance to the treatment.

Vitamins

Vitamin D

Vitamin D independently and/or with calcium, has been identified by epidemiologic and experimental studies as preventing colorectal cancer.[1,2,23] It inhibits cellular proliferation and promotes cellular terminal differentiation. Because of the hypercalcemia that natural vitamin D can induce, there is little clinical evidence available to prove its therapeutic usefulness. New analogues of vitamin D have been synthesized that are without its hypercalcemic effects, but maintain its antineoplastic properties. No results from large long-term clinical studies are available.[1]

β-carotene, vitamin A, and other retinoids

These vitamins inhibit cellular proliferation and induce terminal cellular differentiation in experimental models.[1] Their antioxidant properties help trap organic free radicals, deactivate excited oxygen molecules, and so prevent tissue damage. They have a beneficial effect on promoting differentiation of myeloid and squamous cells. However, short-term clinical studies have not clearly demonstrated a beneficial effect on adenoma recurrence or colorectal cancer incidence. Further analyses of these studies illustrate the complexity of chemoprevention. A significant reduction of adenoma recurrence was shown to occur in persons who kept to a low-fat, high-fiber fruit and vegetable diet and were not chronic alcohol drinkers or tobacco smokers; conversely, promotion of adenoma recurrence occurred in those who did not.[26] In addition, significant side effects have been reported to occur with retinoids, which limit their usefulness.

Folic acid

Folic acid is important for normal cellular function and DNA methylation, which helps maintain genetic stability.[1,2,27] As pointed out in Chapter 4, global hypomethylation is common in the elderly, and there is epidemiologic evidence that colorectal adenomas and cancers are more common in those persons having a low folate intake and especially if also chronic alcohol drinkers.[1,2,27] An observation was made that ulcerative colitis patients, who often have a low vegetable and fruit intake, were more likely to have colorectal cancer if taking salazopyrine (a medication known to reduce blood levels of folic acid).[28] A retrospective study of taking folic acid supplements demonstrated a reduced risk for dysplasia in these patients.[28] However, to confuse the issue, there is experimental evidence in animals that folic acid can potentiate the effects of giving a carcinogen to the animal.[27] There are no published large-scale chemopreventive studies in humans that prove its usefulness as an anticancer agent. In the United States and Canada, folic acid has already been added to flour and cereals so as to supplement its inadequate dietary intake in the general population and minimize birth defects.

Multivitamin and mineral preparations

The antioxidant vitamins C and E have the biochemical potential and epidemiologic evidence to be useful anticarcinogens, and this is also true for selenium.[2,29,30] There is no conclusive evidence from intervention studies in humans that each, individually, has an important chemopreventive role to play. For this reason, they have often been given together, or with other supplements such as β-carotene and calcium, in adenoma intervention trials. The short-term results have not been consistently beneficial or convincing, but they are unlikely to be harmful.[1,2,30]

Analysis of a very large group of persons taking multivitamin preparations for various durations of time showed a significant reduction of colorectal cancer occurring in those taking multivitamins (including folic acid), especially if taken for 10 or more years.[31,32] Based on long-term studies of diet and colon cancer incidence in large US populations, it was suggested to routinely supplement the United States diet with a multivitamin preparation.[33] This suggestion probably reflects the perceived difficulties in changing established dietary habits of a Western population (see Chapter 4).

Bioactive chemicals

Some purified active principles found in fruits, vegetables, cereals, and spices are believed to have anticancer properties (see also Chapter 4). Many such compounds or chemicals are searched for, identified, and extracted from their natural sources. The evidence for their value was initially based on local beliefs, clinical impressions and some epidemiologic evidence. The strongest epidemiologic anticancer evidence is probably for green tea or soybeans, as their intake in the Japanese population has been long term and extensive, whereas in Europe the drinking of red wine has been associated epidemiologically with a reduced risk of cardiovascular disease and for cancer (the detrimental effects of alcohol, as related to large-bowel cancer, are discussed in Chapter 2).

These active principles have been evaluated in cancer cell cultures and experimental studies in animals. They include perillyl alcohol and limonene from citrus fruits, resveratrol from red grapes, diallyl disulfide from garlic, lycopene from tomatoes, curcumin from turmeric, flavanols from green tea, isoflavones such as genistein from soybeans, dithiolthiones from cruciferous vegetables, squalene from olive oil, and ferulic and phytic acids from rice bran.[1,2,34–42]

Genistein

The well-published genistein has a molecular structure similar to the steroid estrogen, and is therefore termed a phytoestrogen. In experimental studies its modes of action are at multiple sites and also include inhibition of proliferation, promotion of apoptosis, and inhibition of angiogenesis, as well as an antiestrogen effect. Its anti-cancer effect is in both hormonal-dependent cancers (such as breast cancer) and colon cancer. The epidemiologic evidence for its preventing colorectal cancer is not as convincing as for the hormone-dependent neoplasia.[39]

Fish oil

The long-chain *n*-3 fatty acids found in fish oils are also taken as a food supplement. Their consumption is associated with a lower risk for major cancers.[43] The pathways of action are quite numerous, pointing to the benefit of promoting fish consumption or at least taking *n*-3 fatty acids.

Which chemopreventive agent to choose?

The drug needs to be a medication or food additive that can be taken over the long term, without significant side effects, having clinically proven cancer-preventive properties, easy to take, and cheap (Tables 5.1 and 5.4). The risk–benefit ratio must always be borne in mind when deciding if a chemopreventive agent needs to be used.

From the list of medications, the COX-2 inhibitors have been best evaluated. However, they still need long-term studies to be proven effective in preventing most colorectal cancer and with minimal side effects. In addition, there has been a suggestion that their therapeutic benefit may be improved by combination therapy with drugs acting through different pathways, for example celecoxib with DFMO.[2,4,44,45] The NO–NSAIDs may prove to provide an even better risk–benefit ratio. It is very likely that they will initially be made available for use in persons at substantially increased risk for colorectal neoplasia.[2,4] These include persons with a strong family history of colorectal

Table 5.4 *Examples of chemopreventive agents being evaluated and their efficacy in preventing colorectal neoplasia*[a]

Agents	Mechanism of action	Evidence of efficacy		Safety
		Experimental	Clinical	
NSAIDs	Inhibit proliferation	Good	Good	Moderate
Other pharmaceuticals	Antioxidants Correct genetic damage Inhibit proliferation Promote apoptosis	Good	No completed trials Good initial clinical results in patients at high risk for neoplasia	Variable
Fiber	Interaction with intraluminal contents	Good	Low	Good
Calcium	Inhibits proliferation	Good	Modest	Good
Vitamins and minerals	Antioxidants Correct genetic damage Inhibit proliferation	Moderate	Inconsistent	Good
Bioactive chemicals	Antioxidants Correct genetic damage Inhibit proliferation	Good	Only epidemiologic evidence No completed trials	Good

[a] See text for further details.

cancer or personal history of advanced adenoma. These medications are expensive. For example, using US costs, it was concluded that colorectal screening was cheaper than COX-2 inhibition therapy, even when there was a family history of cancer.[46]

For women, the decision to take postmenopausal replacement hormones, if only estrogens, is individual. The side effects and long-term risks for other malignancies as well as cardiovascular disease need to be considered. If they are taken, then the risk for large-bowel cancer is reduced.

Based on the evidence from soybean ingestion, green tea, and fish consumption, their active principles are worthy of further studies in humans at risk for colorectal cancer. In the meantime, foods enriched with calcium and folic acid would seem to be useful, at a minimal risk for side effects. Along with multivitamin preparations, they are most useful in persons having an inadequate and/or unbalanced Western diet.

References (*Reviews and general articles)

1. *Corpet DE, Tache S, Chemoprevention of colorectal cancer—database of effective agents and diets ranked by potency. A systematic review of experimental studies (men, rats, mice), http://www.inra.fr/reseau-nacre/sci-memb/corpet/indexan.html, accessed on 13/07/2004.
2. *Hawk ET, Umar A, Viner JL, Colorectal cancer chemoprevention—an overview of the science. Gastroenterology 2004; 126: 1423–47.
3. *Kelloff GJ, Sigman CC, Johnson KM et al, Perspectives on surrogate end points in the development of drugs that reduce the risk of cancer. Cancer Epidemiol Biomark Prev 2000; 9: 127–37.
4. Kelloff GJ, Schilsky RL, Alberts DS et al, Colorectal adenomas: a prototype for the use of surrogate end points in the development of cancer prevention drugs. Clin Cancer Res 2004; 10: 3908–18.
5. Thun MJ, Calle EE, Namboodiri MM et al, Risk factors for fatal colon cancer in a large prospective study. J Natl Cancer Inst 1993; 85: 581–2.
6. Martinez ME, O'Brien TG, Fultz KE et al, Pronounced reduction in adenoma recurrence associated with aspirin use and a polymorphism in the ornithine decarboxylase gene. Proc Natl Acad Sci 2003; 100: 7859–64.
7. Sandler RS, Aspirin prevention of colorectal cancer: more or less? Ann Intern Med 2004; 140: 224–5.
8. Koutsos MI, Shiff SJ, Rigas B, Can nonsteroidal anti-inflammatory drugs be recommended to prevent colon cancer in high-risk elderly patients? Drugs Aging 1995; 6: 421–5.
9. Imperiale TF, Aspirin and the prevention of colorectal cancer. N Engl J Med 2003; 378: 879–80.
10. Einspahr JG, Krouse RS, Yochim JM et al, Associations between cyclooxygenase expression and colorectal adenoma characteristics. Cancer Res 2003; 63: 3891–3.
11. Dannenberg AJ, Zakim D, Chemoprevention of colorectal cancer through inhibition of cyclooxygenase-2. Semin Oncol 1999; 26: 499–504.
12. *Cruz-Correa M, Hylind LM, Romans KE et al, Long-term treatment with sulindac in familial adenomatous polyposis. A prospective cohort study. Gastroenterology 2002; 122: 641–5.
13. Babbar N, Ignatenko NA, Casero RA et al, Cyclooxygenase-independent induction of apoptosis by sulindac sulfone is mediated by polyamines in colon cancer. J Biol Chem 2003; 278: 47762–75.
14. *Rigas B, Kalofonos H, Lobovics E et al, NO-NSAIDS and cancer: promising novel agents. Dig Liver Dis 2003; 35(Suppl 2): S27–34.
15. Fiorucci S, Del Soldato P, NO-aspirin: mechanism of action and gastrointestinal safety. Dig Liver Dis 2003; 35(Suppl 2): S9–19.
16. *Eaden J, Review article: the data supporting a role for aminosalicylates in the chemoprevention of colorectal cancer in patients with inflammatory bowel disease. Aliment Pharmacol Ther 2003; 18(Suppl 2): 15–21.
17. Allgayer H, Review article: mechanisms of action of mesalazine in preventing colorectal carcinoma in inflammatory bowel disease. Aliment Pharmacol Ther 2003; 18(Suppl 2): 10–14.
18. Hess LM, Krutzcsch MF, Guillen J et al, Results of a phase 1 multiple-dose clinical study of ursodeoxycholic acid. Cancer Epidemiol Biomarkers Prev 2004; 13: 861–7.
19. Love RR, Jacoby R, Newton MA et al, Randomized placebo-controlled trial of low-dose alpha-difluoromethylornithine in individuals at risk for colorectal cancer. Cancer Epidemiol Biomark Prev 1998; 7: 989–92.
20. Corpet E, Parnaud G, Delverdier M et al, Consistent and fast inhibition of colon carcinogenesis by polyethylene glycol in mice and rats given various carcinogens. Cancer Res 2000; 60: 3160–4.
21. *Chlebowski RT, Wactawski-Wende J, Ritenbaugh C et al, Estrogen plus progestin and colorectal cancer in postmenopausal women. N Engl Med 2004; 350: 991–1004.
22. Jacobs ET, Giuliano AR, Roe DJ et al, Intake of supplemental and total fiber and risk of colorectal

adenoma recurrence in the wheat bran fiber trial. Cancer Epidemiol Biomark Prev 2002; 11: 906–14.
23. *Grau MV, Baron JA, Sandler RS et al, Vitamin D, calcium supplementation, and colorectal adenomas: results of a randomized trial. J Natl Cancer Inst 2003; 95: 1765–71.
24. Rozen P, Lubin F, Papo N et al, Calcium supplements interact significantly with long-term diet while suppressing rectal epithelial proliferation of adenoma patients. Cancer 2001; 91: 833–40.
25. Miller GD, Anderson JJB, The role of calcium in prevention of chronic diseases. J Am Coll Nutr 1999; 18: 371S–2S.
26. Steck-Scott S, Forman MR, Sowell A et al, Carotenoids, vitamin A and risk of adenomatous polyp recurrence in the polyp prevention trial. Int J Cancer 2004; 112: 295–305.
27. *Kim Y-I, Role of folate in colon cancer development and progression. J Nutr 2003; 133: 3731S–9S.
28. Lashner BA, Provencher KS, Seidner DL et al, The effect of folic acid supplementation on the risk for cancer or dysplasia in ulcerative colitis. Gastroenterology 1997; 112: 29–32.
29. Combs GF Jr, Gray WP, Chemopreventive agents: selenium. Pharmacol Ther 1998; 79: 179–92.
30. *Patterson RE, Kristal AR, Newhouser ML, Vitamin supplements and cancer risk. Epidemiologic research and recommendations, In: Primary and Secondary Preventive Nutrition (Bendich A, Deckelbaum RJ, eds). Totowa, NJ: Humana Press, 2000: 21–43.
31. *Giovannucci E, Stampfer MJ, Colditz GA et al, Multivitamin use, folate, and colon cancer in women in the Nurses' Health Study. Ann Intern Med 1998; 129: 517–24.
32. Jacobs EJ, Connell CJ, Chao A et al, Multivitamin use and colorectal cancer incidence in a US cohort: does timing matter? Am J Epidemiol 2003; 158: 621–8.
33. *Willet WC, Stampfer MJ, Rebuild the food pyramid. Sci Am 2003; 288: 64–71.
34. Crowell PL, Prevention and therapy of cancer by dietary monoterpenes. J Nutr 1999; 129: 775S–8S.
35. Fleischauer AT, Poole C, Arab L, Garlic consumption and cancer prevention: meta-analysis of colorectal and stomach cancers. Am J Clin Nutr 2000; 72: 1047–52.
36. *Clinton SK, Lycopene: chemistry, biology, and implications for human health and disease. Nutr Rev 1998; 56: 35–51.
37. Huang M-T, Newmark HL, Frenkel K, Inhibitory effects of curcumin on tumorigenesis in mice. J Cell Biochem 1997; 27(Suppl): 25–34.
38. *Katiyar SK, Mukhtar H, Tea in chemoprevention of cancer: epidemiologic and experimental studies (Review). Intl J Oncol 1996; 8: 221–8.
39. Booth C, Hargreaves DF, Hadfield JA et al, Isoflavones inhibit intestinal epithelial cell proliferation and induce apoptosis in vitro. Br J Cancer 1999; 80: 1550–7.
40. Hecht SS, Chemoprevention of cancer by isothiocyanates, modifiers of carcinogen metabolism. J Nutr 1999; 129: 768S–74S.
41. Rao CV, Newmark HL, Reddy BS, Chemopreventive effect of squalene on colon cancer. Carcinogenesis 1998; 19: 287–90.
42. Mori H, Kawabata K, Yoshimi N et al, Chemopreventive effects of ferulic acid on oral and rice germ on large bowel carcinogenesis. Anticancer Res 1999; 19: 3775–8.
43. *Larsson SC, Kumlin M, Ingelman-Sundberg M et al, Dietary long-chain n–3 fatty acids for the prevention of cancer: a review of potential mechanisms. Am J Clin Nutr 2004; 79: 935–45.
44. Jacoby RF, Cole CE, Tutsch K et al, Chemopreventive efficacy of combined piroxicam and difluoromethylornithine treatment of Apc mutant Min mouse adenomas, and selective toxicity against Apc mutant embryos. Cancer Res 2000; 60: 1864–70.
45. Wagenaar-Miller RA, Hanley G, Shattuck-Brandt R et al, Cooperative effects of matrix metalloproteinase and cyclooxygenase-2 inhibition on intestinal adenoma reduction. Br J Cancer 2003; 88: 1445–52.
46. *Ladabaum U, Scheiman JM, Fendrick AM, Potential effect of cyclooxygenase-2-specific inhibitors on the prevention of colorectal cancer: a cost-effectiveness analysis. Am J Med 2003; 114: 546–54.

6 Who are at risk from familial colorectal cancer and how can they be managed?

Paul Rozen, Bernard Levin, Graeme P Young

Introduction

The etiology of most cases of colorectal cancer is related to diet and lifestyle habits (see Chapters 2 and 4). However, in about 15–20% of the cases, there is a family history of colorectal cancer and/or other malignancies (Figure 6.1). This includes a small number (<5%) where there is a recognizable dominant familial risk factor, whereas in a larger number (>10%) there is a familial clustering of cancers and/or adenomatous polyps, which could be from a genetic susceptibility due to undefined genetic perturbations, shared environmental-lifestyle risk factors, or an interaction between these two etiologies. This interaction is probably responsible for a large proportion of 'sporadic' colorectal cancer; however we don't recognize this clinically. References 1–4 provide an overview of the clinical features discussed below.

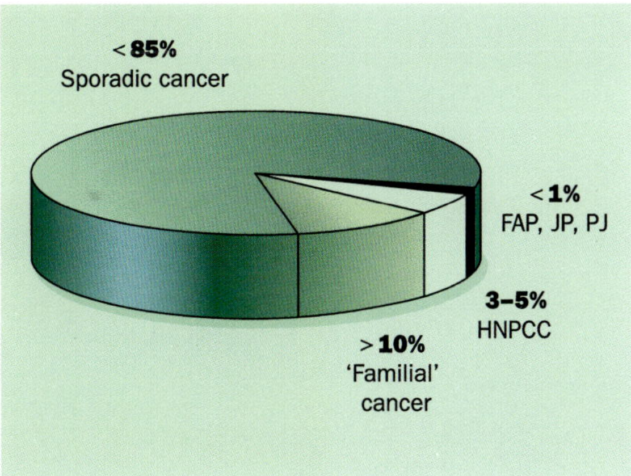

Figure 6.1 *Relative and approximate contributions of familial causes to the incidence of colorectal cancer: FAP, familial adenomatous polyposis; JP, familial juvenile polyposis; PJ, Peutz–Jeghers syndrome; HNPCC, hereditary non-polyposis colorectal cancer (Lynch syndrome).*

How to identify individuals and families at risk for colorectal cancer?

Asking a simple question, 'has anyone had cancer in your family?', can quite easily identify these families. An affirmative answer leads to the follow-up questions, 'Who has had cancer—parents, siblings or children (first-degree relatives); grandparents, grandchildren, uncles, aunts (second-degree relatives); cousins?; Where did these tumors occur—colon, breast, ovary, etc?, and 'At what age did these occur?'. If asking these simple questions becomes routine, then they are not time-consuming and can identify individuals and families at risk for common malignancies (Table 6.1). Answers that cause the physician to suspect a familial risk factor include cancers occurring before the age of 50–55 years, several cancers occurring in the same individual and/or cancers occurring in two or more first or second-degree relatives. These 'alarm' answers demand a more detailed cancer pedigree (Figure 6.2a).

Table 6.1 *Questions to ask for ascertaining familial cancer risk*

Has anyone had **cancer** in your family?
If **affirmative** . . .

- **Who** had cancer?
- **Where** was their cancer?
- At what **age** did it occur?

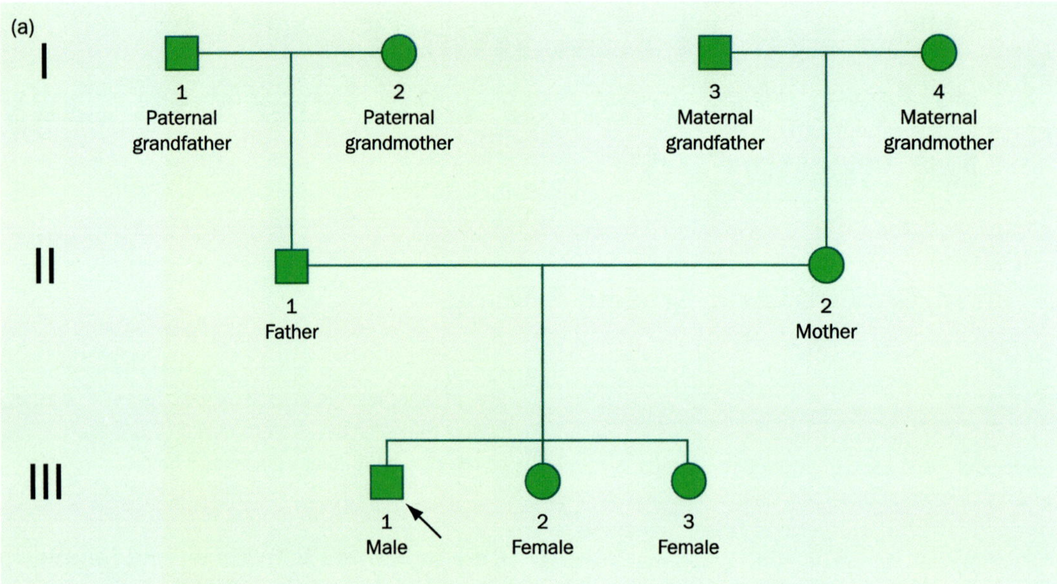

Figure 6.2 *(a) A basic pedigree. The arrow indicates the person who comes for consultation (called 'propositus' or 'proband'). Squares are males, circles females. The Roman numbers on the left indicate generations. The two females in the generation of the propositus are his sisters. Maternal and paternal aunts and uncles are added as necessary.*

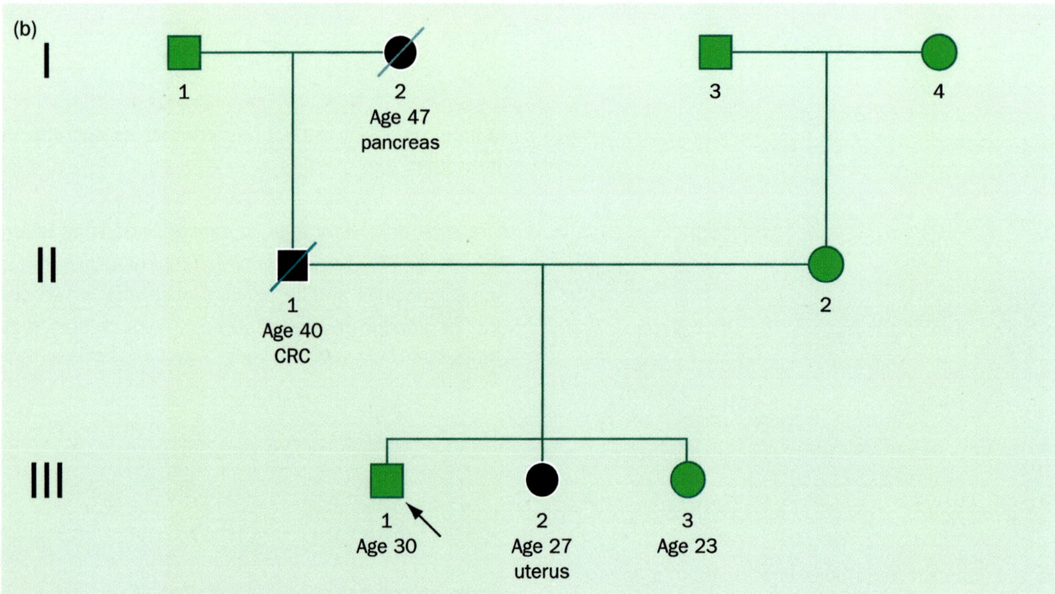

Figure 6.2 *(b) A pedigree suggestive of the Lynch syndrome: three generations of early-onset cancers compatible with this condition. The filled-in symbols indicate that the person is diseased; the line through the symbol indicates that the patient died. The symptomatic sister of the propositus needs genetic consultation and diagnosis; all three siblings need colonoscopy and follow-up as if they are mutation carriers, until proven otherwise.*

It is often useful to identify a family 'mentor(s)' who either knows the family's history or is willing and acceptable to the family to list the relatives and make initial contact with them so as to obtain permission for further questions and to obtain some medical information. This is then followed up by a sympathetic medical interviewer, who, by telephone, can ask directed questions and obtain written permission to obtain medical records, pathology reports, discharge summaries, or death certificates. A more detailed family pedigree can then be drawn-up by a trained medical interviewer or experienced family physician or consultant, or referred to a genetic counselor or medical geneticist. This pedigree allows the visualization of the pathways of inheritance and patterns of disease (organ-specific or distribution of neoplasia among organs) that may be consistent with a specific genetic disorder (Figure 6.2b).

How to classify families at risk for colorectal cancer?

These families fall into three categories, in descending order of risk for cancer. The first group has the smallest number of cases, and includes those individuals having recognizable genetic syndromes; their lifetime risk for cancer ranges from 70 to 100%. The second is a larger group having a strong familial history of colorectal cancer and/or other neoplasia, but not initially identifiable as belonging to a defined syndrome; their cancer risk is intermediate. The third and largest number includes the first-degree relatives of persons who have had sporadic colorectal neoplasia; their lifetime risk is 10–20%. The lifetime risk for colorectal cancer of most 'westernized' populations, without such family or personal histories, is about 5% (Tables 6.2a,b).

The defined genetic syndromes

Many years of astute clinical observations and recent progress in cancer genetics have defined easily recognizable but uncommon cancer syndromes, as those with or without antecedent multiple large-bowel polyps of adenomatous or other histologic types. The number of polyps,

Table 6.2a *Life-long risk for colorectal cancer in a 'westernized' population at average, increased, and high risk*

Risk group	Lifelong risk
Average[a]	1:20
Increased[b]	1:5–10
High[c]	1:2

[a] No family history of colorectal neoplasia.
[b] Family history of colorectal neoplasia, but not belonging to a defined dominant syndrome (see Tables 6.6 and 6.7).
[c] Family history of a dominant syndrome (see Table 6.2b).

Table 6.2b *Classifying causes of familial risk for colorectal cancer and their relative contributions to the total colorectal cancer burden in a 'westernized' population*

Defined genetic syndromes	Contribution to cancer burden	Lifelong risk for cancer
• With many adenomatous polyps		
– Familial adenomatous polyposis	< 1%	80–100%
• With hamartomatous polyps		
– Familial juvenile polyposis	≪ 1%	~ 50%
– Peutz–Jeghers syndrome	≪ 1%	
• Without multiple adenomatous polyps		
– Lynch syndrome	3–5%	≥ 70%
– Ethnic-specific and other susceptibility polymorphisms	? %	≥ 10%
Undefined familial risk		
• First-degree relatives of colon cancer or adenoma patients[a]	> 10%	10–20%

[a] see Table 6.6

their histology, and the clinical manifestations of the disease, which almost always includes extracolonic involvement, help classify the syndromes.[2–4]

Familial syndromes characterized by intestinal polyposis

These syndromes are classified clinically as having multiple adenomatous polyps or non-neoplastic, hamartomatous or hyperplastic polyps (Figure 6.3).

Familial adenomatous polyposis (FAP)

This condition is described in detail, as it illustrates the overall clinical problem of familial cancer.[1,2,5]

The classical clinical definition of FAP is based on finding more than 100 colonic adenomatous polyps. This is a dominant, autosomal (not sex-related) condition that occurs in one of 5–10 000 births. The polyps usually appear at the time of adolescence and thereafter increase in numbers; if the patient is an affected carrier, the polyps are usually found by the age of 40 years. Colonic cancer occurs almost inevitably and at an earlier than usual age,

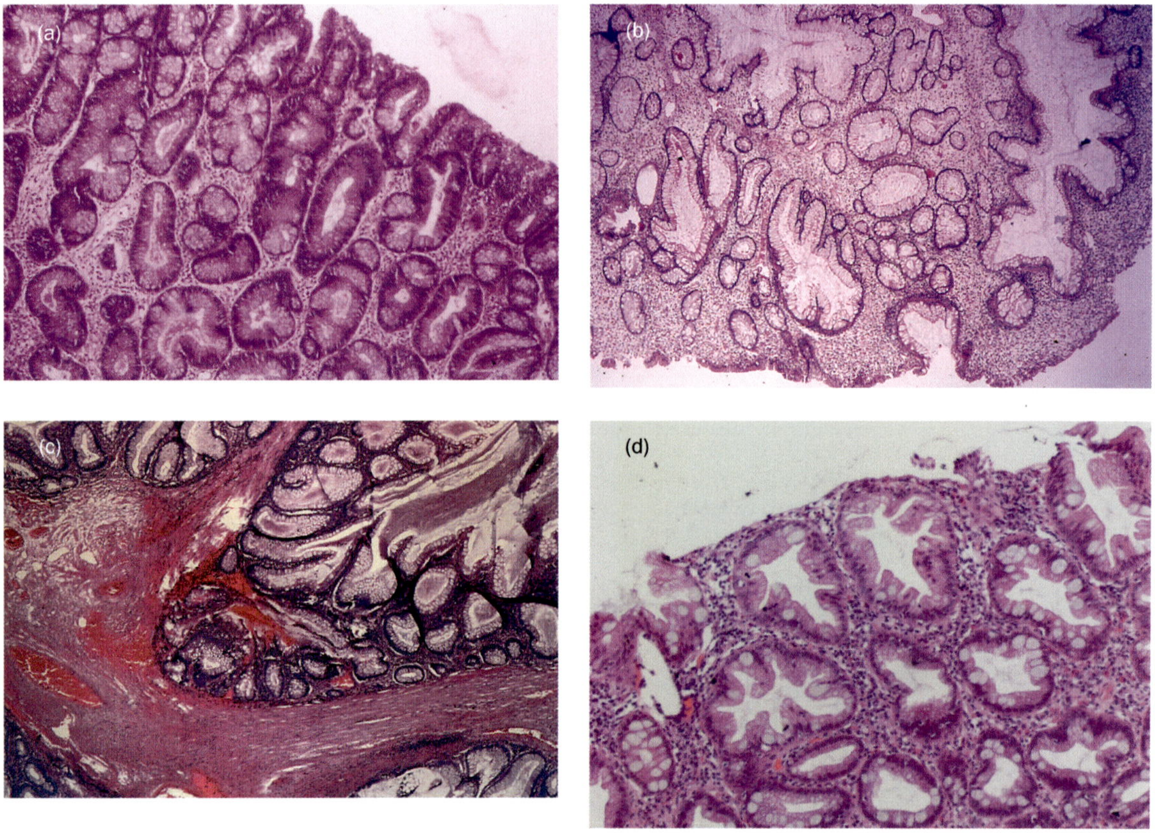

Figure 6.3 *(a) Section from a typical adenomatous polyp. Note the tubular morphology of the crypts; the dark-stained elongated nuclei are indicative of mild dysplasia. (b) Section from a juvenile polyp. These are red, round, smooth, or lobulated polyps. Microscopically, they are characterized by cystic dilatation of mucus-containing glands lined by normal epithelium. There is often dense stomal cellularity. (c) Section from a Peutz–Jeghers polyp. The histologic appearance of this hamartomatous polyp is similar to that of normal mucosa, other than the typical presence of bands of smooth muscle in the lamina propria. (d) In the hyperplastic polyp, the typical 'saw-tooth' or 'serration' of non-dysplastic epithelial cells is indicative of continuous cellular proliferation without normal cellular loss ('apoptosis'). There is usually increased cellularity of the stroma. (Figures provided by Dr E Brazowski, Tel Aviv, Israel.)*

but only rarely before the age of 20 years.[5,6] There are extracolonic gastrointestinal manifestations of disease, which include gastric polyps (mostly non-adenomatous 'fundic gland' polyps) and small-bowel adenomas, both of which rarely require intervention. However, duodenal adenomas, especially those on or around the papilla of Vater, may grow to a large size, undergo progressive dysplasia, and become invasive carcinomas (Figure 6.4).[5] Extraintestinal manifestations include subcutaneous masses, osteomas and dental abnormalities—none of which are malignant—and soft-tissue ('desmoid') tumors in the mesentery or areas of scars or abdominal wall that are benign but locally can form life-threatening masses. Gardner described the presence of these extraintestinal lesions and this phenotypic variant is named after him.[3] Retinal pigmented spots, (CHRPE or congenital hypertrophy of the retinal pigment epithelium) are found in a number of cases, but are not diagnostic of FAP. Other rare lesions include thyroid or liver (in babies) or brain tumors.

The genetic etiology of FAP has been identified as a mutation occurring on chromosome 5q in the area of the *APC* gene.[4] About one-third of these cases are new mutations, i.e. there is no evidence that the disorder was inherited.[5] Many different mutations have been identified in this large gene and, in general, there is a correlation between the genetic site and severity of clinical manifestation.[5–9] Laboratory success in identifying the mutation is about 70–90%, depending on the sophistication of their technique, but requires the DNA of an affected patient.[4,10–12] Its identification is important so as to be used as a screening test for possible mutation carriers in the asymptomatic family members at risk.[5,12]

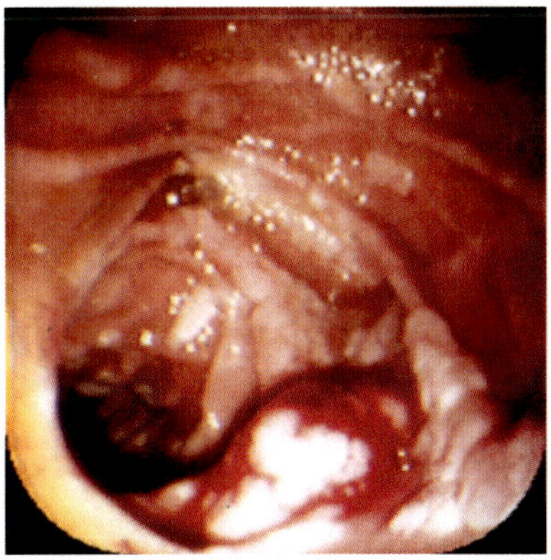

Figure 6.4 *Large bleeding duodenal adenoma in a FAP patient. Small flat adenomas are seen in the adjacent mucosa. Following multiple biopsies and endoscopic ultrasonography, the polyp was removed by mucosectomy and the surrounding polyps destroyed by argon plasma coagulation.*

Diagnosis

Diagnosis is essentially dependent on the clinical suspicion of the physician and, whenever possible, it should be confirmed by genetic analysis. Because the clinical manifestations can be minimal, the referral for costly FAP DNA analysis is very much dependent on in-depth clinical evaluation of the patient and family history.[9] Genetic testing of children at risk is performed just before or at puberty, when the diagnosis becomes of clinical relevance. The proven mutation-negative child can then be left without further investigation. The mutation-positive child (or all children, if no mutation can be identified in the FAP patient, or if no patient is available for testing) is best seen by the examining gastroenterologist. The child or youth is given an explanation about the necessity for an intrarectal examination. At the first examination, it is best to do a brief and minimal flexible sigmoidoscopy with directed and random biopsies. A painful or psychologically traumatic endoscopy reduces the chances to have cooperation for a more complete examination in the future. The child or young adult should be seen and followed up by the one physician with whom the patient feels comfortable. The child is easily frightened and anxious, especially when the family history of cancer and operations are discussed. Once the youth's confidence is obtained, then, at about the age of completing secondary schooling, a baseline colonoscopic examination should be performed. This might be needed earlier if there are symptoms or multiple polyps found at sigmoidoscopy or there was a family history of colorectal cancer at an early age.[2,5,6]

Recently, it has become apparent that the clinical features may not be 'classical', and there may be relatively few or even no large-bowel adenomas at the time of endoscopic examination, or they may occur only in the proximal colon. These patients are older than usual for FAP, develop cancer at a later age, and mostly do not have extracolonic disease. This condition has been called 'attenuated' FAP. In this context, when FAP is suspected, colonoscopy is therefore the best way to pursue the diagnosis.[7–9] The adenomas may be small and flat or may be intramucosal, and are therefore identified by taking multiple random biopsies or by dye-staining and/or using a magnifying colonoscope. Histologically, these are called 'microadenomas' or appear as ' flat' adenomas (Figure 6.5).[13]

The treating physician needs to be aware that the clinical manifestations of FAP may vary between family members and between branches of that extended, but affected family (Table 6.3):[8] so, a one-time clinical examination does not necessarily exclude FAP. If genetic testing is unavailable, then the at-risk family members must continue to be under close systematic clinical and endoscopic follow-up.

As stated, large-bowel endoscopy is the most important clinical examination. However, the disease is lifelong and there are multiple clinical manifestations.[2,5] An annual physical examination includes an evaluation for soft tissue, bone, or abdominal masses. Abdominal ultrasound examination, gastroduodenoscopy, and colonoscopy are performed before elective surgery of the colon (Table 6.4).

Treatment

Treatment is by surgical removal of the large intestine, before cancer occurs. The usual age for this is the late teens or early twenties.[2,5] As this is usually an elective procedure the timing can be arranged so as to be least inconvenient, e.g. during vacation before starting studies or a new job. For girls, it is sometimes best arranged either before marriage or after pregnancies, as there is a signifi-

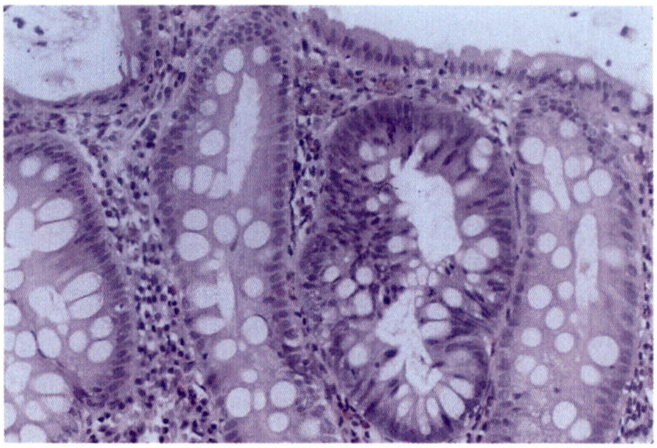

Figure 6.5 *Intramucosal microadenoma. Note the appearance of dark-stained and elongated dysplastic nuclei in a distorted crypt that does not protrude above the surrounding normal surface epithelium.*

Table 6.3 *Phenotypic variations in familial adenomatous polyposis*

- Between families having the same site of mutation (interfamilial variation)
- Between members of same family (intrafamilial variation)

Assumption: unrecognized modifying genes and/or genetic–environmental interactions

Table 6.4 *Screening for familial adenomatous polyposis*[a]

Diagnosis
- *DNA testing, pre or postnatal:* Useful in > 70% of cases. If it is positive or not available, then:
- Flexible sigmoidoscopy at age 10–12 years with random mucosal biopsies
- Colonoscopy with random biopsies at age 18–20 years; repeated every 2 years
- Retinal examinations to identify CHRPE[ab]
- Panoramic X-rays of face for osteomas[ab]

Follow-up
- Physical examination, yearly
- US or CT or MRI of abdomen, yearly[ab]
- Rectal surveillance, every 3–12 months, if ileorectal anastomosis was performed
- Pouch surveillance every 1–2 years
- Gastroscopy or duodenoscopy, alternating every 1–3 years

[a] CHRPE, congenital hypertrophy of the retinal pigment epithelium; CT, computed tomography; MRI, magnetic resonance imaging; US, ultrasound
[b] Elective tests.

cant loss of fecundity after pouch operation.[14] The elective surgery can be further delayed if there is good rapport with a compliant patient and the polyps are sparse and not large.[5,8,15] The most common reasons for delaying surgery are a desire to complete a study program or the family. This requires careful clinical and colonoscopic annual follow-up.

The surgical treatment is usually removal of the entire large bowel, with or without stripping the remaining rectal mucosa down to the dentate line and forming an internal pouch from the small intestine (Figure 6.6).[2,5,16] This is usually a two-stage procedure with a temporary diverting ileostomy. However, there are medical centers that perform this in one stage, and by laparoscopy, which is obviously more convenient for the patient but problematic if there is an anastomotic leak. In a few cases, where there are sparse rectal polyps, a low ileorectal anastomosis is performed, leaving rectal mucosa for careful biannual endoscopic follow-up.[9,17,18]

Follow-up

It is essential that annual follow-up continues after the surgical procedures are completed, including physical examination, abdominal ultrasound (US), and computed tomography (CT) or magnetic resonance imaging (MRI) if there is a suspected desmoid tumor.[5,19] Upper endoscopy with a gastroscope, alternating with a side-viewing duodenoscope, should be performed every 1–3 years in order to identify peri- and ampullary duodenal adenomas.[5,18,19] These polyps should be ablated endoscopically before they reach a large size and/or become invasive cancers (see Figure 6.4 and Table 6.4). The gastric polyps are usually non-neoplastic fundic gland polyps, but dysplasia, adenomas, and even gastric cancer have been reported.[5,20]

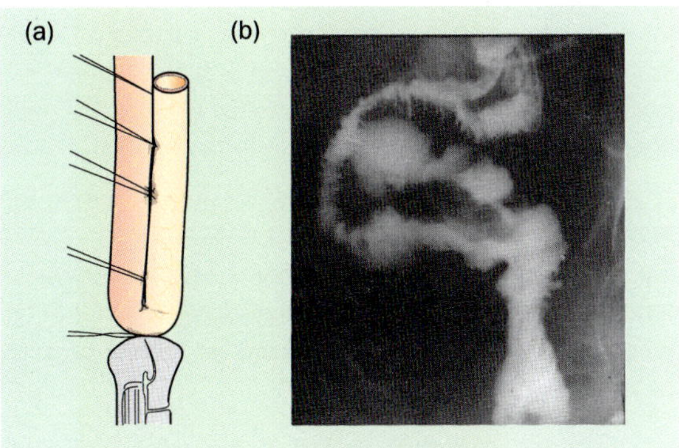

Figure 6.6 *(a) Schematic illustration of a 'J-pouch', formed from the distal small intestine and attached to the anal sphincter; the shorter limb of the 'J' acts as a fecal reservoir. (b) An X-ray demonstration of this pouch. (Figures provided by Dr A Deutsch, Petach Tikva.)*

Postoperatively, there is always some disturbance of bowel habits and even control of bowel function. This is least after an ileorectal anastomosis, worst after mucosectomy to the dentate line and pouch formation, and intermediate after stapled anastomosis and leaving a small cuff of rectal mucosa above the dentate line.[16,17] Consequently, it is important to see the patients postoperatively and reassure them that bowel function will improve with time and explain how to best adapt to the change. This usually requires a change in diet and appropriate medications to manage symptoms.

The pouch and anastomosis should be examined every 1–2 years, looking for neoplasia that may require endoscopic treatment or even further surgery.[2,5,21–23]

Chemoprevention

There are no agreed upon chemopreventive recommendations for FAP patients with an intact colon.[24] However, nonsteroidal anti-inflammatory drugs (NSAIDS)—including the selective cycloxygenase-2 (COX-2) inhibitors—suppress adenoma growth and provide supplemental treatment to endoscopic polypectomy if there is an intact rectum postcolectomy or duodenal adenomas.[5] The treatment can be in the form of suppositories or medications by mouth. However, there are case reports of rectal cancer occurring even without polyp growth.[25] So, in some cases, this is only a temporizing treatment before definitive surgery (see Chapter 5). There is now US Food and Drug Administration (FDA) approval to use the selective COX-2 inhibitor celecoxib as a supplemental preoperative treatment, for reducing the adenomatous polyp burden, even in the intact colon of FAP patients (Figure 6.7). Its longer-term usefulness and use in children remain to be evaluated.[26,27] A major problem with celecoxib chemoprevention is the large dosage needed and subsequent high cost of chronic therapy.

There is no established chemopreventive or therapeutic protocol for desmoid tumors. It is usually best not to operate upon them, as they are not always possible to completely remove and any surgical procedure can stimulate further growth or recurrence. In some cases, desmoid tumors regress or do not progress in size. Desmoids

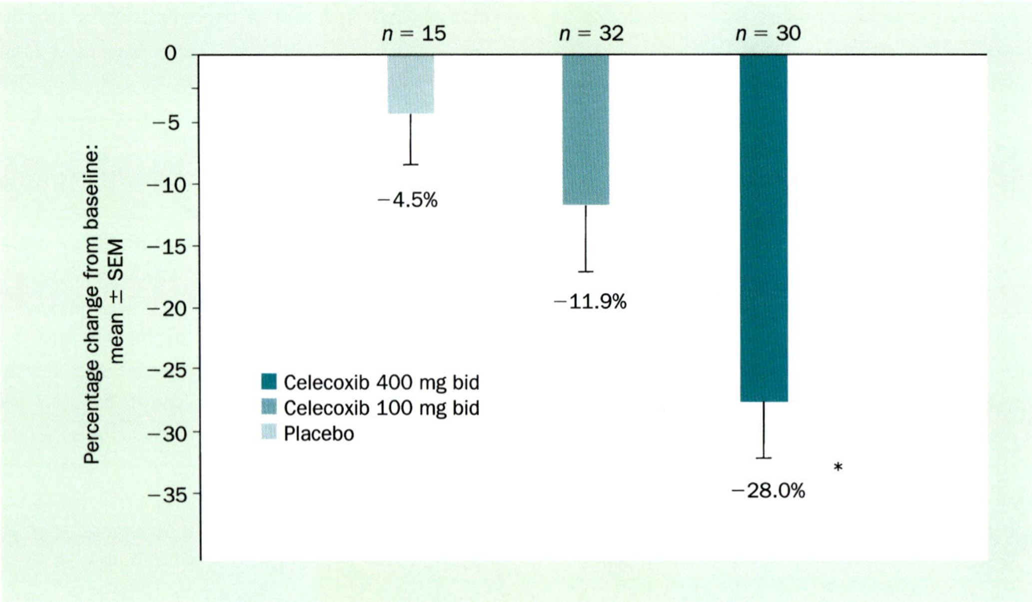

Figure 6.7 *Change in the number of colorectal polyps in FAP patients receiving placebo or celecoxib (Celebrex) for 6 months. The reduction in polyp burden was highly significant (*p = 0.003 vs placebo) with the dosage of 400 mg twice a day. Figure derived from reference 26 and published with permission of the authors.*

occurring in the abdominal wall may require surgical removal if bulky. However, antiestrogens (such as tamoxifen) and NSAIDs (such as celecoxib) are tried when there is evidence of a desmoid, before they become large and/or endanger a surrounding organ. They have been found useful in high dosage.[5,28] There are also case reports of success with other medications.[5]

Prognosis and support

After colectomy, FAP patients may die from rectal cancer (if an ileorectal anastomosis was performed), or desmoid tumors, or duodenal cancers, or from other rare complications.[18] Otherwise, they have a good prognosis and quality life. Patients need lifelong medical and emotional support. There are often intrafamilial crises if the marriage partner has not been prepared adequately by a genetic counselor. Affected children who have not been adequately counseled may develop antagonistic feelings towards the disease-transmitting parent and they may need help from a child psychologist who understands the medical problem.[5]

Other adenomatous polyposis syndromes

It has become apparent that other genetic disorders can also manifest with multiple, but usually less than 100 polyps. Mutations of both *MYH* gene alleles on chromosome 1 can explain a proportion of the older FAP-like patients who do not have a mutation of the *APC* gene.[29] As this condition is recessive (not dominant, as is FAP), both of these genes must be mutated (homozygote state) before becoming clinically apparent; this requires that both parents were asymptomatic carriers of the mutation. The pedigree will therefore indicate that the polyposis appeared in a quarter of the siblings, and only in that one generation. The risk of colorectal cancer in heterozygotes might also be slightly increased.

The hamartomatous polyposis syndromes

Including familial juvenile polyposis and Peutz–Jeghers syndrome, hamartomatous polyposis syndromes must be differentiated from FAP, as their clinical manifestations, genetic diagnosis, treatment, follow-up, and prognosis are different.[2–4,30] The essential diagnostic element is the polyp histology (see Figure 6.3b). An experienced gastrointestinal histopathologist is needed for making this differential diagnosis. Even so, there may still be some confusion in classification, as the histology may show a 'mixed' picture, which includes adenomatous and other histologic types. These may be part of the hereditary mixed polyposis syndrome or dysplastic changes occurring in the progression of the hamartoma to malignancy.[30–32]

Familial juvenile polyposis

Sporadic colonic juvenile polyps are a common finding in infants, sometimes causing symptoms, but usually occurring without a family history of polyps or cancer. The familial syndrome is uncommon, and there the polyps can be found not only in the colon but also in the stomach and small intestine. The incidence is much lower than FAP. The clinical features may also include non-gastrointestinal lesions, and these have led to the subclassification into other syndromes: Cowden, Bannayan–Ruvalcaba–Riley, and Gorlin.[2–4,30] This, and the different mutations that have been identified led to the realization that familial juvenile polyposis is a heterogeneous condition: i.e. different mutations can cause the appearance of juvenile polyps and the various other clinical manifestations.[33] Mutations causing syndromes having juvenile polyps have been identified on chromosomes 6, 9, 10, and 18. Identifying the particular mutation is difficult, but, if successful, it becomes a useful screening test for that particular family.[3,4,33] In contrast to FAP, there is no description of a new mutation occurring spontaneously.

It has been estimated that in familial juvenile polyposis, there is a 50% lifetime risk for cancer, including a 15% risk for colon cancer.[30,32] The patients and their affected first-degree relatives need repeated routine physical examination and upper and lower endoscopy. Small-bowel radiologic examination, capsule endoscopy, and enteroscopy need to be performed if there is a suspicion of small-bowel polyps. Whenever possible, endoscopic polypectomy should be performed repeatedly, and surgery delayed until the clinical features, the number of polyps, and their dysplastic changes require surgical intervention. The surgical procedure should be tailored to answer the clinical needs, since, in contrast to FAP, where definitive surgery is recommended because of the high risk for colorectal cancer and where each surgical procedure can lead to adhesions and desmoid tumors, this is not the case in familial juvenile polyposis.[30,34] Intraoperative enteroscopy will then be useful to identify and treat small bowel lesions.[35] These familial juvenile polyps, in contrast to sporadic juvenile polyps, strongly express COX-2 (Figure 6.8).[36] It is still not proven that chemoprevention with COX-2 inhibitors will be of long-term help.

Peutz-Jeghers syndrome

This is an uncommon genetic disorder, having about one-third of the incidence of FAP. Genetically, this syndrome has a high degree of penetrance, and, in many cases, the mutation has been found on chromosome 19.[3,4,37] However, clinically it is easily identified by the pigmented spots that appear on the lips and other mucous membranes such as the buccal mucosa, nail beds, conjunctiva, palms, and soles.[2] The pigmentation can be identified during infancy, but may fade away by early adulthood. The polyps have a characteristic histology and are not neoplastic; however, dysplasia can occur and leads to cancer (see Figure 6.3c). The polyps can occur throughout the gastrointestinal tract and even in other organs. The clinical

(a)

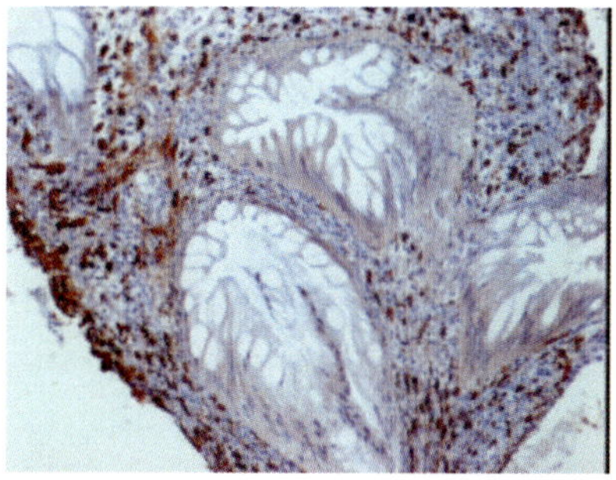

(b)

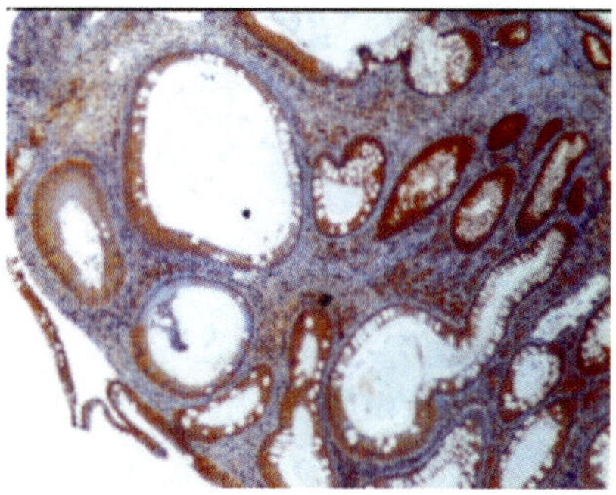

Figure 6.8 *Sporadic juvenile polyp, showing dilated crypts and dense stromal cellularity. COX-2: staining of stromal cells (brown). (b) Familial juvenile polyp stained for COX-2: staining of both epithelial and stromal cells (brown). (Figures provided by Dr E Brazowski, Tel Aviv.)*

complaints are often related to gastrointestinal tract polyps, causing obstruction or bleeding.

The risk for cancer in the gastrointestinal tract and elsewhere is high by early mid-adulthood. Cancers occur in the gastrointestinal tract, pancreas, breasts, uterus, ovaries, and testes.[2–4,37] Because of the pleomorphic manifestations and sites of neoplasia, repeated medical examinations are needed, starting from early adulthood. These include physical examination, breast and gynecologic, testicular examinations, and abdominal US. Other tests include gastrointestinal endoscopy to identify and remove polypoid lesions, small-intestinal radiologic examination, capsule endoscopy, and enteroscopy to examine the small intestine especially when surgery is performed. These polyps also express COX-2 and are suppressed by COX-2-inhibiting drugs.[38]

Other non-adenomatous polyposis syndromes

These include *hyperplastic polyposis* and the *Cronkhite–Canada syndrome*, both having a risk for colorectal cancer. A few hyperplastic polyps are commonly found in the rectum, and are not associated with neoplasia (see Figure 6.3d). However, there are an increasing number of reports of patients with multiple hyperplastic polyps, with or without a family history of these polyps and/or colorectal cancer. These polyps are often large and proximal to the rectosigmoid. They probably undergo dysplasia and are recognized as serrated adenomas with a risk for cancer (see Chapter 8).[39]

The Cronkhite-Canada syndrome is rare, not familial, and sometimes transient. There are typical dermatologic features and gastrointestinal polyposis. The polyps' histology has features of juvenile, hyperplastic, serrated adenomas, and there is a risk for gastrointestinal adenocarcinoma.[40]

Familial syndromes not characterized by many intestinal polyps

Adenomatous polyps can occur in these conditions, but they are usually few in number as compared to the polyposis syndromes.

Hereditary non-polyposis colorectal cancer (HNPCC)—Lynch syndrome

Probably the most commonly occurring defined genetic syndrome, HNPCC contributes about 2–5% of all colorectal cancer (see Figure 6.1).[1,41,42] The incidence varies from country to country, depending on the presence of 'founder mutations', stability of the population and sophistication of technique used for data ascertainment.[41,42] Warthin recognized it as a cause of familial cancer, but Henry Lynch defined its clinical features and recognized its clinical importance as an example of familial cancer that could be helped by early recognition and surgical treatment.[1] The occurrence of polyps is more frequent than expected, but less than polyposis.[41] Thus, the synonym 'Lynch syndrome' is now preferred.

Lynch syndrome is a dominant disorder with a high degree of penetrance, although 'skipped generations' can occur. The genetic pathway to neoplasia is uniquely different from that of sporadic large-bowel cancer. The commonest mutations occur on chromosomes 2 (*MSH2*), 3 (*MLH1*), but uncommon mutations also occur elsewhere, that allow 'naturally occurring' errors in chromosome replication to remain uncorrected, and this is termed 'defective mismatch repair' (see Chapter 3). This defective pathway allows cancer to appear relatively quickly, through rapidly advancing adenomas, in young adulthood.[1,3,43,44] This defective pathway is germline in the Lynch syndrome, but it can also be somatic (occurring locally) and is responsible for about 15% of sporadic colorectal cancers (see Chapter 3).

The cancer commonly occurs in the colon without the appearance of multiple precursor adenomatous polyps being noted—hence its name. However, adenomatous polyps are found, and they are frequently highly dysplastic.[3,43,44] There is a high likelihood of cancer appearing in other gastrointestinal and non-gastrointestinal organs, with or without colonic involvement.[1,3] These include the small intestine, pancreas, ovary, uterus, prostate, urinary tract, skin, and brain, and a higher risk for breast cancer and stomach cancer in some families.

In this syndrome, the appearance of a brain tumor is called the 'Turcot syndrome'. The concurrent occurrence of sebaceous tumors of the skin and a small bowel and/or other tumors is called the 'Muir-Torre syndrome' (Figure 6.9).[1]

Diagnosis

As there is no diagnostic phenotype or easily performed screening test, the initial diagnosis is clinical by obtaining a cancer pedigree suggesting this syndrome (see Figure 6.2b).[1] This has been defined as two generations with cancer involving three or more relatives from the same family, one of whom should be younger than 50 years of age, one

(a) (b)

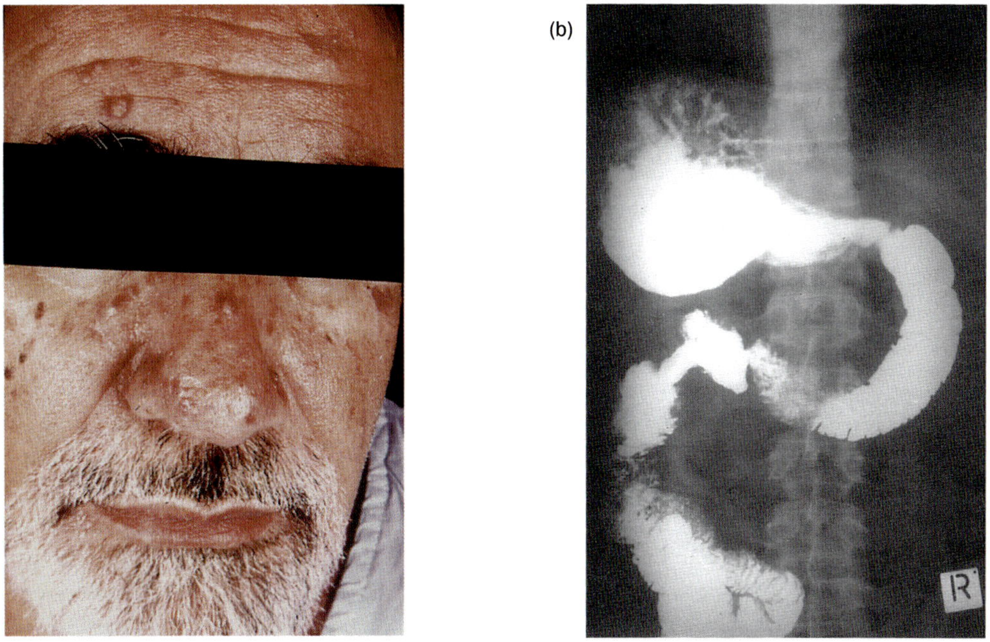

Figure 6.9 *Muir–Torre syndrome. Multiple sebaceous adenomas on the face of a patient having a typical HNPCC family history. (b) Upper gastrointestinal X-ray of the same patient, demonstrating a postduodenal narrowing due to a cancer of the small intestine.*

of the cancers should be of the colon and the others might be of the other Lynch syndrome target organs. This is referred to as 'modified Amsterdam criteria'.[45] There are affected families that do not completely fulfill these clinical criteria due to the small size of the family, genetic–genetic interactions, or having uncommon mutations.[46,47] FAP needs to be excluded, as sometimes it is difficult to clinically differentiate the Lynch syndrome from attenuated FAP.[1]

The identification of the actual mutation is difficult due to the large number of genetic sites at risk. If found, it is obviously very useful as a screening test of the relatives at risk. However, there are other indirect tests that can help in classifying the cancer case as probably belonging to this syndrome and to localize the genetic site of the responsible mutation. Microsatellites are the repetitive sequences of DNA that are found in the chromosome between coding areas of the gene. The genetic disturbance in HNPCC allows a disorder of these sequences to remain uncorrected and this can be detected and quantified. The finding of a significant degree of microsatellite instability (MSI) in the tumor tissue itself ('MSI-high') is consistent with the pathogenetic pathway of the Lynch syndrome. This test is not cheap but is now becoming more readily available. It can be performed on the patient's DNA or tumor tissue after DNA extraction.[3] The criteria to define MSI-high, MSI-low, or MSI-stable were established at a US National Institutes of Health (NIH) Workshop held in Bethesda, Maryland. These are referred to as 'Bethesda criteria', and they also include a broader set of clinical criteria for examining the presence of MSI.[48] In addition, there are now cheaper immunohistochemical tests to stain the tumor tissue and indicate if chromosome 2 or 3 is intact or not (mutated): if either were not intact, this would be consistent with a mutation such as *MLH1*, *MSH2*, or *MSH6* in that chromosome. This could be somatic and just in the tumor, or it could be a germline mutation, indicating the possibility of HNPCC (Figure 6.10).[3,49] This is a useful, simple, and inexpensive initial screening test. Both the MSI and immunohistochemical tissue tests will not exclude the possibility of sporadic colorectal cancer occurring due to a somatic mutation.

Screening and post operative follow-up

As neoplasia can appear in early adult life and genetic testing may not be available or is not informative, it is

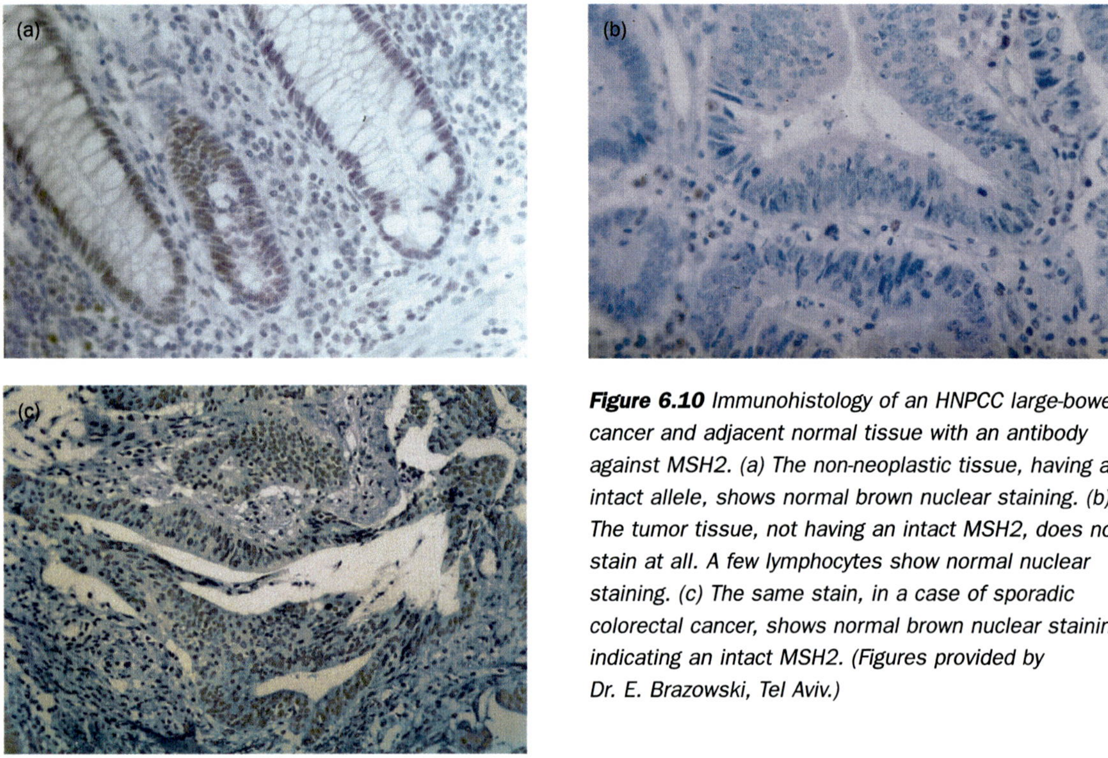

Figure 6.10 *Immunohistology of an HNPCC large-bowel cancer and adjacent normal tissue with an antibody against MSH2. (a) The non-neoplastic tissue, having an intact allele, shows normal brown nuclear staining. (b) The tumor tissue, not having an intact MSH2, does not stain at all. A few lymphocytes show normal nuclear staining. (c) The same stain, in a case of sporadic colorectal cancer, shows normal brown nuclear staining indicating an intact MSH2. (Figures provided by Dr. E. Brazowski, Tel Aviv.)*

usually recommended to start screening in the early twenties.[1] There is also an advantage in getting the at-risk young relatives used to periodic examinations before they get diverted into other activities and responsibilities. The annual protocol should include a complete system review and physical examination; tests include a urine examination, abdominal and pelvic (in females) US examination, and gynecologic and breast examinations and a colonoscopic examination at least every 2 years, even after subtotal colectomy.[1,50,51] As two-thirds of Lynch syndrome colorectal neoplasia occurs proximal to the rectosigmoid, colon screening should be by total colonoscopy. If the family history is indicative of neoplasia in other target organs, e.g. stomach, then these should also be included in the screening protocol.[1] This protocol of targeted screening has been shown to be cost-effective in reducing mortality from large-bowel cancer (Table 6.5).[1,52,53]

Treatment

At present there is no clinical evidence that preventive dietary treatment changes the risk for neoplasia in these patients. However, there is epidemiologic and experimental evidence for the neoplasia promoting effects of cigarette smoking, alcohol intake, and cooking-induced heterocyclic amines with MSI-high status, and conversely the protective effect of vitamin C on mismatch-repair deficient cell lines.[54,55] So, it would seem prudent to advise a

Table 6.5 *Screening and follow-up of Lynch syndrome (HNPCC) patients*

Start screening from age 20 years, or 10 years less than the youngest first-degree cancer relative

- Physical examination, yearly
- Fecal occult blood testing, yearly (alternating with colonoscopy)[a]
- Colonoscopy every 2 years, and also if after partial colonic resection
- Ultrasound, abdominal, and gynecologic examination, yearly[a]
- Urine tests, yearly[a]
- Breast screening
- DNA tests (useful in ~40%)

[a] Elective tests

healthy lifestyle and dietary habits. There are no positive results available of chemopreventive trials in HNPCC patients. Only some HNPCC tumors express COX-2, but their fibroblast cell lines do so strongly, and so it remains to be seen if they would be responsive to NSAID chemoprevention.[56,57]

If large-bowel adenomatous polyps are identified, then the treatment is by polypectomy.[58] In the case of cancer, and because of the high incidence of metachronous neoplasia, the recommendation is for an extended resection so as to remove much of the target organ at risk, but also to maintain the quality of life.[51] As neoplasia can recur, the final result might be ileorectal or ileoanal anastomosis and pouch.[50,59] If the woman patient is menopausal and/or there is a family history of uterine-ovarian cancer, then a preventive oophorectomy and hysterectomy are recommended at the time of colonic surgery, especially as gynecological surveillance is relatively insensitive.[60] If colonoscopic screening of a proven mutation carrier is technically difficult and/or becomes a physical or psychological burden, prophylactic subtotal colectomy might be considered.

There is some clinical and experimental evidence that HNPCC tumors are relatively resistant to 5-fluorauracil (5–FU).[61,62] However, their cell lines are more sensitive to cisplatin and irinotecan.[63] To date, there has not been a policy decision to routinely adapt the choice of chemotherapy to the MSI status of the tumor.

Prognosis

It has been demonstrated that identification of mutation carriers—or even those just having the clinical criteria for HNPCC—and their prospective systematic clinical screening will reduce their mortality from large-bowel cancer.[58] Even those persons who have had a colorectal cancer treated have a longer survival than those having the same stage of sporadic cancer.[1,64]

Other defined genetic susceptibility conditions

A widely prevalent, but low-penetrant *polymorphism (I1307K)* of the *APC* gene on chromosome 5, leading to susceptibility for colorectal neoplasia, has been identified in Jews of European origins, Ashkenazi Jews, who are an ethnic group at risk for cancer.[3,65] This leads to an unstable *APC* gene and allows cancer to occur in a slightly higher than expected rate in carriers with a family history of colorectal neoplasia.[66] Its clinical use as a marker of risk has not been established. Similar low-penetrance, but highly prevalent susceptibility mutations, will probably be found in other ethnic groups or extended families at risk for colorectal cancer.

Another condition is the *hereditary mixed polyposis syndrome*, which is also described in Ashkenazi Jews. This is a dominant condition, with the occurrence of hyperplastic, atypical juvenile, adenomatous polyps, having a risk for colorectal cancer. The mutation has been localized to chromosome $15q_{13-14}$, but not yet identified. The importance of this condition in the general population is not yet established.[31]

There is some epidemiologic evidence of risk for colorectal cancer occurring in breast cancer patients, and vice versa (see Chapter 2). A low-penetrance breast cancer susceptibility mutation (*CHEK2 1100delC*) has also been associated with risk for colorectal cancer in these patients.[67]

Relatives of colorectal neoplasia patients

Both retrospective analyses and prospective screening studies demonstrated that first-degree relatives of 'sporadic' colorectal cancer or adenoma patients are at risk for the same neoplasia. Paradoxically, even though they are the largest group at risk for familial colorectal cancer, they are the least well understood (see Figure 6.1). It is assumed that these cancers result from the interaction between genetic susceptibility and environmental-lifestyle risk factors.[68]

The degree of risk depends on the age of diagnosis of the patient's neoplasm, the number of relatives affected with colorectal neoplasia, and the age of the investigated relative.[69] The range of risk, by strength of family history, can be seen in Tables 6.6 and 6.7.[69] The younger asymptomatic proband is at the highest risk; the risk remains elevated but relatively lower in the aging proband. The adult descendants at risk often have a higher degree of compliance for screening than do the patients' siblings, and they should all be encouraged to do so. The recommended screening protocol is dependent on the estimated degree of risk for colorectal cancer, and is shown in Table 6.8.[70]

Relatives should be recommended to follow a cancer-preventive diet and lifestyle (see Chapter 4). Epidemiologic

Table 6.6 Lifetime risk ratios for proband with a family history of colorectal cancer[a]

Neoplasia patient	Relative risk for colon cancer in first-degree relative
One parent with cancer	3–4
One sibling with cancer	3–7
First-degree relative with adenomatous polyp	3–4
First-degree relative aged < 60 years with adenoma	3.6
First-degree relative aged > 70 years with adenoma	1.4
Family history of colon cancer, proband with adenoma	3

[a] Derived from reference 69.

Table 6.7 Cumulative risk (%) of cancer for probands who have a first-degree relative with colon cancer as compared to the risk in a control population[a]

Age of proband (years)	Age of colon cancer relative		Control
	< 55 years	> 55 years	
	Risk for colon cancer (%)		
29	—	—	—
39	0.2	0.1	0.0
49	0.9	0.5	0.1
59	2.8	1.0	0.6
69	5.0	2.2	1.3
79	8.4	4.4	2.4

[a] Derived from reference 69.

studies have demonstrated that this has the potential to halve their risk for colorectal cancer.[71,72]

Genetic-environmental interactions and chemoprevention

As already discussed in the sections on FAP and HNPCC, the clinical manifestations of disease can vary from family to family and even within families. This may be due to the presence of modifying genes and/or interactions with the environment, especially diet and lifestyle.[8,67,68,71,72] Diet and lifestyle are closely related to the etiology and prevention of colorectal neoplasia. At present, it would seem prudent to recommend a 'healthy' diet and lifestyle to patients at risk for colorectal neoplasia (see Chapters 4 and 5).[24,72]

There is evidence that aspirin reduces the risk for sporadic large-bowel cancer and risk for recurrent adenomatous polyps. Based on this, large-scale studies were performed in adenoma patients using COX-2 inhibitors. However, as yet, there is no consensus to promote the routine use of aspirin or any other NSAID to prevent this neoplasm because of their side effects and/or also because of their costs. Calcium supplements will also reduce the risk for recurrent adenomatous polyps (see Chapters 4 and 5). Chemoprevention will modify the polypoid expression of adenomas in FAP and the hamartomatous polyps, but as yet there are no definitive published results of chemopreventive trials in these patients with an intact colon, or in HNPCC patients.

Table 6.8 Screening protocol for first-degree relatives of sporadic colorectal cancer or adenoma patients

Start screening from age 40 years, or 5–10 years less than the youngest neoplasia relative

- **One relative aged < 55 years with neoplasia, or more than one relative of any age**
  - Colonoscopy every 5 years
  - Fecal occult blood, yearly between colonoscopies[a]
- **One relative aged ≥ 55 years with neoplasia:**
  - Fecal occult blood, yearly and flexible sigmoidoscopy, every 5 years or
  - Colonoscopy, every 5 years[a]
  - Fecal occult blood, yearly between colonoscopies[a]

[a] Elective tests.

Sociolegal aspects of familial cancer and counseling

The identification of an affected high-risk patient with or without an identified genetic mutation can lead to guilt, anxiety, cancer phobia, denial, and refusal to cooperate.

These patients and their families need a sympathetic treating physician who understands the complexity of their condition and can provide clear advice.[1,3,73,74] However, a geneticist or genetic counselor is needed prior to genetic testing, and they are especially important when dealing with prenuptial young adults.[1,3] Not involving the future spouse can lead to extreme strains on intrafamilial relationships when the medical condition and risk for cancer in the patient and children become known. Children may need help from a psychologist who understands the medical problem, especially if they need to undergo a potentially traumatic or mutilating procedure such as creation of a stoma. As many of the patients may be underage, informed consent from the parents must be obtained for all genetic testing and other invasive procedures.[75] It is usually recommended and required that a geneticist and not the treating physician obtain this informed consent.

Medical records need to be available and information transferable when needed and allowed by local law. However, medical secrecy must also be maintained. The information is not only relevant to the affected patient but also to his or her immediate family and even to future descendants. This leads to ethical dilemmas, and patients, for personal or religious reasons, may even refuse to provide a family history or undergo diagnostic procedures.[76] A more common and difficult problem occurs when the affected patient refuses to allow the information to be provided to the unsuspecting immediate family at risk.[76] Another common problem is that identification of an asymptomatic person at risk and needing diagnosis and follow-up could lead to loss of job and medical and life insurances.[76–79] These fears inhibit the patients' cooperation. There is no simple answer to these problems, and they will need to be addressed by legislation.[80]

Physician compliance

This issue is rarely addressed. Medical students, family physicians, internists, surgeons, gastroenterologists, gynecologists, and oncologists must be educated about the importance of obtaining a simple family cancer history.[81,82] This can lead to the identification of a family at risk for colorectal cancer who may require investigation and careful follow-up by a protocol appropriate to their disease and risk.[83,84] Courts of law have now recognized that the failure to obtain a relevant family history and instructing the family on their risk can be considered medical negligence.[85,86] However, it is not clear how this can be done without the affected patient's consent.

References (*Reviews and general articles)

1. *Lynch HT, de la Chapelle A, Hereditary colorectal cancer. N Engl J Med 2003; 348: 919–32.
2. *Hyer W, Beveridge I, Domizio P et al, Clinical management and genetics of gastrointestinal polyps in children. J Pediatr Gastroenterol Nutr 2000; 31: 469–79.
3. *Grady WM, Genetic testing for high-risk colon cancer patients. Gastroenterology 2003; 124: 1574–94.
4. *Cohen Jr MM, Molecular dimensions of gastrointestinal tumors: some thoughts for digestion. Am J Med Genet 2003; 122A: 303–14.
5. Rozen P, Samuel Z, Rabau M et al, Familial adenomatous polyposis at the Tel Aviv Medical Center: demographic and clinical features. Fam Cancer 2001; 1: 75–82.
6. Eccles DM, Lunt PW, Wallis Y et al, An unusually severe phenotype for familial adenomatous polyposis. Arch Dis Child 1997; 77: 431–5.
7. Friedl W, Caspari R, Sengteller M et al, Can *APC* mutation analysis contribute to therapeutic decisions in familial adenomatous polyposis? Experience from 680 FAP families. Gut 2001; 48: 515–21.
8. Rozen P, Samuel Z, Shomrat R et al, Notable intrafamilial phenotypic variability in a kindred with familial adenomatous polyposis and an *APC* mutation in exon 9. Gut 1999; 45: 829–33.
9. *Burt RW, Leppert MF, Slattery ML et al, Genetic testing and phenotype in a large kindred with attenuated familial adenomatous polyposis. Gastroenterology 2004; 127: 444–51.
10. Marsh DJ, Theodosopoulos G, Howel V et al, Rapid mutation scanning of genes associated with familial cancer syndromes using denaturing high-performance liquid chromatography. Neoplasia 2001; 3: 236–44.
11. Gavert N, Yaron Y, Naiman T et al, Molecular analysis of the *APC* gene in 71 Israeli families: 17 novel mutations, Hum Mutat 2002; 19: 664. Online citation: Mutation in Brief #508 (2002) http://www.interscience.wiley.com/humanmutation/pdf/mutation/508.pdf
12. Bapat B, Noorani H, Cohen Z et al, Cost comparison of predictive genetic testing versus conventional clinical screening for familial adenomatous polyposis. Gut 1999; 44:698–703.

13. Kubota O, Kino I, Depressed adenomas of the colon in familial adenomatous polyposis. Histology, immunohistochemical detection of proliferating cell nuclear antigen (PCNA), and analysis of the background mucosa. Am J Surg Pathol 1995; 19: 318–27.
14. *Olsen KØ, Juul S, Bülow S et al, Female fecundity before and after operation for familial adenomatous polyposis. Br J Surg 2003; 90: 227–31.
15. *Phillips, RKS, Spigelman AD, Can we safely delay or avoid prophylactic colectomy in familial adenomatous polyposis? Br J Surg 1996; 83: 769–70.
16. Remzi FH, Church JM, Bast J et al, Mucosectomy vs. stapled ileal pouch–anal anastomosis in patients with familial adenomatous polyposis: functional outcome and neoplasia control. Dis Colon Rectum 2001; 44: 1590–6.
17. van Duijvendijk P, Slors JF, Taat CW et al, Functional outcome after colectomy and ileorectal anastomosis compared with proctocolectomy and ileal pouch–anal anastomosis in familial adenomatous polyposis. Ann Surg 1999; 230: 648–54.
18. *Galle TS, Juel K, Bülow S, Causes of death in familial adenomatous polyposis. Scand J Gastroenterol 1999; 34: 808–12.
19. Burke CA, Beck GJ, Church JM et al, The natural history of untreated duodenal and ampullary adenomas in patients with familial adenomatous polyposis followed in an endoscopic surveillance program. Gastrointest Endosc 1999; 49: 358–64.
20. Shimoyama S, Aoki F, Kawahara M et al, Early gastric cancer development in a familial adenomatous polyposis patient. Dig Dis Sci 2004; 49: 260–5.
21. Thompson-Fawcett MW, Marcus VA, Redston M et al, Adenomatous polyps develop commonly in the ileal pouch of patients with familial adenomatous polyposis. Dis Colon Rectum 2001; 44: 347–53.
22. *Church J, Burke C, McGannon E et al, Risk of rectal cancer in patients after colectomy and ileorectal anastomosis for familial adenomatous polyposis. A function of available surgical options. Dis Colon Rectum 2003; 46: 1175–81.
23. Baixauli J, Delaney CP, Wu JS et al, Functional outcome and quality of life after repeat ileal pouch–anal anastomosis for complications of ileoanal surgery. Dis Colon Rectum 2004; 47: 2–11.
24. *Hawk E, Lubet R, Limburg P, Chemoprevention in hereditary colorectal cancer syndromes. Cancer 1999; 86 (Suppl): 2551–63.
25. *Cruz-Correa M, Hylind LM, Romans KE et al, Long-term treatment with sulindac in familial adenomatous polyposis: a prospective cohort study. Gastroenterology 2002; 122: 641–5.
26. Steinbach G, Lynch PM, Phillips RKS et al, A randomized, double-blind, placebo-controlled study of celecoxib, cyclooxygenase-2 inhibitor, in family adenomatous polyposis. N Engl J Med 2000; 26: 1946–52.
27. Phillips RK, Wallace MH, Lynch PM et al, A randomized, double blind, placebo controlled study of celecoxib, a selective cyclooxygenase 2 inhibitor, on duodenal polyposis in familial adenomatous polyposis. Gut 2002; 50: 857–60.
28. Hansmann A, Adolph C, Vogel T et al, High-dose tamoxifen and sulindac as first-line treatment for desmoid tumors. Cancer 2004; 100: 612–20.
29. *Lipton L, Tomlinson I, The multiple colorectal adenoma phenotype and *MYH*, a base excision repair gene. Clin Gastroenterol Hepatol 2004; 2: 633–8.
30. Rozen P, Samuel Z, Brazowski E et al, An audit of familial juvenile polyposis at the Tel Aviv Medical Center: demographic, genetic and clinical features. Fam Cancer 2003; 2: 1–7.
31. Rozen P, Samuel Z, Brazowski E, A prospective study of the clinical, genetic, screening and pathologic features of a family with hereditary mixed polyposis syndrome. Am J Gastroenterol 2003; 98: 2317–20.
32. *Jass JR, Williams CB, Bussey HJR et al, Juvenile polyposis—a precancerous condition. Histopathology 1988; 13: 619–30.
33. Houlston R, Bevan S, Williams A et al, Mutations in DPC4 (SMAD4) cause juvenile polyposis syndrome, but only account for minority of cases. Hum Mol Genet 1998; 7: 1907–12.
34. Scott-Conner CEH, Hausmann M, Hall TJ et al, Familial juvenile polyposis: patterns of recurrence and implications for surgical management. J Am Coll Surg 1995; 181: 407–13.
35. Rodriguez-Bigas MA, Penetrante RB, Herrera L et al, Intraoperative small bowel enteroscopy in familial adenomatous and familial juvenile polyposis. Gastrointest Endosc 1995; 42: 560–4.
36. Brazowski E, Rozen P, Misonzhnick-Bedny F et al, Characteristics of familial juvenile polyps expressing cyclooxygenase-2. Am J Gastroenterol 2005; 100: 130–8.
37. Lim W, Shah B, Murday V et al, Further observations on *LKB 1/STKII* status and cancer risk in Peutz–Jeghers syndrome, Br J Cancer 2003; 89: 308–13.
38. Udd L, Katajisto P, Rossi DJ et al, Suppression of Peutz–Jeghers polyposis by inhibition of cyclooxygenase-2. Gastroenterology 2004; 127: 1030–7.
39. *Jass JR, Serrated adenoma of the colorectum. Curr Diag Pathol 2002; 8: 42–9.
40. Yashiro M, Kobayashi H, Kubo N et al, Cronkhite–Canada syndrome containing colon cancer and serrated adenoma lesions. Digestion 2004; 69: 57–62.
41. Salovaara BR, Loukola A, Kristo P et al, Population-based molecular detection of hereditary nonpolyposis colorectal cancer. J Clin Oncol 2000; 18: 2193–200.
42. Samowitz WS, Curtin K, Lin HH et al, The colon cancer burden of genetically defined hereditary nonpolyposis colon cancer.

Gastroenterology 2001; 121: 830–8.
43. de Jong AE, Morreau H, van Puijenbroek M et al, The role of mismatch repair gene defects in the development of adenomas in patients with HNPCC. Gastroenterology 2004; 126: 42–8.
44. Rijcken FEM, Hollema H, Kleibeuker JH, Proximal adenomas in hereditary non-polyposis colorectal cancer are prone to rapid malignant transformation. Gut 2002; 50: 382–6.
45. *Vasen HF, Watson P, Mecklin JP et al, New clinical criteria for hereditary nonpolyposis colorectal cancer (HNPCC, Lynch syndrome) proposed by the International Collaborative Group on HNPCC. Gastroenterology 1999; 116: 1453–6.
46. Peltomäki, P, Gao X, Mecklin J-P, Genotype and phenotype in hereditary nonpolyposis colon cancer: a study of families with different vs. shared predisposing mutations. Fam Cancer 2001; 1: 9–15.
47. Wagner A, Hendriks Y, Meijers-Heijboer EJ et al, Atypical HNPCC owing to *MSH6* germline mutations: analysis of a large Dutch pedigree. J Med Genet 2001; 38: 318–22.
48. Umar A, Boland CR, Terdiman JP et al, Revised Bethesda Guidelines for hereditary nonpolyposis colorectal cancer (Lynch syndrome) and microsatillite instability. J Natl Cancer Inst 2004; 96: 261–8.
49. Stormorken AT, Müller W, Lemkemeyer B et al, Prediction of the outcome of genetic testing in HNPCC kindreds using the revised Amsterdam criteria and immuno-histochemistry. Fam Cancer 2001; 1: 169–73.
50. Rodriguez-Bigas MA, Vasen HFA, Pekka-Mecklin J et al, Rectal cancer risk in hereditary nonpolyposis colorectal cancer after abdominal colectomy. Ann Surg 1997; 225: 202–7.
51. *de Vos tot Nederveen Cappel WH, Nagengast FM, Griffioen G et al, Surveillance for hereditary nonpolyposis colorectal cancer: a long-term study on 114 families. Dis Colon Rectum 2002; 45: 1588–94.
52. *Vasen HFA, van Ballegooijen M, Buskens E et al, A cost-effectiveness analysis of colorectal screening of hereditary nonpolyposis colorectal carcinoma gene carriers, Cancer 1998; 82: 1632–7.
53. Reyes CM, Allen BA, Terdiman JP et al, Comparison of selection strategies for genetic testing of patients with hereditary nonpolyposis colorectal carcinoma. Effectiveness and cost-effectiveness. Cancer 2002; 95: 1848–56.
54. Wu AH, Shibata D, Yu MC et al, Dietary heterocyclic amines and microsatellite instability in colon adenocarcinomas. Carcinogenesis 2001; 22: 1681–4.
55. Glaab WE, Hill RB, Skopeck TR, Suppression of spontaneous and hydrogen peroxide-induced mutagenesis by the antioxidate ascorbate in mismatch repair-deficient human colon cancer cells. Carcinogenesis 2001; 22: 1709–13.
56. Sinicrope FAA, Lemoine M, Xi L et al, Reduced expression of cyclooxygenase 2 proteins in hereditary nonpolyposis colorectal cancers relative to sporadic cancers. Gastroenterology 1999; 117: 350–8.
57. Cutler NS, Graves-Deal R, LaFleur BJ, Stromal production of prostacyclin confers an antiapoptotic effect to colonic epithelial cells. Cancer Res 2003; 63: 1748–51.
58. *Jarvinen HJ, Aarnio M, Mustonen H et al, Controlled 15-year trial on screening for colorectal cancer in families with hereditary non-polyposis colorectal cancer. Gastroenterology 2000; 118: 829–34.
59. Van Dalen R, Church J, McGannon E et al, Patterns of surgery in patients belonging to Amsterdam-positive families. Dis Colon Rectum 2003; 46: 617–20.
60. *Dove-Edwin I, Boks D, Goff S et al, The outcome of endometrial carcinoma surveillance by ultrasound scan in women at risk of hereditary nonpolyposis colorectal carcinoma and familial colorectal carcinoma. Cancer 2002; 94: 1708–12.
61. Ribic CM, Sargent DJ, Moore MJ et al, Tumor microsatellite-instability status as a predictor of benefit from fluorouracil-based adjuvant chemotherapy for colon cancer. N Engl J Med 2003; 349: 247–57.
62. Carethers JM, Smith EJ, Behling CA. et al, Use of 5–fluorouracil and survival in patients with microsatellite-unstable colorectal cancer. Gastroenterology 2004; 126: 394–401.
63. Fallik D, Borrini F, Boige V et al, Microsatellite instability is a predictive factor of the tumor response to irinotecan in patients with advanced colorectal cancer. Cancer Res 2003; 63: 5738–44.
64. Gryfe R, Kim H, Hsieh ETK et al, Tumor microsatellite instability and clinical outcome in young patients with colorectal cancer. N Engl J Med 2000; 342: 69–77.
65. Barchana M, Liphshitz I, Rozen P, Trends in colorectal cancer incidence and mortality in the Israeli Jewish ethnic populations. Fam Cancer 2004; 3: 207–14.
66. Rozen P, Naiman T, Strul H et al, Clinical and screening implications of the I1307K *APC* variant in Israeli Ashkenazi Jews. Evidence for a founder effect. Cancer 2002; 94: 2561–8.
67. Meijers-Heijboer H, Wijnen J, Vasen H et al, The *CHEK2* 1100delC mutation identifies families with a hereditary breast and colorectal cancer phenotype. Am J Hum Genet 2003; 72: 1308–14.
68. Ishibe N, Freedman AN, Understanding the interaction between environmental exposures and molecular events in colorectal carcinogenesis. Cancer Invest 2001; 19: 524–39.
69. *Offit K, Brown K, Quantitating familial cancer risk: a resource for clinical oncologists. J Clin Oncol 1994; 12: 1724–36.
70. Schoenfeld PS, Fincher RK for the Military Colorectal Cancer Screening Trials Group, Colonoscopic

surveillance of patients with a family history of colon cancer and a history of normal colonoscopy: Is a five-year interval between colonoscopies appropriate? Clin Gasroenterol Hepatol 2003; 1: 310–14.

71. Ulrich CM, Kampman E, Bigler J et al, Colorectal adenomas and the C677T *MTHFR* polymorphism: evidence for gene-environmental interaction? Cancer Epidemiol Biomark Prev 1999; 8: 659–68.
72. Fernandez E, Gallus S, LaVecchia C et al, Family history and environmental risk factors for colon cancer. Cancer Epidemiol Biomark Prev 2004; 13: 658–61.
73. Braithwaite D, Emery J, Walter F et al, Psychological impact of genetic counseling for familial cancer: a systematic review and meta-analysis. J Natl Cancer Inst 2004; 96: 122–33.
74. Hadley DW, Jenkins J, Dimond E et al, Genetic counseling and testing in families with hereditary nonpolyposis colorectal cancer, Arch Intern Med 2003; 63: 573–82.
75. Kodish ED, Testing children for cancer genes: the rule of earliest onset. J Pediatr 1999; 135: 390–5.
76. Vernon SW, Gritz ER, Peterson SK et al, Intention to learn results of genetic testing for hereditary colon cancer. Cancer Epidemiol Biomark Prev 1999; 8: 353–60.
77. Wilcke JTR, Seersholm N, Kok-Jensen A et al, Transmitting genetic risk information in families: attitudes about disclosing the identity of relatives. Am J Hum Genet 1999; 65: 902–9.
78. McEwen JE, McCarty K, Reilly PR, A survey of medical directors of life insurance companies concerning use of genetic information. Am J Hum Genet 1993; 53: 33–45.
79. Rodriguez-Bigas M, Vasen HFA, O'Malley L et al, Health, life and disability insurance and hereditary nonpolyposis colorectal cancer. Am J Hum Genet 1998; 62: 736–37.
80. Lynch PM, Jurisprudential considerations in the evaluation and screening of high-risk patients. In: Secondary Prevention of Colorectal Cancer (Rozen P, Winawer SJ, eds). Basel: Karger, 1986: 55–63.
81. Schroy III PC, Barrison AF, Ling BS et al, Family history and colorectal cancer screening: a survey of physician knowledge and practice patterns. Am J Gastroenterol 2002; 97: 1031–6.
82. Barrison AF, Smith C, Oviedo J et al, Colorectal cancer screening and familial risk: a survey of internal medicine residents' knowledge and practice patterns. Am J Gastroenterol 2003; 98: 1410–16.
83. Stoffel EM, Garber JE, Grover S et al, Cancer surveillance is often inadequate in people at high risk for colorectal cancer. J Med Genet 2003; 40: e54(http//www.jmedgenet.com/cgi/content/full/40/5/e54).
84. Wideroff L, Freedman AN, Olson L et al, Physician use of genetic testing for cancer susceptibility: results of a national survey. Cancer Epidemiol Biomarkers Prev 2003; 12: 295–303.
85. *Lynch HT, Paulson J, Severin M et al, Failure to diagnose hereditary colorectal cancer and its medicolegal implications. A hereditary nonpolyposis colorectal cancer case. Dis Colon Rectum 1999; 42: 31–5.
86. Feld AD, Malpractice risks associated with colon cancer and inflammatory bowel disease. Am J Gastroenterol 2004; 99: 1641–4.

7 How should we follow up premalignant conditions?

Bernard Levin, Paul Rozen, Graeme P Young

Introduction

It is important to define with some precision the appropriate follow-up of patients at increased risk who have premalignant lesions of the colon and rectum. Such follow-up principally involves colonoscopic surveillance. Whereas it is critical to detect neoplastic lesions at an early, preinvasive stage, cost containment is another goal of a defined policy because of the expense of such surveillance. Recent advances in our understanding of the biology of colonic carcinogenesis enhance our surveillance strategies. This chapter will focus on a discussion of follow-up after removal of colorectal adenomas, endoscopic surveillance of patients with chronic inflammatory bowel disease, and women with a history of gynecologic cancer.

Follow-up after removal of colorectal adenomas

For a description of how polyps are classified, see Table 7.1 and Figure 7.1.

By definition, adenomatous epithelium is neoplastic and all adenomas exhibit some degree of dysplasia. Dysplasia may be classified as mild (low grade), moderate, or severe (high grade). The degree of cytologic atypia and glandular architectural distortion determine the grade of dysplasia. At clinical discovery, approximately 5% of adenomas contain high-grade dysplasia and 2.5% contain invasive cancer. The correct term for a lesion with invasive cancer is adenoma-containing adenocarcinoma.[1] Predominant villous histology, severe dysplasia, and size ≥1 cm are all associated with an increased risk of cancer within the adenoma and are sometimes referred to as 'advanced pathology'.[2] The relationship between size and degree of dysplasia is illustrated in Table 7.2.

In countries with a high or intermediate risk for colorectal cancer, the incidence of colonic adenomas increases with age. In the United States and other Western countries at autopsy adenomas are found in 30–50% of individuals older than 60 years of age. In Hawaii, the incidence of colorectal cancer among people of Japanese descent is extremely high and parallels the high prevalence rate of adenomas. Other US and European populations have

Table 7.1 *Classification of large-bowel non-cancerous polypoid lesions and their relative malignant potential*

Mucosal lesion	Malignant potential
Neoplastic[a]	
Tubular adenoma	+
Tubular villous adenoma	++
Villous adenoma	+++
Non-neoplastic	
Hyperplastic polyp	−
Serrated adenoma[b] (mixed hyperplastic and adenomatous polyp)	+
Juvenile polyp (polyposis)[b]	−/+++
Peutz–Jeghers polyps[b]	−/+
Inflammatory polyp	−
Submucosal lesion	
Lipoma	−
Carcinoid	−/+
Colitis cystic profunda	−

[a] The larger the adenoma, the more the villous elements, the greater the risk for cancer.
[b] The greater the number of adenomatous elements occurring in this non-neoplastic polyp, the greater the risk for cancer. See also Chapter 6.

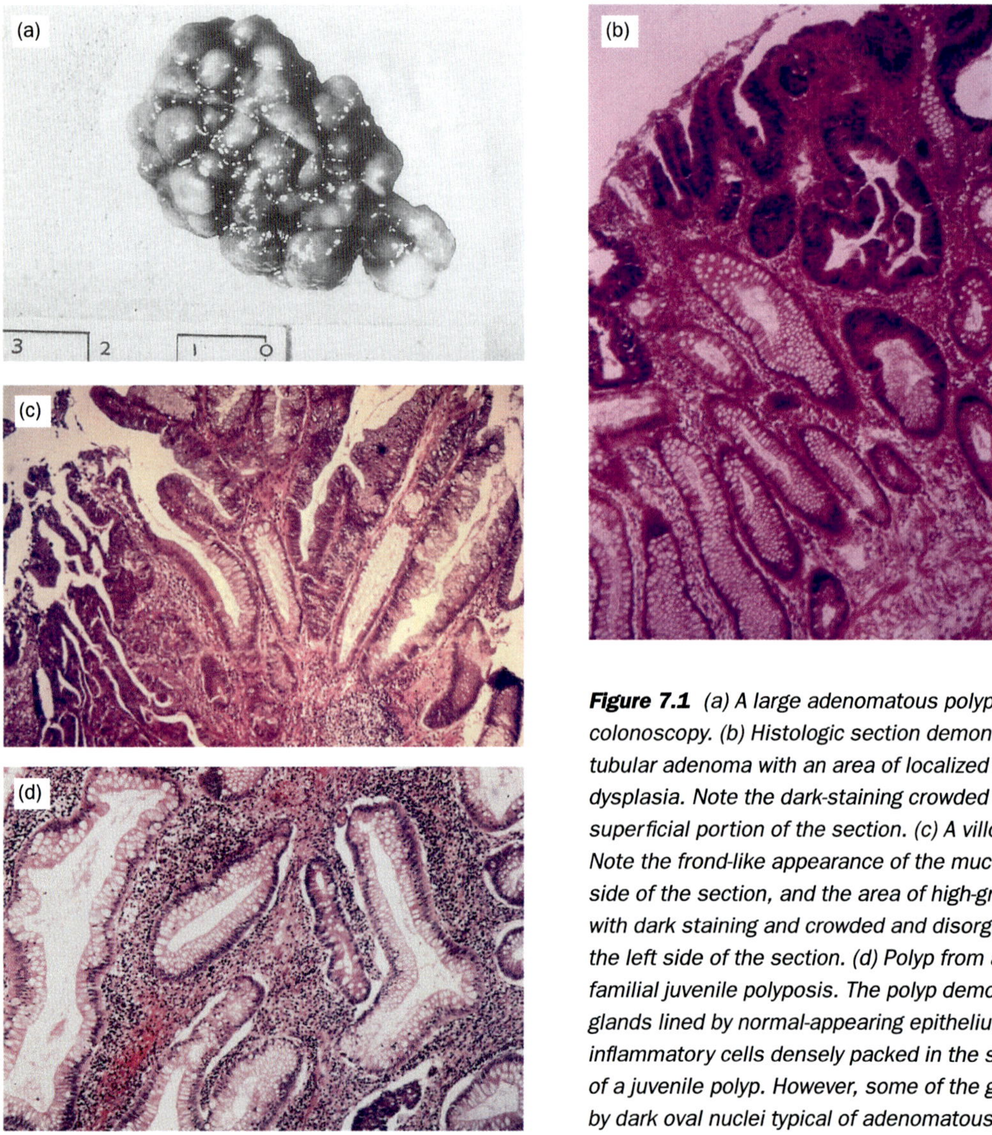

Figure 7.1 *(a) A large adenomatous polyp removed at colonoscopy. (b) Histologic section demonstrated a tubular adenoma with an area of localized high-grade dysplasia. Note the dark-staining crowded nuclei in the superficial portion of the section. (c) A villous adenoma. Note the frond-like appearance of the mucosa on the right side of the section, and the area of high-grade dysplasia with dark staining and crowded and disorganized nuclei on the left side of the section. (d) Polyp from a patient with familial juvenile polyposis. The polyp demonstrates dilated glands lined by normal-appearing epithelium with inflammatory cells densely packed in the stroma, typical of a juvenile polyp. However, some of the glands are lined by dark oval nuclei typical of adenomatous changes.*

comparable prevalence rates of adenoma. In contrast, a 5% prevalence of adenomas was found in Cali, Columbia (Table 7.3).[3] In a recent clinical study of over 3000 US Army veterans (96% men) whose mean age was 63 years, colonoscopic examination showed one or more neoplastic lesions in 38% of the patients, an adenoma with a diameter of at least 10 mm or a villous adenoma in 8%, an adenoma with high-grade dysplasia in 2%, and invasive cancer in 1%.[4] Because of the high prevalence of adenomas in some Western countries but not in others (including Israel), the management of adenomas, and especially post-polypectomy surveillance, has substantial economic implications. Fortunately, there is considerable experience and information available from the US population, upon which to base recommendations for similar populations.[5]

Important in the development of a strategy for surveillance is an understanding of the biology of adenomas. Few adenomatous polyps progress to cancer; the rate is estimated at about 2.5 polyps per 1000 per year.[2] The transformation occurs over many years. Estimates are based

Table 7.2 *High-grade dysplasia found in adenomas removed by colonoscopy, by size and histology (n = 3371)*[a]

Histology	Size (cm)		
	<0.5	0.6–1.0	>1.0
Tubular	0.7%	2.7%	7.4%
Tubulovillous	14.7%	19.6%	31.7%
Villous	20.0%	17.6%	35.0%

[a]Adapted from reference 2.

largely on indirect evidence such as observations on biopsied polyps that are not removed and their transformation to cancer over a period of 10–15 years. Another line of evidence derives from data on mean age of people with early adenomatous polyps and those with colorectal cancer. The average age difference was 18 years.

Encouraging evidence related to the effectiveness of post-polypectomy colonoscopic surveillance derives from the US National Polyp Study, a cohort of 1418 patients who had undergone complete colonoscopy and removal of one or more adenomatous polyps from the colon. These individuals were followed for an average of 5.9 years per patient. After adjusting for adenoma size, age, and sex, rates of cancer were 76–90% lower than expected in comparison with three reference groups

Table 7.3 *Prevalence of adenomas in selected autopsy studies*[a]

Study location	Years	Prevalence (%)	
		Men	Women
USA			
Hawaii	1969–1984	64	57
New Orleans	1970–1975	36	20
New York	1960	40	37
Europe			
Oslo, Norway	1974–1976	40	33
Liverpool, UK		37	29
Asia			
Akita, Japan	1970–1973	38	24
Hong Kong	1985	19	34
South America			
Cali, Colombia		6.0	5.0

[a]Modified from reference 3 with permission.

(Figure 7.2). Another long-term follow-up of colorectal cancer occurring in post-polypectomy patients showed a lower reduction in colorectal cancer incidence.[6] These results of incomplete protection against colorectal cancer are only partially explained by missed lesions; they also

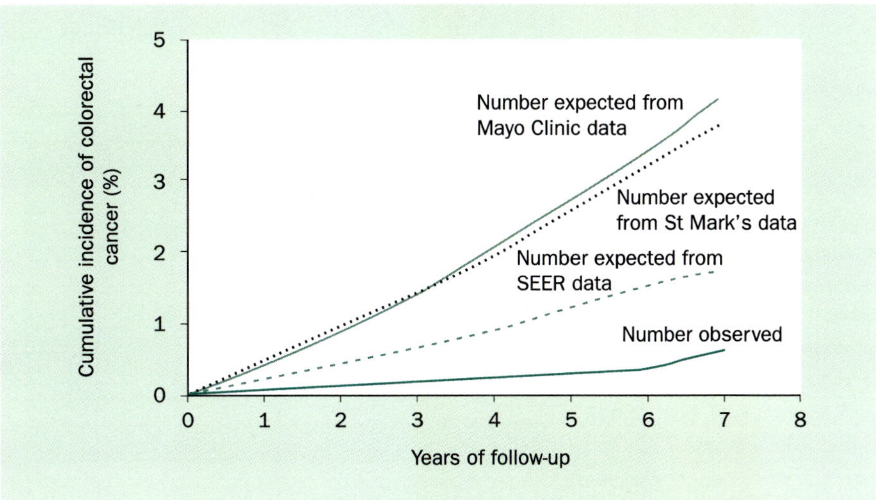

Figure 7.2 *Cumulative observed incidence of colorectal cancer in the US National Polyp Study cohort was significantly less than that estimated to occur in two reference populations. (Reproduced with permission from Winawer SJ et al,*[7] *©1993 Massachusetts Medical Society. All rights reserved.)*

point to a contribution of the non-polypoid pathway to carcinogenesis.

The investigators in the National Polyp Study determined the optimal frequency of surveillance in patients who had undergone prior polypectomy and who were randomized to undergo surveillance colonoscopy either at 1 and 3 years or only 3 years after polypectomy.[7] The two groups showed no difference in the proportion of detection of adenomatous polyps with advanced pathology: 3.3% in both groups; 95% confidence interval (CI) 0.8–5.3%. These data suggest that the first follow-up screen after polypectomy can be deferred for 3 years. A longer follow-up interval of 6 years has been proposed for subjects other than those who have three or more adenomas at initial colonoscopy or who are 60 years of age or over and have a first-degree relative with colorectal cancer.[5] Similar conclusions have been reached by other investigators.[8] In an analysis of the National Polyp Study using the MISCAN-COLON model, it was suggested that regression of adenomas may be an important aspect of the natural history.[9]

Clinical significance of distal adenomas

In a British study, 1618 patients were treated for rectosigmoid adenomas using rigid sigmoidoscopy.[10] These patients were not initially followed up and the study retrospectively assessed their long-term risk of developing colorectal cancer. The study was performed in the precolonoscopy era. The risk of subsequent colon cancer was increased 1.7–fold when a single adenoma was detected and 4.8–fold if multiple adenomas were present, but it was not increased when only a single small (≤1 cm) tubular adenoma was detected. Recently, investigators determined the risk of advanced proximal neoplasia, defined as a polyp ≥1 cm or with predominant villous features, or a polyp with high-grade dysplasia or cancer, among persons with distal neoplastic polyps.[11] The prevalence of advanced proximal neoplasia among patients with no distal polyps was 1.5%. Among patients with distal tubular adenomas and those with advanced distal polyps, the prevalence of advanced proximal neoplasia was 7.1% and 11.5%, respectively. Age over 50 years and male sex increased the risk of advanced proximal neoplasia 3.5–fold. Based on these findings and other data, colonoscopy is advised for patients with a distal adenoma of any size found at flexible sigmoidoscopy.[12] In the United States, the PLCO (Prostate, Lung, Colorectal and Ovarian Cancer Screening) trial is a randomized controlled, multicenter community study. A recent study from this group examined the yield of adenomas and cancers in the distal colon, found by repeat flexible sigmoidoscopy, 3 years after a negative examination. The incidence of adenoma or cancer in the distal colon was 3.1%. One-quarter of the individuals with adenomas had advanced adenomas and six distal colon cancers were detected for an advanced distal lesion detection rate of 0.8%. Although it cannot be determined whether these lesions were missed at the initial flexible sigmoidoscopy, or whether they developed over the 3-year observation period examination, the authors note that 80% of those with advanced distal adenomas had lesions detected in a portion of the colon that had been adequately examined at the initial sigmoidoscopy. However, the yield for cancer and advanced adenomas 3 years after a negative sigmoidoscopy was one-fourth to one-third of what was detected at the initial endoscopic examination 3 years earlier.[13]

Reports from Japan have shown that 'flat adenomas' are more likely to contain carcinoma or severe dysplasia than sessile adenomas of similar size.[14] Flat lesions can be defined endoscopically and histologically. Histologically, the dysplastic tissue does not protrude above the mucosal surface or the dysplastic tissue is no more than twice the thickness of the mucosa (Figure 7.3). Endoscopically, these lesions are usually less than 1 cm in diameter, and have a non-exophytic flat-topped shape, sometimes with a

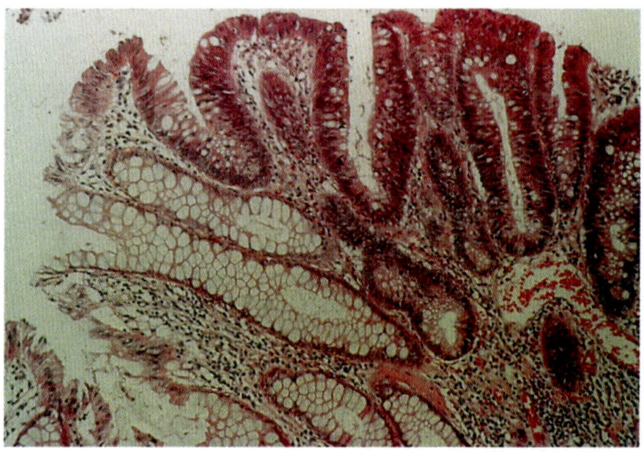

Figure 7.3 *Photomicrograph of a 'flat' adenoma, which appears to be in the same plane as the surrounding mucosa.*

central red-colored depression. In a British series of asymptomatic persons undergoing flexible sigmoidoscopy, the incidence was 1 in 1000.[15] In a recent study also from the UK, flat adenomas and carcinomas had high malignant potential compared to protuberant (polypoid/sessile) lesions and had a propensity to develop in the right hemicolon.[16]

In the United States, current evidence suggests that clinically important flat lesions with a high malignant potential are unlikely to be frequently overlooked. For example, in the National Polyp Study, the incidence of diminutive adenomas was 0.9%.[17]

Hyperplastic polyps and serrated adenomas

More attention has been focused recently on an alternative pathway of colorectal cancer development, namely a hyperplastic polyp-serrated adenoma–adenoma sequence.[18] Sporadic hyperplastic polyps are considered to be nonneoplastic lesions, but recent observations on multiple, large, and proximal hyperplastic polyps have challenged this concept. Genetic alterations that are frequent in colorectal carcinoma, such as *K-ras* mutations and microsatellite instability, have been reported in some of these polyps. These genetic abnormalities are also present in serrated adenomas. Admixtures of these lesions occur; the serrated adenoma/mixed hyperplastic adenomatous polyp is uncommon and is characterized by the saw-toothed architectural features of a hyperplastic polyp but with the presence of epithelial dysplasia. In addition, it has been recently shown that methylation of CpG islands, a molecular defect commonly found in colorectal cancer, is frequently found in serrated adenomas and mixed lesions.[19] Follow-up strategies for individuals in whom these lesions are found have not been well defined. At present, they should be managed as for adenomatous polyps (see also Chapter 6).

Adenomas in hereditary non-polyposis colorectal cancer

The adenoma–carcinoma sequence in hereditary nonpolyposis colorectal cancer (HNPCC) seems to be accelerated (less than 3 years), as illustrated by the relatively frequent occurrence of cancers within the first few years after an endoscopically clean colon ascertained by colonoscopy.[20] In addition, high-grade dysplasia and villous architecture are well described in these lesions. Recent evidence suggests that these polypoid lesions are mostly found in the right colon, are often large, and display the mismatch repair defect from the earliest stages of development. Immunochemical staining for microsatellite instability seems advisable for large adenomas with high-grade dysplasia in those patients under 50 years of age (see also Chapter 6).[21]

Colonoscopic surveillance

The following management guidelines for surveillance of adenomatous polyps have been developed by the National Health and Medical Research Council of Australia.[22] Colonoscopic surveillance should be implemented:

- at 3 months following piecemeal removal, or excision of a malignant adenoma, or a large adenoma that may have been excised incompletely
- within 1 year following incomplete or possible inadequate examination, e.g. in a subject with multiple adenomas
- at 3 years for subjects with high-grade dysplasia, villous changes in adenomas or three or more adenomas, or in those aged 60 or older with a first-degree relative with colorectal cancer
- at 4–6 years in subjects without the preceding risk factors.

These recommendations are similar to those suggested by the US Multisociety Task Force on Colorectal Cancer (Table 7.4).[5]

Future developments

For individuals who are prone to adenoma recurrence, chemopreventive measures may be useful to reduce the risk of recurrence.[23] Examples of such agents include curcumin, folic acid, aspirin, statins, calcium, and nonsteroidal anti-inflammatory drugs (NSAIDs). Clinical trials of these compounds are in progress in Europe, Australia, Israel, Asia, and North and South America. It is premature to recommend any specific chemopreventive intervention at this time (see also Chapter 5). The risks and benefits of such interventions need to be carefully defined for the individual patient. In all cases, preventive dietary and lifestyle recommendations should be given (see Chapter 4).

Table 7.4 Follow-up after colonoscopic polypectomy

Colonoscopic findings	Follow-up required
• Piecemeal removal Adenoma containing adenocarcinoma	3 months
• Multiple adenomas or possibly inadequate examination	12 months
• High-grade dysplasia Villous changes in adenoma Three or more adenomas	36 months
• Single, tubular adenoma	48–72 months

Chronic inflammatory bowel disease

Introduction

Among all patients diagnosed with a large-bowel carcinoma, about 1% give an antecedent history of ulcerative colitis or Crohn's disease. The management of those at risk poses a challenge for both patient and physician. Specific guidelines for Crohn's disease have not been established: this discussion will focus predominantly on ulcerative colitis.

Clinical features

In a patient with long-standing ulcerative colitis, the patient or physician may attribute symptoms such as rectal bleeding, abdominal cramping, or diarrhea to colitis and the diagnosis of carcinoma may be missed until far advanced.

Risk factors

The two best-established risk factors for developing colorectal cancer in ulcerative colitis are anatomic extent of colonic involvement and duration of disease. Patients with extensive colitis (disease proximal to the splenic flexure) are at greatest risk, whereas those who have only proctitis do not have an increased risk of cancer.[24] Patients with left-sided disease are also at intermediate increased risk.[25]

Colorectal cancer is rare when the duration of pancolitis is less than 8 years. The risk begins to rise above that of the general population after about 8–10 years of the disease. Although earlier retrospective reports from specialty referral centers had reported higher cancer rates, current estimates from population-based studies indicate that the cumulative incidence is 5–10% after 20 years' disease duration and 12–20% after 30 years.[24] Contrary to earlier views, age at onset does not seem to be an independent risk factor, but young patients are more likely to have pancolitis, and over the ensuing years, be more susceptible to cancer than those with more limited disease.[25,26]

Clinicopathologic features

The macroscopic appearances are heterogeneous and include strictures, nodules, plaques, and irregular polypoid masses.[27] Some cancers arise in totally flat mucosa and may be detected only by chance. Fixed colonic strictures should be regarded with suspicion, and have been reported to harbor cancer in 24–40% of cases (Figure 7.4). Multiple synchronous colorectal cancers occur much more frequently in inflammatory bowel disease than in the general population.[27] Microscopically, mucinous adenocarcinomas are twice as common in ulcerative colitis compared with sporadic cancers.

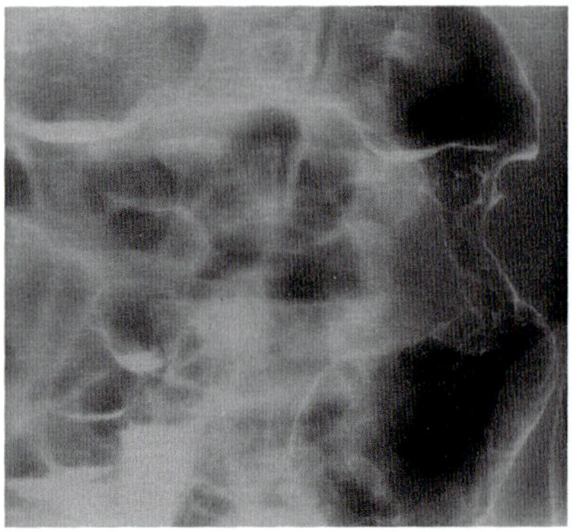

Figure 7.4 *Radiograph demonstrating a colonic stricture and synchronous cancers in a patient with ulcerative colitis. Note the lack of haustra, which is typical of long-standing and extensive colitis.*

Pathogenesis of cancer in ulcerative colitis

Although there is little difference between the overall and stage-adjusted survival rates of cancer in chronic ulcerative colitis and in the general population, the early diagnosis of cancer is an important goal. Both sporadic colorectal cancer and colitis-associated large-bowel cancer arise from dysplastic precursors. Sporadic colorectal cancer usually arises from an adenomatous polyp, whereas colitis-associated cancer typically arises from flat dysplasia or a dysplasia-associated lesion or mass (DALM). Dysplasia is defined as an unequivocal neoplastic alteration of the large-bowel epithelium confined within the basement membrane in which it arises; regenerative and reactive changes resulting from inflammation are excluded. The nomenclature and criteria for assessment of dysplasia have been standardized.[28] Examples of dysplastic changes are illustrated in Figure 7.5.

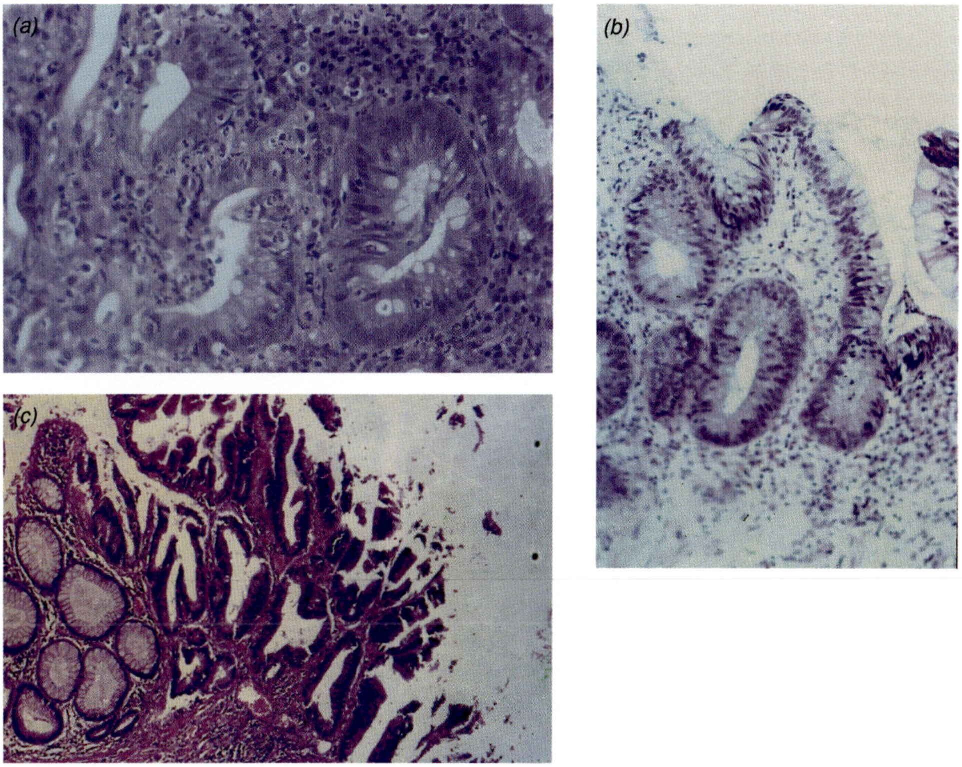

Figure 7.5 *Photomicrographs of dysplastic changes occurring in chronic ulcerative colitis. (a) A screening biopsy taken at random from a patient with longstanding, extensive, and mildly active ulcerative colitis. The crypts are distorted and the epithelial cells have hyperchromatic stratified nuclei. There is dense stromal inflammation, which enters the glands (cryptitis). This regenerative atypia cannot be easily differentiated from low-grade dysplasia; thus, this case is classified as indeterminate dysplasia, probably negative. (b) A screening biopsy taken from the rectum of a patient with longstanding, extensive, but quiescent ulcerative colitis. The crypts' lining cells have hyperchromatic stratified nuclei, which are also seen in the surface epithelial cells. There is relatively little stromal inflammation. This was classified as low-grade dysplasia. Endoscopy repeated a few months later demonstrated a small nodular mass in the rectum, which on repeated biopsies demonstrated high-grade dysplasia. Colectomy was performed, and the final diagnosis was adenocarcinoma that did not invade through the entire rectal wall. (c) Screening biopsy from a patient with longstanding, extensive ulcerative colitis in clinical remission. A small, elevated irregular lesion was identified at endoscopy. On the left side of the figure, the crypts are slightly distorted and are lined with dark-staining basal nuclei, compatible with ulcerative colitis in remission. On the right side, there are distorted glands with a villiform appearance, and the dark-staining nuclei are stratified, compatible with high-grade dysplasia.*

Patient management

The management possibilities for patients at increased risk for colorectal cancer include prophylactic proctocolectomy and/or periodic endoscopic surveillance together with medical management (see also Chapter 5). An onset of total ulcerative colitis in childhood or adolescence may convey a high enough risk to warrant prophylactic surgery as an alternative to facing a lifelong program of colonoscopic surveillance. Moreover, advances in surgical technique imply that a permanent stoma can be avoided in most elective cases by creating an ileoanal J-pouch (see Chapter 6). Surgical removal of the large bowel must be based on individual considerations, such as age, intractability of symptoms, psychologic factors, and ease of access to continued medical care, including regular colonoscopic surveillance. Even an elective ileostomy will provide better quality of life than chronic disease requiring constant use of medications that also impair health. Particularly in young patients, the quality of life after proctocolectomy is extremely good. For optimal results, an experienced colorectal surgical team should perform surgical management, whether pouch construction or ileostomy.

In Denmark, a proactive policy of intensive chronic medical therapy with 5-aminosalicylic acid (5-ASA) preparations and surgery for medical treatment failures has removed the increased risk for colorectal cancer. In their population, after a median 19 years follow-up, the risk of cancer was no different than for the general population.[29]

Surveillance in practice

The rationale for cancer surveillance in ulcerative colitis is based on the assumption that dysplasia is a reliable marker for pre-neoplasia or cancer and that surveillance detects cancer at an earlier stage, hence improving survival. The aim of surveillance is to intervene before the development of cancer. Cancer surveillance is a continuous process of clinical evaluation and investigation.[30] Colonoscopy is used initially during the early years of the disease to determine the extent of colonic involvement; subsequently, annual surveillance colonoscopies are performed in those with 8–10 years of symptoms and extensive colitis (extending to involvement of the hepatic flexure). For those with colitis confined to the left side of the colon, surveillance should begin 12 years after onset of symptoms. Multiple biopsies are obtained at 10–12 cm intervals throughout the colon, including the cecum, ascending colon, hepatic flexure, splenic flexure, sigmoid, and rectum. Approximately 30–35 biopsies are obtained during this procedure. At least two-thirds of neoplasms or dysplastic changes occur in the rectosigmoid. For this reason, if annual colonoscopy is difficult to arrange or is unacceptable to the patient, a compromise in which annual flexible sigmoidoscopy is replaced by colonoscopy every second year may be preferable to infrequent surveillance.[30] In Table 7.5, the histologic findings and clinical actions recommended are summarized. Methylene-blue chromoendoscopy has been demonstrated to facilitate the detection of intraepithelial neoplasia in chronic ulcerative colitis compared to conventional colonoscopy, and may be used more widely in the future.[31] A normal appearing colonoscopy is associated with a non-increased risk for colorectal cancer.[32]

A management algorithm is presented in Figure 7.6. If no dysplastic changes are found, surveillance is repeated at 1- to 2-year intervals. In the presence of indefinite dysplasia, colonoscopy should be repeated in 6 months. High-grade dysplasia (HGD), whether it occurs in a mass lesion or in flat mucosa, is considered an indication for colectomy. The cancer risk is also high enough to warrant colectomy if low-grade dysplasia (LGD) is found in a mass lesion. When LGD is detected in flat mucosa, the high risk of progression to HGD or cancer warrants a policy of early colectomy. Some recommend a repeat colonoscopy 3–6 months later to confirm the presence of LGD before proceeding with removal of the colon. If the presence of LGD is not confirmed, yearly surveillance is continued. Key to all colonoscopic surveillance is reliance on an expert gastrointestinal pathologist for interpretation of the mucosal biopsies and correlation with clinical findings. This is particularly crucial when making decisions about the management of HGD or LGD.

Adenomas in the ulcerative colitis patient

In patients who do not have pancolitis, an adenoma may arise within the proximal, normal colonic mucosa. Such adenomas may be either pedunculated or sessile, and should be managed as they would in a patient without colitis. If a sessile adenoma arises within bowel involved by the colitic process, it cannot reliably be differentiated from a dysplastic mass, and a colectomy may be the most prudent clinical action. When a pedunculated adenoma arises in a colon involved by colitis, the adjacent and remote mucosa should be sampled during colonoscopic polypectomy. If there is no evidence of dysplasia beyond the

Table 7.5 *Biopsy classification of dysplasia in inflammatory bowel disease and recommended clinical action in the course of endoscopic surveillance*

Pathologic findings[a]	Recommended clinical action
• Negative for dysplasia	
Normal mucosa	Continue periodic surveillance
Inactive colitis	Continue periodic surveillance
Active colitis	Treat colitis
• Indefinite for dysplasia	Repeat surveillance in 6 months
• Positive for dysplasia	
Low-grade dysplasia	Proctocolectomy, or repeat biopsies in 3–4 months, colectomy if confirmed
High-grade dysplasia	Proctocolectomy
• Sessile lesion (dysplasia-associated mass)	Proctocolectomy
• Polypoid adenomas in non-dysplastic epithelium	Colonoscopic polypectomy

[a] Classification derived from reference 28.

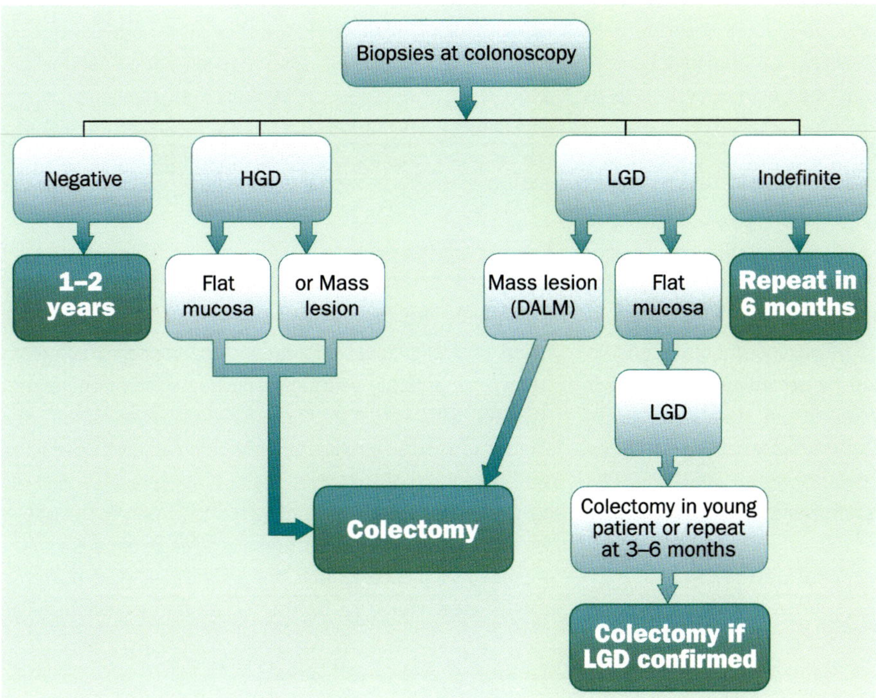

Figure 7.6 *Patient management algorithm in chronic ulcerative colitis surveillance. HGD, high-grade dysplasia; LGD, low-grade dysplasia; DALM, dysplasia-associated lesion or mass.*

adenoma, no further action is needed. If dysplasia is present elsewhere, a colectomy is recommended.[5,33] Recently, a more conservative approach to the management of sporadic adenoma-like dysplastic lesions occurring in ulcerative colitis has been suggested. This approach depends heavily on the availability of expert endoscopic and gastrointestinal pathologic consultation.[33, 34]

Patients with an ileorectal anastomosis

Patients with an ileorectal anastomosis and a history of chronic ulcerative colitis remain at risk for the development of rectal cancer. For this reason, the procedure has fallen out of favor. In the presence of a retained rectal segment, frequent periodic endoscopic surveillance with multiple biopsies should be performed according to the previous guidelines.

Sclerosing cholangitis and cholangiocarcinoma

Primary sclerosing cholangitis has been reported in both ulcerative colitis and Crohn's disease. Patients with ulcerative colitis and sclerosing cholangitis have an increased risk of developing colorectal cancer and also a risk of developing cholangiocarcinoma in either the extrahepatic or intrahepatic biliary tract. The disease may be clinically silent for a lengthy period, with the gradual onset of nonspecific symptoms. Magnetic resonance cholangiopancreatography is being used with increasing frequency to establish the diagnosis.

Effectiveness of surveillance

Randomized controlled trials on the effectiveness of surveillance in patients with long-standing ulcerative colitis have not been conducted. A summary of prospective cohort studies from both the United States and Europe suggests that the percentage of advanced colon cancers with bad outcome is reduced by surveillance to 35%.[35] Cancers tend to be detected at an earlier stage in patients who are undergoing surveillance, and these patients have a better prognosis; however, lead-time bias could contribute to this apparent benefit.

Chemoprevention of colorectal cancer in ulcerative colitis

A possible protective role for NSAIDs in the chemoprevention of colorectal neoplasia in ulcerative colitis has long been of interest.[29] The most promising results on the role of 5-ASA compounds are derived from a case-control study in the UK, where the use of mesalamine (5-ASA) was associated with a >90% reduction in risk, whereas sulfasalazine was associated with a 59% reduction in risk. All other 5-ASA agents failed to demonstrate a benefit.[34–36]

Studies on folate supplementation in chronic ulcerative colitis have not indicated a definite benefit, although biologic plausibility exists.[34]

Use of ursodeoxycholic acid has been demonstrated in a placebo-controlled trial in individuals with primary sclerosing cholangitis to be associated with a 74% decrease in the risk of developing cancer or dysplasia.[34,37] This promising lead warrants further study.

Future developments

More accurate and better methods of surveillance are needed. Based on recent findings, genomic instability and microsatellite instability occur early on in the course of dysplasia development and may afford an opportunity for earlier diagnosis on biopsy.[38] The potential role of molecular marker detection in the stool is under investigation in the non-colitic population and may be applicable in the future to surveillance.[39]

Recently, advances in biomedical optics are being applied to enhance sensitivity and specificity of conventional diagnostic endoscopy for the detection of dysplastic lesions in early cancer. These techniques include autofluorescence imaging, light-scattering spectroscopy, chromoendoscopy, and optical coherence tomography with real-time Doppler capabilities. Such techniques may facilitate detection of premalignant lesions in chronic ulcerative colitis.[40]

Crohn's disease

Cancer of the large bowel

There is a significantly increased incidence of colorectal cancer in patients with extensive colonic involvement. Patients with long-standing anorectal involvement also appear to be at significantly increased risk of developing anal or rectal malignancies. Although dysplasia is well recognized, surveillance in patients with Crohn's disease of the large bowel may be technically difficult because of the presence of strictures and fistulous disease. If possible, surveillance should be performed as for ulcerative colitis.

Cancer of the small bowel

Small-bowel cancer in the general population is extremely rare, but is more common in patients with Crohn's disease of the small bowel, particularly in association with fistulous disease and bypassed loops of bowel. There is a long latent period between disease onset and cancer (mean of 18 years). In Crohn's disease, two-thirds of cancers occur in the ileum whereas in the general population small-bowel tumors are more evenly distributed throughout the small intestine. In the future, video capsule endoscopy may facilitate surveillance of the small bowel; however, there is the danger of impaction in strictures.[41]

Women with breast and gynecologic cancer

Meta-analyses have suggested that women with prior ovarian or endometrial cancer have an increased relative risk of subsequent colorectal cancer. This risk is greater than the relative risk of 1.1 (95% CI = 0.99–1.31) for colorectal cancer in women with prior breast cancer.[42,43] There is no increased risk of colorectal cancer in women with cervical cancer.[44] Analysis of data from the SEER (Surveillance, Epidemiology, and End Results) Program in the United States has demonstrated that the increased risk of colorectal cancer is confined to women diagnosed with endometrial cancer before age 50 or ovarian cancer before age 65 years.[44] The respective relative risks are as follows: for those with ovarian cancer below 50 years old, 3.67 (95% CI 2.74–4.88); for those with ovarian cancer above 50 years old, 1.52 (95% CI 1.25–1.83); and for those with endometrial cancer below 50 years old, 3.9 (95% CI 2.73–4.17). In approaching risk assessment in women with prior endometrial or ovarian cancer, a detailed family history should be obtained to identify kindreds with an established genetic syndrome such as HNPCC, and appropriate screening measures can then be implemented (see Chapter 6). If the woman was diagnosed with endometrial cancer at <50 years old or ovarian cancer at <64 years old and the family history does not meet or approach criteria for HNPCC, then a colonoscopy at 3- to 5-year intervals is advised. The basis for this recommendation is that the relative risk of colorectal cancer in such patients is comparable to the risk in first-degree relatives of patients diagnosed with colorectal cancer or with adenomas at a young age.[45]

For patients diagnosed with ovarian cancer over 64 years old and endometrial cancer after age 50, average-risk screening approaches are adequate.

Future developments

As risk models are developed, it is likely that surveillance recommendations will be increasingly refined so that only the most cost-effective and beneficial approaches are selected.

References (*Reviews and general articles)

1. *Hamilton SR. Pathology and biology of colorectal neoplasia: In: Prevention and Early Detection of Colorectal Cancer (Young GP, Rozen P, Levin B, eds), London: WB Saunders, 1996; 3–21.
2. *O'Brien MJ, Winawer SJ, Zauber AG et al, The National Polyp Study: patient and polyp characteristics associated with high grade dysplasia in colorectal adenomas. Gastroenterology 1990; 98: 371–9.
3. Peipins LA, Sandler RS, Epidemiology of colorectal adenomas. Epidemiol Rev 1994; 16: 273–97.
4. Lieberman DA, Weiss DG, Bond JH et al, Use of colonoscopy to screen asymptomatic adults for colorectal cancer. N Engl J Med 2000; 343: 162–8.
5. *Winawer S, Fletcher R, Rex D et al, Colorectal cancer screening and surveillance: clinical guidelines and rationale. Gastroenterology 2003; 124: 544–60.
6. Church TR, Mandel JS, Bond JH et al, Colorectal cancer incidence reduction due to polyp removal: results from the Minnesota Trial. Gastroenterology 2003; 124 (Suppl 1): A55.
7. Winawer SJ, Zauber AG, O'Brien MJ et al, Randomized comparison of surveillance intervals after colonoscopic removal of newly diagnosed adenomatous polyps. N Engl J Med 1993; 328: 901–6.
8. Noshiswani K, von Stolk R, Rybicki L et al, Adenoma size and number are predictive of adenoma recurrence. Gastrointest Endosc 2000; 51: 433–7.
9. Loeve F, Boer R, Zauber AF et al, National Polyp Study data: evidence for regression of adenomas. Intl J Cancer 2004; 111: 633–9.
10. Atkin WS, Morson BC, Cuzick J, Long-term risk of colorectal cancer after excision of rectosigmoid adenomas. N Engl J Med 1992; 26: 658–62.
11. Imperiale TF, Wagner DR, Lin CY et al, Risk of advanced proximal neoplasms in asymptomatic adults according to the distal colorectal findings. N Engl J Med 2000; 343: 169–74.
12. Rex DK, Chak A, Vasuveda R et al, Prospective determination of distal colon findings in average risk patients with proximal colon cancer. Gastrointest Endosc 1999; 49: 27–30.

13. Schoen RE, Pinsky PF, Weissfeld JL et al. Results of repeat sigmoidoscopy 3 years after a negative examination. JAMA 2003; 290: 41–8.
14. Mitooka H, Fujimora T, Maeda S, Minute flat depressed neoplastic lesions of the colon detected by contrast chromoscopy using an indigo carmine capsule. Gastrointest Endosc 1995; 41: 453–9.
15. Hart AR, Kudo S, MacKay EH, et al, Flat adenomas exist in asymptomatic people: important implications for colorectal cancer screening programmes. Gut 1998; 43: 229–31.
16. Hurlstone SP, Cross SS, Adam I et al, Prospective clinicopathologic and endoscopic evaluation of flat and depressed colorectal lesions in the United Kingdom. Am J Gastroenterol 2003; 98: 2543–9.
17. Winawer SJ, Zauber AG, Ho MN et al, Prevention of colorectal cancers by colonoscopic polypectomy. N Engl J Med 1993; 329: 1977–81.
18. Higuchi T, Jass JR, My approach to serrated polyps of the colorectum. J Clin Pathol 2004; 57: 682–6.
19. Park S-J, Rashid A, Lee J-H et al, Frequent CpG island methylation in serrated adenomas of the colorectum. Am J Pathol 2003; 162: 815–22.
20. Rijeken FEM, Hollema H, Kleibuker JH, Proximal adenomas in hereditary non-polyposis colorectal cancer are prone to rapid malignant transformation. Gut 2002; 50: 382–6.
21. DeJong A, Morreau H, Van Puijenbroek M et al, The role of mismatch repair gene defects in the development of adenomas in patients with HNPCC. Gastroenterology 2004; 126: 42–8.
22. *National Health and Medical Research Council, Australia, Clinical Practice Guidelines. The Prevention, Early Detection and Management of Colorectal Cancer, 1999.
23. *Hawk ET, Levin B, Colorectal cancer prevention. J Clin Oncol 2005; 23: 378–91.
24. *Eaden JA, Abrams KR, Mayberry JF, The risk of colorectal cancer in ulcerative colitis: a meta-analysis, Gut 2001; 49: 526–35.
25. Ekbom A, Helmick C, Zack M et al, Ulcerative colitis and colorectal cancer. A population-based study. N Engl J Med 1990; 323: 1228–33.
26. Ahsgren L, Jonsson B, Sterling R et al, Prognosis after early onset of ulcerative colitis: a study from an unselected patient population. Hepatogastroenterology 1993; 40: 467–70.
27. Harpaz N, Talbot IC, Colorectal cancer in idiopathic inflammatory bowel disease. Semin Diagn Pathol 1996; 13: 339–57.
28. Riddell RH, Goldman H, Ransohoff DF et al, Dysplasia in inflammatory bowel disease: standardized classification with provisional clinical applications. Hum Pathol 1983; 14: 931–68.
29. Winther KV, Jess T, Langholz E et al, Long-term risk of cancer in ulcerative colitis: a population-based cohort study from Copenhagen County. Clin Gatroenterol Hepatol 2004; 2: 1088–95.
30. Lennard-Jones JE, Prevention of cancer mortality in inflammatory bowel disease. In: Prevention and Early Detection of Colorectal Cancer (Young GP, Rozen P, Levin B, eds). London: WB Saunders, 1996: 217–38.
31. Kiesslich R, Fritsch J, Holtmann M et al, Methylene blue-aided chromoendoscopy for the detection of intraepithelial neoplasia and colon cancer in ulcerative colitis. Gastroenterology 2003; 124: 880–8.
32. Rutter MD, Saunders BP, Wilkinson KH et al, Cancer surveillance in longstanding ulcerative colitis: endoscopic appearances help predict cancer risk. Gut 2004; 53: 1813–6.
33. *Odze RD, Farraye FA, Hecht JL et al, Long-term follow-up after polypectomy treatment for adenoma-like dysplastic lesions in ulcerative colitis. Clin Gastroenterol Hepatol 2004; 2: 534–41.
34. *Itzkowitz SH, Harpaz N, Diagnosis and management of dysplasia in patients with inflammatory bowel diseases. Gastroenterology 2004; 126: 1634–48.
35. *Mpofu C, Watson AJ, Rhodes JM, Strategies for detecting colon cancer and/or dysplasia in patients with inflammatory bowel disease. Cochrane Database Syst Rev 2004; (2): CD000279.
36. Eaden J, Abrams K, Ekbom A et al, Colorectal cancer prevention in ulcerative colitis: a case-control study. Aliment Pharmacol Ther 2000; 14: 145–53.
37. Pardi DS, Loftus EV, Kremos W et al, Ursodeoxycholic acid as a chemopreventive agent in patients with ulcerative colitis and primary sclerosing cholangitis. Gastroenterology 2003; 124: 889–93.
38. Willenbucher RF, Aust DE, Chang CG et al, Genomic instability is an early event during the progression pathway of ulcerative-colitis-related neoplasia. Am J Pathol 1999; 154: 1825–30.
39. Traverso G, Shuber A, Levin B et al, Detection of APC mutations in fecal DNA of patients with colorectal tumors. N Engl J Med 2002; 346: 311–20.
40. *Dacosta RS, Wilson BC, Marcon NE, Optical techniques for the endoscopic detection of dysplastic colonic lesions. Curr Opin Gastroenterol 2005; 1: 70–9.
41. *Keroack M, Video capsule endoscopy. Curr Opin Gastroenterol 2004; 20: 474–81.
42. Schoen RE, Weissfeld JL, Kuller LH, Are women with breast, endometrial or ovarian cancer at increased risk for colorectal cancer?, Am J Gastroenterol 1994; 89: 835–42.
43. *Eisen GM, Sandler RS, Are women with breast cancer more likely to develop colorectal cancer? Critical review and meta-analyses. J Clin Gastroenterol 1994; 19: 57–63.
44. Weinberg DS, Newtschaffer CJ, Tophan BA, Risk for colorectal cancer after gynecologic cancer. Ann Intern Med 1999; 131: 189–93.
45. St John DJB, McDermott FT, Hopper JL et al, Cancer risk in relatives of patients with common colorectal cancer. Ann Intern Med 1995; 118: 785–90.

8 How should we screen for early colorectal neoplasia?

Graeme P Young, Paul Rozen, Bernard Levin

Introduction

The biology of colorectal cancer (CRC) provides opportunities for preventive strategies based on early detection of curable cancer or removable adenoma. The process of cancer development (as described in Chapter 3) consists of multiple steps; some events (especially development of polypoid adenomas and occult bleeding, but also shedding of cell components) are recognizable clinically at premalignant stages. The process extends over a considerable period of time, possibly as long as 10 or more years in non-familial cancers. Figure 8.1 shows in diagrammatic form how various forms of tests can be applied to the stages of tumorigenesis.

From the perspective of healthcare policy, CRC meets the requirements of the World Health Organization (WHO) for suitability for screening.[1] Screening for CRC first became feasible when Greegor described the use of the guaiac-based fecal occult blood test (G-FOBT) for early detection.[2]

Although countries around the world are increasingly embracing screening in one way or another (see Preface and Chapter 1), some primary care practitioners remain pessimistic about the ability of screening to reduce mortality.[3,4] This is largely due to a misunderstanding of the interactive and obligatory relationship between clinical practice and public health programs, including population-based screening. It is important that a screening test directed at healthy people has an impact that is measurable at the population level.[1] Healthy people are inherently reluctant to undergo invasive and inconvenient tests for screening, such as colonoscopy, without strong motivation. Indeed, proposing invasive methods for screening should be tempered by the knowledge that a minority, only about 4–7%, will develop CRC.

Screening for CRC occurs in several settings—screening that applies to the individual and screening that applies to the population. The imperatives for each are different, and each has its place, although to varying degrees, in different countries and settings.

The traditional approach to screening has consisted of a face-to-face meeting between the individual and a health professional (primary care practitioner, nurse, or specialist)—this is sometimes referred to as '*case-finding*' or individualistic screening. It may be initiated by the individual or the physician. Here, the person can be assessed for symptoms and level of risk. What is offered is done in the context of counseling. Duty of care and doing what is best for the patient drives the decision-making and cost-effectiveness tends not to be a consideration.

Population screening is becoming increasingly organized and implemented. It seeks, through a standardized and usually impersonal approach, to engage individuals in at least some form of preventive activity—in effect, doing anything is better than doing nothing. If one seeks to have impact on CRC outcomes at the population level, simplicity, acceptability, feasibility, and low initial cost with proven cost-effectiveness are key factors. Many thousands will be tested in a short time frame, often without ability to ascertain presence of symptoms or to profile risk through a counseling process.

Test specificity has been a major consideration in population screening.[5] But now, as we see a trend to recommend screening by colonoscopy itself, specificity for any type of FOBT is seen as being less of an issue than is sensitivity.[6] Ability to detect advanced adenomas, not only cancer, is increasingly considered to be important.

Screening of healthy people is ultimately an important issue for the community as a whole, especially where healthcare costs are shared across the community as in

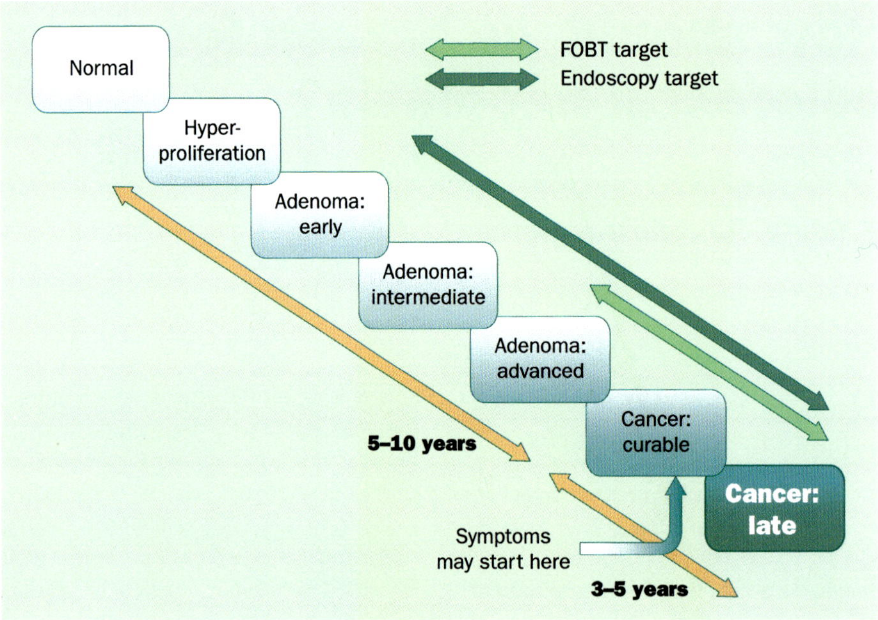

Figure 8.1 *The stages of colorectal tumorigenesis, their approximate duration, relationship to symptom onset, and likelihood of detection by clinical screening methods. Adenoma: early, intermediate, advanced, refers to progressive changes in size, amount of villous elements and/or degree of dysplasia. The immunochemical fecal occult blood test (FIT) is more likely than a guaiac FOBT to identify the advanced polyp.*

Canada, Australia, Western Europe, and Israel.[7] This chapter will therefore address screening from both the population and personal perspectives.

The screening program

Screening can be defined as an ongoing process directed at asymptomatic individuals that has the goal of reducing morbidity and mortality from CRC.

Where the general population is the starting point, the process must:

1. be able to identify those in whom screening is not appropriate
2. be able to identify those who need individualized surveillance and/or genetic testing
3. have its potential value and adverse effects explained to participants in an informed manner
4. have its outcomes continually monitored
5. be able to be resourced and afforded by those who manage the healthcare system
6. be made attractive to those lacking interest or motivation.

Where the individual is the starting point, the same principles apply, except that the last point is much less of an issue and more easily managed. Furthermore, the strategy is not so much to achieve participation with any test (any test being better than none at all), but rather to ensure that the best test is undertaken.

Screening is a stepwise process (Table 8.1). At each step, a judgment is based on likelihood of outcomes and should be justifiable on the basis of evidence. Thus, we will analyze each step from operational and outcome perspectives.

There are two main choices for the program at the point where a test is offered:

- **One-step screening:** here the definitive test, colonoscopy, is offered.
- **Two-step screening:** here, a simpler test is offered first, e.g. FOBT; those with a positive result then proceed on to colonoscopy. This serves to direct colonoscopic resources to those with a higher risk of neoplasia than implied by the one-step process.

Table 8.1 *The screening process*[a]

- **Invite** participation in a screening program by targeting those at risk for colorectal cancer:
  - use either a personalized approach within a healthcare environment, or
  - use a mass population approach with wide coverage of the population
- For those with **high risk factors** (colorectal symptoms, family history or personal history of relevant colorectal disease), provide access to an individualized prevention strategy
- Provide a **safe, effective, acceptable** and **affordable** screening test in one of two main ways:
  - the two-step process: perform a simple test such as a fecal occult blood test (FOBT) to establish risk and select who moves on to colonoscopy
  - the one-step process: perform colonoscopy
- Facilitate **compliance** with any necessary diagnostic and therapeutic follow-up
- Offer **rescreening** at the appropriate interval, having more accurately identified risk status
- **Monitor** adequacy of participation, quality of tests and clinical procedures, and the outcomes of the program

[a] Adapted from reference 7.

Targeting individuals at risk

In an industrialized or westernized country, everyone over 50 years of age is considered to be at least at 'average risk'; i.e. at sufficiently high probability of having CRC to justify screening for it on the grounds of cost-effective outcome (see Figure 2.5). As an example, the prevalence of CRC in the state of Victoria (Australia) in a population aged 25–50 years old is 0.016%, compared with 0.2% for those in the next 25-year age span (50–75 years old), i.e. they are 12 times more likely to have colorectal cancer. So, age 50 years old is the generally accepted starting point in the absence of any other risk factors and is the recommendation of the American Cancer Society and most other international authorities.[8–10]

However, any unselected population will include subjects with symptoms who require diagnostic assessment and who are not suitable for population screening. There will also be those of above-average risk who require an individualized approach to surveillance (see Chapters 6 and 7). They will usually not be apparent when the target population is defined, unless screening is being managed through a physician or medical interviewer. Table 8.2 summarizes these points.

The screening offer and participation

As described above, the initial offer of screening can take various forms: mass population, screenee-initiated, and physician-initiated (Table 8.3).[11]

The latter two forms of screening are sometimes referred to as 'case-finding' and are discussed later in the chapter. Mass population-based screening is by nature impersonal, but is likely to be systematic in its approach and more likely to improve outcomes at the population level if large numbers participate.

Table 8.2 *Targeting individuals at risk*

- **Average risk** people are those aged ≥50 years old in a Western or westernizing country: these require at least a basic screening program such as a fecal occult blood test (FOBT)
- Those at **higher risk** have:
  - symptoms possibly due to colorectal cancer, especially rectal bleeding
  - at least one first degree relative with colorectal neoplasia
  - a personal history of colorectal neoplasia or chronic inflammatory bowel disease
    - They should be given a personalized assessment and, in many instances, be offered more intensive surveillance

Table 8.3 *Methods and contexts for offering screening*

- **Mass** (population-based) screening:
  - initiated by a healthcare system or insurance
  - is impersonal but is systematic and of wide impact
  - participation is as much a key to success as is the type of test done – 'doing anything is better than nothing'
  - simplicity, acceptability, feasibility, and low initial cost with proven cost-effectiveness are key factors
- **Individualized** screening (case-finding):
  - initiated by screenee or physician
  - is ad hoc and not necessarily of wide impact, but ensures appropriate attention to personal situation
  - allows personal evaluation for symptoms and risk factors (see Table 8.2).
  - what is done is offered within a counseling context
  - duty of care drives the choice of the optimal test

When screening is offered, whether from a central coordinating facility in a population program or within the context of case-finding, it should:

1. Optimize access to the screening process, e.g. include diagrammatic instructions and simple language, or even include translations for immigrant populations.
2. Simplify and maximize participation, e.g. provide the stool-sampling device and any dietary instructions needed (see also the subsequent section on acceptability of screening tests), and simplify scheduling of a procedure with minimal waiting time.
3. Explain the potential benefit of participation: i.e. reduction in mortality from bowel cancer in the participants.
4. Identify the outcomes and subsequent action required: i.e. a positive test requires diagnostic follow-up, whereas a negative test has its limitations of sensitivity.
5. Explain the risks: i.e. missed cancers or complications of colonoscopy. It is important to indicate that the screening test is a selection process for colonoscopy that directs colonoscopy to those more likely to have cancer; it might not identify everyone with neoplasia!
6. Encourage ongoing, future systematic participation.
7. Obtain informed consent.[12]

The goal of the offer is to get the highest possible participation rate, as curable lesions (asymptomatic cancers and adenomas) will only be found in those who undertake testing.

Organizing a screening program

Organization of a screening program can be at various levels: by a government health authority, by preventive health personnel within a health maintenance organization (HMO), or by the practitioner. The first such organization is illustrated by the model of national mammography screening programs that are being implemented in Western European and Scandinavian countries. There are examples of large-scale CRC screening programs of this type that are also being performed (see Chapters 1 and 10). If such an organizational framework were in place as for breast cancer screening, it might be cost–beneficial to utilize it also for a similar national CRC screening program.[13] It is important not to provide a competing service that might be perceived by women as being less relevant for them and who may be under the impression that breast and cervical cancer screening is their priority and only necessary preventive examinations. An added benefit of enrolling the female partner, who is often responsible for family health practices, may be that she can then persuade the male partner to also participate in such a preventive program. This has been one of the points emphasized in the recent US public health campaign for CRC screening.

Another possible model for organizing CRC screening is by a large group practice, which may be multidisciplinary or a single subspecialty, usually gastroenterologists. They may be providing medical services for a defined geographic area or subcontracting a medical insurance or servicing large places of work. CRC screening, added to the standard medical services provided, might be offered as an incentive to join that medical service, or to obtain a service contract. Lastly, in many medical systems, including those of countries having a high risk for CRC, the individual primary care physician takes full responsibility for preventive medical practices in adults.[7] This is also discussed in detail in Chapter 10.

Screening test options and their features

The screening test is a key element of a screening program; those being offered the test must be prepared to take it, and in doing so it should increase the chance of detecting a curable neoplastic lesion (see Figure 1.7). The test should be sensitive (i.e. it should detect most affected individuals) and specific (i.e. it should not subject healthy persons to excessive anxiety or extra testing) (see Table 1.4).

Screening methods that might be considered for use are summarized in Table 8.4, which also shows what each is capable of detecting.

Correct usage is vital to success. The biology of bleeding from neoplasia dictates both the correct usage of FOBTs and their efficacy. The anatomic distribution of colorectal neoplasias (cancer or adenoma) determines the usefulness of the sigmoidoscopic screening.

Symptoms and digital rectal examination

The classic clinical presentations of colorectal cancer are described in Chapter 1.

Performance of a digital rectal examination in those over 50 years old seems prudent as part of any physical examination and certainly as part of a work-up for rectal bleeding. It should be performed before inserting an endoscope and should include examination of the prostate.

Performing an in-office G-FOBT has been common practice and some have suggested that performing FOBT as part of a digital rectal examination may be better than not doing it at all.[14] However, usually only one sample rather than the recommended two or three is obtained. The patient has rarely undertaken dietary preparation, which increases the risk of false positives, and there is always the concern that digital rectal examination will generate minor trauma and so lead to a false-positive result and hence an unnecessary colonoscopy.[15] Only recently has FOBT, as part of a digital rectal examination, been evaluated in a large group of asymptomatic subjects.[16] They found that sensitivity for neoplasia was much better if 3-day sampling was performed compared to a single in-office test (sensitivity was only 4.9% when collected in this manner). We do not recommend screening based on digital sampling of stool as part of a rectal examination.

Table 8.4 *Screening test options*[a]

Method	Purpose
Digital rectal examination	Tactile examination of rectum within reach of finger
G-FOBT	Detects blood in feces originating from entire GI tract through chemical detection of heme, with maximum sensitivity of about 0.5 g Hb/g stool
Immunochemical FOBT (FIT)	Detects blood in feces originating from colon/rectum by immunochemical detection of hemoglobin at sensitivity of about 50–100 μg Hb/g stool
Flexible sigmoidoscopy	Visual detection of cancer and adenoma within reach of instrument
Colonoscopy	Visual detection of cancer and adenoma within reach of instrument
Barium enema	Radiologic (two-dimensional) detection in a clean colon, with or without air contrast
CT colonography	Radiologic (three-dimensional) detection, using complete organ reconstruction based on air–solid interface
Fecal molecular and DNA tests	Biochemical and/or genetic testing of molecular components of cells shed from neoplasms into feces

[a] G-FOBT, guaiac-based fecal occult blood test; FIT, fecal immunochemical test; CT, computed tomography; GI, gastrointestinal; Hb, hemoglobin.

Fecal tests

Fecal tests include tests for components of blood and molecular tests for molecules indicating neoplasia. Most have not been proven practical (because of their complexity) or useful, other than the tests for heme/hemoglobin or for DNA.

Fecal occult blood tests

The fact that microscopic bleeding may arise from curable cancers, and indeed adenomas, provides the basis for screening using an FOBT.[11,17] However, the biology of bleeding is complex, and for FOBT screening to be effective, these tests must be used properly in a way that maximizes their ability to detect bleeding from neoplasia.

FOBTs have a very real place in screening for CRC.[6] Their value is proven in randomized controlled trials at the population level and they meet WHO requirements (see Chapter 1 and Table 1.5 for details).[1,9]

The following lists the ideal test characteristics, considering the various facets of the screening process:[17]

1. **Sampling:**
   - convenient, without need of attending physician
   - readily performed without need for diet and drug restrictions
   - acceptable, with easy and simple fecal sampling.
2. **Performance:**
   - selective for colorectal bleeding
   - able to select out those most likely to have neoplasia and to whom diagnostic colonoscopic resources are applied.
3. **Tests development:**
   - suitable for mass development of large numbers in a short time
   - subject to ready quality control and objective reading of results with a stable, instrument-readable and preferably quantitative endpoint.

Ability to select out those most likely to have neoplasia is embodied in the pre-test/post-test likelihood ratio or, in more familiar terms, reflects the balance of sensitivity and specificity.[5] Sensitivity facilitates detection of those with significant neoplasia, whereas specificity effectively determines the number of colonoscopy examinations needed.

Types of FOBT: guaiac and immunochemical tests

FOBTs available for screening are based on two principal technologies: chemical tests and immunochemical tests. The major biologic and technologic features of these tests are outlined in Table 8.5 and shown diagrammatically in Figure 8.2.[5,17,18] Key issues for deciding which to use are outlined in Table 8.6. The main brands commercially available are listed in Table 8.7, but it must be emphasized that the levels of evidence supporting use of an individual brand vary greatly.[18]

The *chemical tests* (e.g. Hemoccult II) use guaiac to detect the peroxidase activity of heme (Tables 8.5 and 8.6);[5] hence, the abbreviation G-FOBT. They react to any peroxidases in feces (e.g. those in plant foods and heme in red meat) and are affected by certain chemicals (e.g. vitamin C). Because heme is relatively stable in the gut (although slow degradation occurs in the colon), these tests may detect bleeding from any site, including the stomach. The sample collection device for these tests requires the screenee to take a sample of feces, avoiding contamination by toilet bowl water, and smear feces onto the device. In the laboratory, developing the card to read the qualitative result appears simple (Figure 8.3), but in practice is not always reliably accurate without training.[19] Hemoccult SENSA is deliberately made to be more readable (Figure 8.3) and more sensitive for peroxidase, but this does affect specificity, especially if red meat had not been excluded from the diet before preparing the test.[18] It is now clear that if test development is delayed 72 hours after sampling, the problem of plant peroxidase interference is minimized.[20,21] Thus, dietary restrictions for G-FOBT can be simplified to only exclude red meat and very high-peroxidase foods such as horseradish.

Before the availability of Hemoccult SENSA, rehydration of Hemoccult was tried so as to increase sensitivity, but this has an adverse effect on specificity by activation of plant peroxidases and is no longer recommended.[18,20] To summarize, while of proven efficacy, G-FOBT have the following shortcomings:[17]

- restrictions of diet and drugs are needed to optimize specificity and sensitivity, especially for the sensitive G-FOBT

Table 8.5 Main biologic and technologic features of different types of fecal occult blood tests (FOBTs)

Type[a]	Basis	Stool sampling method	Endpoint
Chemical (G-FOBT)	Guaiac; detects peroxidase	Wooden spatula collects fecal smear for most	• Transient blue blush of color on paper card (subjective and read by eye) • Qualitative only
Immuno-chemical (FIT)	Anti-human hemoglobin antibody	Wooden spatula, probe, spoon, or brush	• Various methods, some subjective and others objective and automated • May be quantitative

[a] G-FOBT, guaiac-based fecal occult blood test; FIT, fecal immunochemical test.

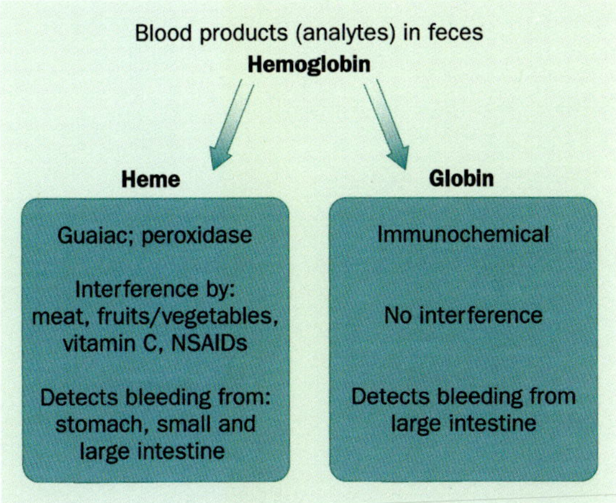

Figure 8.2 *Diagrammatic representation of hemoglobin breakdown in the colonic lumen and the consequences for detection by guaiac-based fecal occult blood test (G-FOBT) and fecal immunochemical test (FIT) technologies. NSAIDs, non-steroidal anti-inflammatory drugs.*

- they generally use spatula sampling of stools, which need to be kept out of contact with toilet bowl water
- they are not selective for colorectal bleeding
- the endpoint can be difficult to read and is transient
- sensitivity for cancer is suboptimal for less sensitive G-FOBT products
- more sensitive G-FOBTs are subject to unpredictably high false-positive rates
- they are not suitable for mass development or reading or quantifying the result.

Fecal immunochemical tests (FITs) use antibodies specific for human globin, so they are not affected by diet (Tables 8.5 and 8.6).[5] Because globin is rapidly degraded by digestive enzymes, these tests are highly selective for occult bleeding of colorectal origin. For some years these tests have been the standard FOBT in Japan and they are now becoming more available in other countries (Table 8.7). Depending on the version of FIT and the manufacturer, improvements in fecal sampling have been made. For instance, Immudia-HemSp, OC-Sensor, MagStream, and Bayer Detect use a probe that is poked into the stool, whereas Hemoccult-ICT uses the stick and smear approach similar to Hemoccult. InSure uses a novel brush method to sample stool immersed in toilet bowl water. They can be office or laboratory hand-developed, using a predetermined standard threshold of hemoglobin to indicate a positive test. Readability is generally simple and reliable (Figure 8.4). Whereas Hemoccult-ICT and InSure use an immunochromatographic method similar to a urine pregnancy test, to give a qualitative result, Immudia-HemSp requires laboratory development using a hemagglutination method. It is beyond the scope of this chapter to explore the technologic details further, but laboratory development is preferred in many countries—especially for mass screening, when many tests must be done and quality assurance is vital.[17,22,23]

There is now an appreciation that automated laboratory development allows for managing large numbers of FOBTs in a standardized manner, namely development and quantification of the fecal hemoglobin level. These include the MagStream-HemSp development of Immudia-HemSp, OC-Sensor development of OC-Hemodia and the InSure test. Latex agglutination FIT can also be quantified.[17,23] For some products, the developing instrument reads a bar code

Table 8.6 Usage and performance issues for different types of fecal occult blood tests (FOBTs)

Type of FOBT	Diet restrictions	Drug interference	Site of detectable occult bleeding	Specificity for neoplasia[d]	Sensitivity for cancer[d]
Chemical (guaiac)	Required: red meats; possibly certain raw plant foods[a].	Vitamin C, possibly NSAIDs[b]	Rectum >colon >stomach (in decreasing order of sensitivity)	90–98%, depending on test brand, sensitivity, and usage	35–80%, with one-time testing Over 90% with repeated testing
Immuno-chemical (FIT)	None required	None	Colon and rectum	Around 95%, depending on what sensitivity level is accepted[c]	70–90%, but data are limited

[a] Delaying development for 72 hours minimizes interference from plant foods and avoids need for their restriction. Red meats must be restricted when using a more sensitive G-FOBT[18]

[b] Low-dose aspirin is not a problem, but therapeutic doses for rheumatic disorders may be so

[c] The tests generally provide a qualitative result, but newer immunochromatographic tests may be quantifiable.

[d] These are indicative estimates only and have been adapted from reference 18.

Table 8.7 Examples of commercially available fecal occult blood tests (FOBTs)

Guaiac-based FOBTs (G-FOBTs)

- Hemoccult II, Haemoccult, and Hemoccult SENSA are registered trademarks of Beckman Coulter, Inc., Primary Care Diagnostics
- Colo-Rectal is a registered trademark of Hoffman LaRoche AG
- Seracult Plus is a registered trademark of Propper Manufacturing Co., Inc.
- HemoFEC is a registered trademark of Boehringer Mannheim GmbH
- ColoScreen is a registered trademark of Helena Laboratories

Fecal immunochemical tests (FITs)

- Immudia-HemSp and MagStream-HemSp[a] are registered trademarks of Fujirebio, Inc., Tokyo, Japan
- Inform[a] and InSure FOBT[a] are registered trademarks of Enterix Australia Pty Limited and Enterix USA Inc., New Jersey
- Bayer Detect[a] is a registered trademark of Bayer Diagnostics, Tarrytown, NY, who are marketing MagStream HemSp
- OC-Hemodia and OC-Sensor[a] are registered trademarks of Eiken, Tokyo, Japan
- Hemolex is a registered trademark of Orion Diagnostica, Espoo, Finland
- Mono-Haem is a registered trademark of Silenus Laboratories
- Hemoccult-ICT (previously marketed as *FlexSure OBT*) and HemeSelect (not marketed) are registered trademarks of Beckman Coulter, Inc., Primary Care Diagnostics
- Clearview Ultra-FOB test is a registered trademark of Wampole Laboratory, USA
- ImmoCARE is a registered trademark of CARE Products, USA
- Instant-View Fecal Occult Blood Test is a registered trademark of ALFA Scientific Designs, USA

[a] These are laboratory-developed quantitative hemoglobin tests. The other tests are office/laboratory-developed tests with inflexible, predetermined levels for hemoglobin detection.

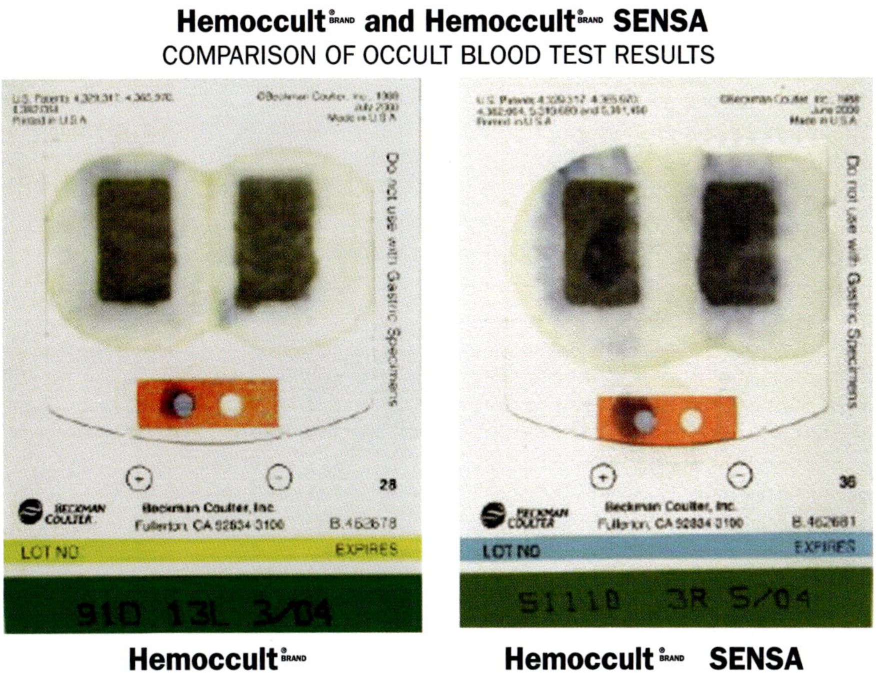

Figure 8.3 *Developed sample cards from Hemoccult II and Hemoccult SENSA (Beckman Coulter Inc.). Note the more easily read Hemoccult SENSA. Blood levels in the stool were the same for each test.*

on the test and so ensures accurate identification of the screenee, prints out the results, and in some can provide a reminder printout for future recall for FOBT. There are internal controls so as to maintain quality control.

InSure is established in the Australian and the US markets where it is also included in Medicare. OC-Sensor is available in Europe, where it has been used as the FOBT for a large-scale screening program in the North of Italy.[23] It is now being evaluated in Israel. MagStream-Bayer Detect is under trial in Australia and Europe.

The advantage of fecal hemoglobin measurement is that it returns full control of sensitivity and specificity to the end-user.[17] By quantifying the fecal hemoglobin level, fewer samples are needed: e.g. in a comparative trial, two InSure samples from two separate stools were more sensitive for colorectal neoplasia than were six G-FOBT samples in 3 days.[18] This improves compliance for preparing FOBTs and reduces costs. In Italy, only one-stool sampling is requested and in Japan two samples.[22,23]

Quantifying the fecal hemoglobin allows the preparation of receiver-operating characteristic curves (ROC), which can be used to establish at what level of fecal hemoglobin colonoscopy is recommended. At the population level, such an approach allows maximizing the test specificity:sensitivity ratio, thereby adapting the colonoscopy rate to the facilities and budget available for screening.

Table 8.6 shows estimates of sensitivity for the different types of the FOBT for blood in feces. As a general rule, FITs are at the more sensitive end of the range, whereas G-FOBT tests vary widely across the range.

Bleeding from colorectal neoplasia

The nature of blood products excreted in feces varies according to the site of bleeding.[5] FITS are advantageous as they are more selective for large bowel bleeding. Whereas fecal blood loss is common in patients with colorectal neoplasia, it is not always outside the normal range of up to 1.5 ml/day and G-FOBTs have difficulty discriminating between normal subjects and cancer-bearing patients.[24,25] Adenomas bleed less than cancers, but recent studies with FIT are confirming early results that it is possible to detect hemoglobin lost from adenomas (Figure 8.5).[5,17]

In patients with neoplasia, the quantity of bleeding from

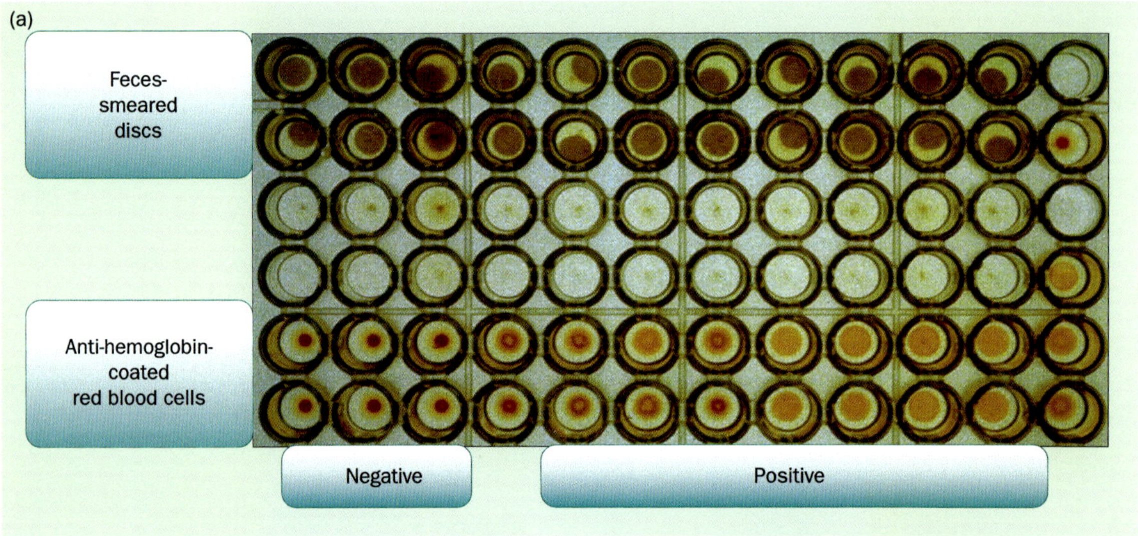

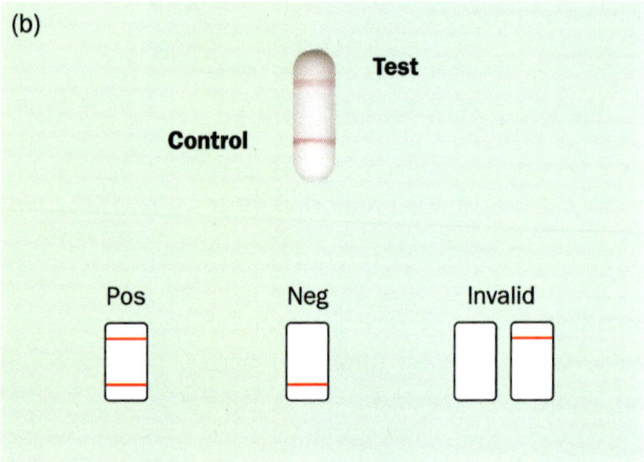

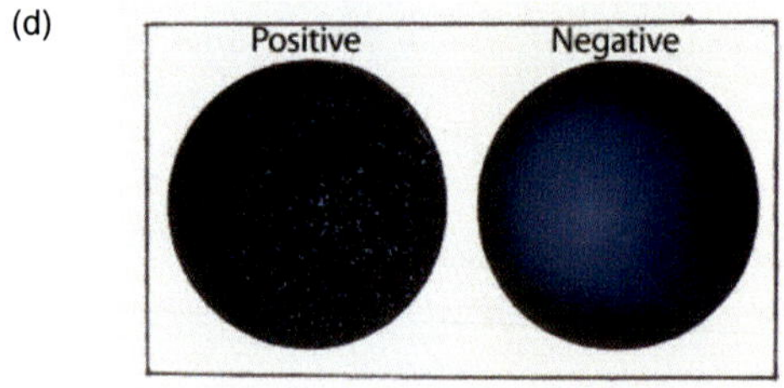

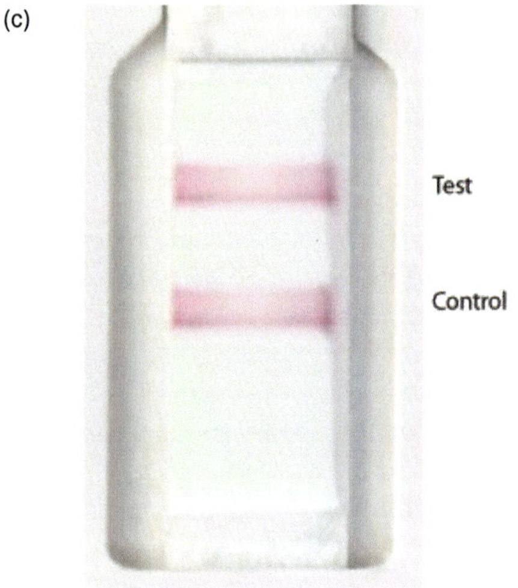

Figure 8.4 *Examples of developed FITs (immunochemical FOBTs).*
(a) Hemagglutination plate for the Immudia-HemSp test, showing positive and negative results.
(b) Positive sample of the Hemoccult-ICT developed by the immunochromatographic method.
(c) Positive sample of the InSure test (Enterix Inc.) developed by the immunochromatographic method.
(d) Latex agglutination results for Hemolex.

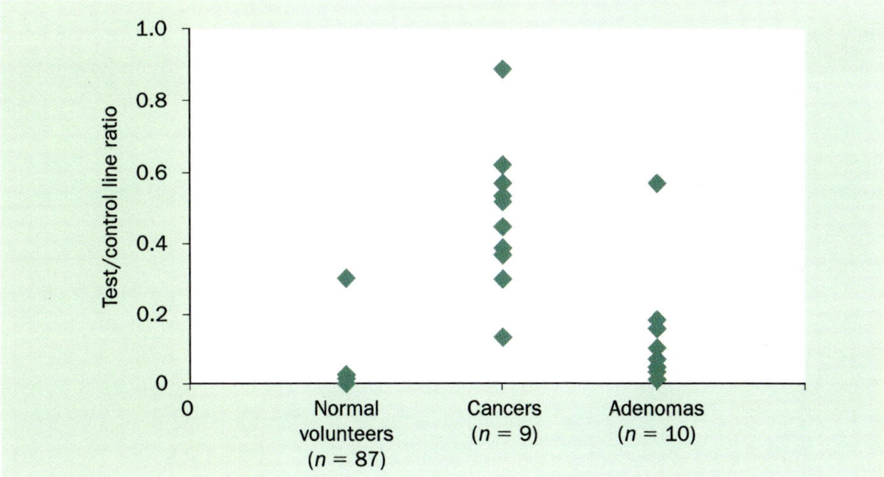

Figure 8.5 *Fecal hemoglobin concentrations in patients with neoplasia. Concentrations are expressed as intensity ratio relative to control line, measured using an adaptation of the InSure test where the endpoint is quantified by an optical device: normal n = 166, cancer n = 22, adenoma n = 18. Each group is significantly different from the other, $p < 0.05$. Note the small overlap between normals and cancer patients and the intermediate levels in those with adenomas. (From reference 17 with permission.)*

cancers varies from day to day, and so it is normally recommended that FOBTs are performed on multiple, usually three, separate stools.[5,25] However, this has been determined using crude blood detection methods (G-FOBT and radiochromium Hb labeling). Recent studies with FIT show that two-day and even one-day testing (which further promotes compliance for testing) is useful, and bleeding might be more consistent than has been thought.[18,22,23,26]

Correct usage of FOBT

When screenees use an FOBT, it is important that they follow the manufacturer's instructions carefully. These usually achieve control of sample size and stability of sample for hemoglobin detection and do not recommend obtaining the sample by digital examination. Dietary restrictions (red meat) should be followed if using a G-FOBT. For G-FOBTs, it is useful to provide a collection device that facilitates stool sampling and avoids contact with toilet water and/or chemical cleaners. The collection device should ideally be disposable in the toilet. The InSure FIT is designed for sampling the stool immersed in toilet bowl water. The screenee should perform stool sampling using the manufacturer's sampling device and stools should be sampled from multiple points at the surface of each stool. The sample should be returned promptly to the doctor or laboratory for development. These issues are summarized in Table 8.8.

Doctor's office or laboratory-based testing?

Although developing and reading the card seems simple (see Figure 8.3), studies have shown that reliability improves with training.[19] Dietary peroxidase interference can be significant and is often not controlled prior to attending a doctor's office and having an FOBT done.[20,21] Furthermore, fewer samples are collected because of decreasing compliance.[17] Office-based testing is now becoming increasingly replaced by laboratory development.

Summary of FOBT technologies

1. Two different types of FOBT are readily available; their requirements are different in practice.
2. Dietary factors and drugs may interfere with G-FOBT. The more sensitive G-FOBT is especially at risk of dietary false-positive results.
3. The type and quantity of blood derivatives in feces vary with site of occult bleeding and FITs are 'colorectal selective'.

4. FOBTs will not completely discriminate between those with and without neoplasia, but FIT does so better than G-FOBT.
5. The manufacturer's recommendations for sampling of stools should be followed closely, and samples should be sent to the office/laboratory in the sampling device and not as whole stools.
6. Contamination of feces by toilet bowl water before sampling should be avoided except for tests designed to sample stools in the bowl.
7. Multiple samples should be taken from the surface of the stool.
8. Samples are best collected by the screenees in their own homes.

Practical points when using a FOBT

G-FOBTs are relatively inexpensive, and there are various manufacturers (see Table 8.7). Published sensitivity for blood and the results of their use in clinical trials are the objective means to decide between the various manufactured G-FOBTs.[18]

Developing an FOBT card seems easy, but there are points to note that will help obtain maximum compliance with their use and quality performance. The first is to overcome the psychologic barrier to manipulating feces. The use of an explanatory video film and/or personal explanation by a nurse practitioner or medical interviewer can help overcome this initial barrier.

In order to facilitate compliance for screening and annual repeated FOBTs, the dietary and medication limitations should be minimized to those absolute necessary. These have been described in this chapter. Similarly, the collection of fecal samples should be as easy and as efficient as possible. This is best done by using a paper collecting device that can be attached to the toilet seat or toilet bowel (Figure 8.6). This allows for easier sampling, avoids contact with toilet water (and chemicals), and allows for disposal of the stools and collecting paper in the toilet. Note that this is not necessarily the best way to collect samples for certain FITs, such as InSure.

Cards must be clearly identified with the screenee's name, etc., and the date of preparation (Figure 8.7). The thinly smeared cards should be left open for a few minutes until air-dried. This minimizes bacterial degradation of fecal hemoglobin and its products. For the same reason, completed cards should be kept in a cool place until returned for development. Special return mailing envelopes are available, but, even so, exposure to high ambient temperatures in an outdoor mailbox should be avoided.

These instructions are also applicable to those FITs that use a sampling methodology similar to G-FOBTs.

Table 8.8 *Important points for correct usage of fecal occult blood tests (FOBTs)*

- Sampling of stools onto the device should be performed by the screenee using the manufacturer's sampling device and following manufacturer's instructions
- Manufacturer's instructions should also be used for storing and transporting samples
- Screenees should avoid straining at stool
- Menstruation, and sampling after endurance sports participation, may give a positive result
- Dietary restrictions should be followed if using a guaiac-based FOBT (G-FOBT) and should be commenced 3 days prior to taking the first sample; avoid taking vitamin C with a G-FOBT
- Do not cease low-dose aspirin prescribed for cardiovascular disorders, but it is prudent to avoid larger doses of anti-inflammatory drugs (G-FOBT only)
- Stools should be sampled from multiple points at the surface of each stool
- Avoid contact of stools with toilet bowl water unless the test is specifically designed to allow this
- Return the samples as quickly as possible for development

(a)

(b)

(c)

(d)

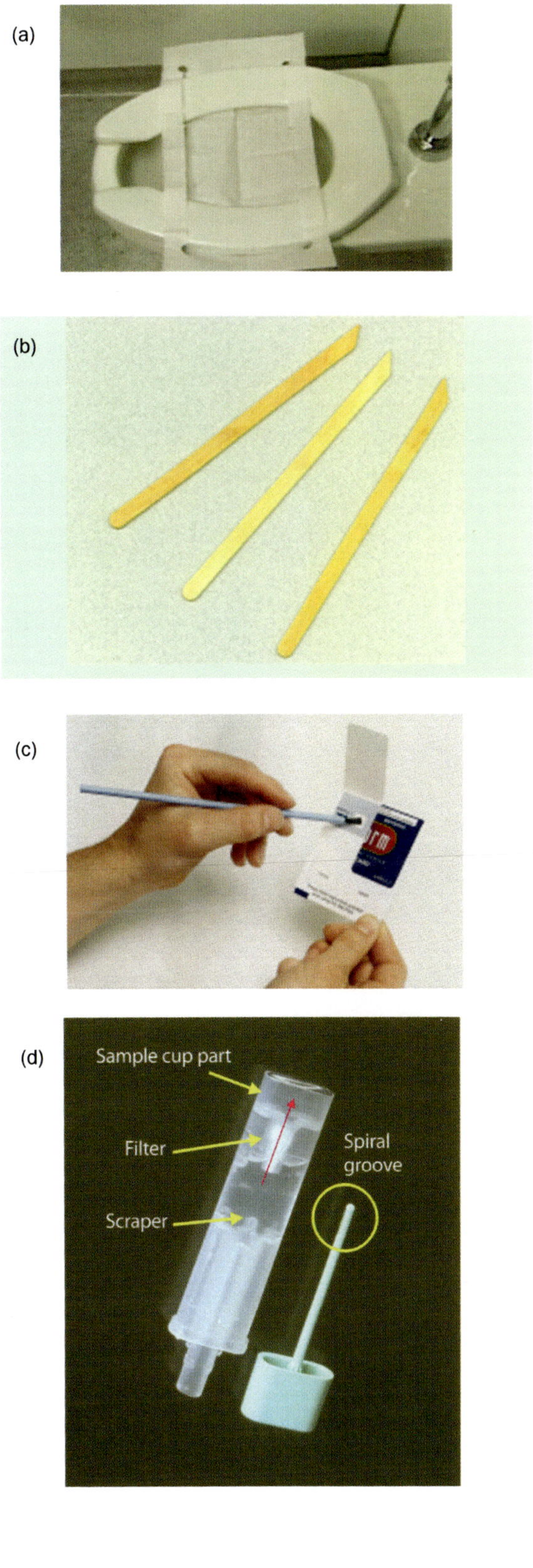

Figure 8.6 *Stool collection devices. (a) Example of stool-collecting device for use with the Hemoccult stick. (b) Hemoccult II sampling sticks as used for sampling stool clear of toilet bowl water. (c) InSure brush used for sampling from toilet bowl water adjacent to stool and for applying sample to card. (d) Probe used for OC-Sensor. The serrations at the tip trap the feces; excess feces is removed when pushing the probe through a scraper, and then a diaphragm, and into the container tube storage fluid.*

Practical points on developing G-FOBT

The G-FOBT is frequently developed and interpreted by non-laboratory-trained personnel. This is undesirable, as there are potential sources of mistakes that can lead to under- or over-reading of the test result. The clinical significance of a false-positive or a false-negative test has been described in Chapter 1 and in this chapter. There are several points to note. Develop the G-FOBT card no sooner than 3 days after preparing the last test so as to allow degradation of vegetable peroxidases, but no later than 14 days after the first test preparation so as to prevent dehydration and loss of sensitivity.[21] Expiry dates of developing agents need to be checked. The test card should have an internal control to demonstrate that the developing agents and the card itself are performing as expected.

Reading the test results is subjective: namely, the identification of a blue color. After applying the developing agent, a timer should be used and the card carefully observed for any transient positive (blue) coloration around the edges, or spreading out from the smeared 'window' (see Figure 8.3). Any blue color, no matter how transient, represents a positive test result. There are several sources of potential error. If the FOBT manufacturer has not maintained quality control of the background paper or cards have not been stored

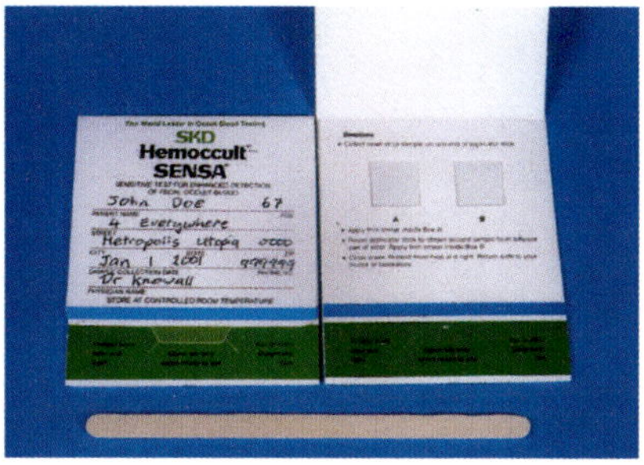

Figure 8.7 *The front of each FOBT card must be filled in with identification data and date. This flap is then opened and stools thinly applied to each of the two 'windows' using the wooden spatula provided.*

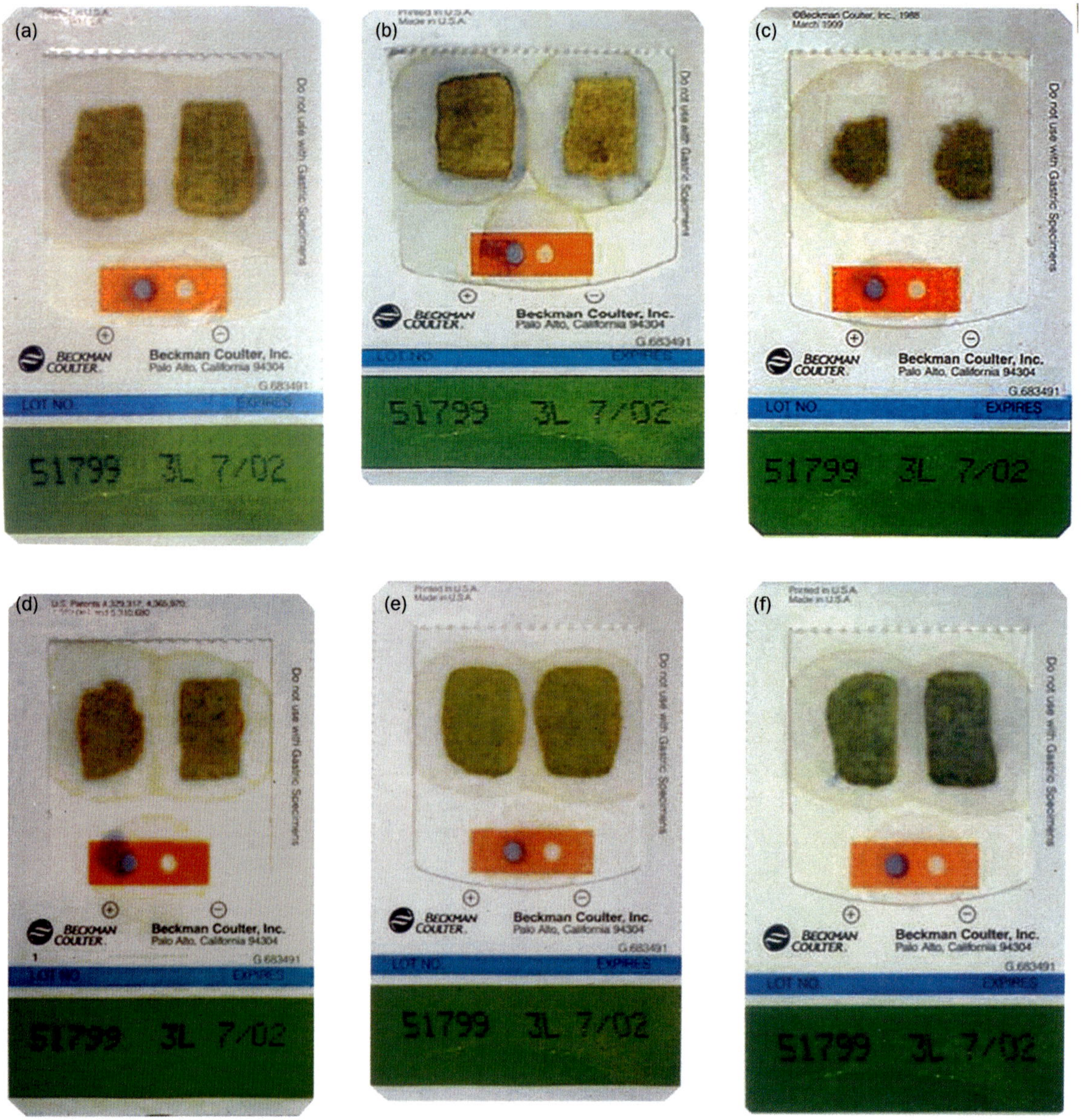

Figure 8.8 *Examples of different guaiac fecal occult blood test (G-FOBT) endpoints. (a) Developed G-FOBT negative for occult blood. Note the blue color of the 'performance' monitor on the lower left and lack of color on the lower right after applying the developing reagent. This indicates the correct performance of the test card and reagents. There is no blue color around the two smeared windows. (b) There is a strong blue color that has leached out around the smeared windows, indicating a positive test. (c) and (d) There is a weak bluish tinge around the smeared windows, still indicating a positive test. (e) Note the greenish tinge of the smeared 'windows' after applying the developing reagent. This is due to bile staining, and as there is no blue color, it is a negative test for blood. (f) After applying the developing reagent, there is both a green tinge due to bile and a surrounding bluish tinge indicating a positive test for blood.*

at the correct temperature, there may be a bluish tinge when wet with the developing agent. Bile staining will give a greenish color, and iron or bismuth give a black color to the smeared stools. Examples of developed FOBTs are given in Figure 8.8, and these illustrate the range of colors that represent positive or negative tests for fecal occult blood when using the guaiac reagent.

For all the above reasons, in order to minimize subjective errors, it is best to have G-FOBT developed in laboratories by experienced technicians.[19] This also allows for quality control, which should be done once or twice a year by providing smeared cards which have had known amounts of blood added to normal feces. This also allows for the evaluation of the technicians for their reading threshold for blood.[21]

Stool molecular and DNA tests

Cells shed from cancers and adenomas are detectable in the stools.[27] Tests that are capable of detecting molecular or genetic events that either cause cancer or else result from development of neoplasia could theoretically be useful in selecting who undergoes colonoscopy.[27]

Because of the molecular heterogeneity of DNA in neoplasms, selecting the best panel of markers is a challenge. A large colonoscopy controlled study demonstrated a sensitivity of stool DNA tests of 51.6% for colorectal cancer.[28] The sensitivity of the DNA panel was significantly better than the G-FOBT (Hemoccult II) prepared at the same time, although their specificities were similar. The present versions of stool DNA tests are costly (in excess of US$500) and require a cumbersome stool collection that needs to be rapidly delivered to the processing laboratory.

It is expected that within the next decade this innovative technology will eventually lead to more specific and simple tests that provide an effective first test in a two-step screening process. The newer stool molecular tests might be based on RNA or protein markers and be less subject to heterogeneity than DNA tests.

Radiology tests

Barium enema

The use of a barium enema as a screening tool has been considered to be a cost-effective strategy (see Chapter 1). Clearly, the quality of the examination and experience of the person interpreting the films is of great importance. The Council of the American College of Radiology has recommended a practice standard that allows detection of 90% of cancers and 80% of polyps larger than 1 cm.[29] This can best be achieved by quality, air-contrast studies.[30]

Radiology is relatively insensitive for small polyps, a characteristic that might well be an advantage if small polyps (<1.0 cm) are not considered to be of high clinical significance.[29] A recent comparison of colonoscopy and double-contrast barium enema for surveillance after polypectomy showed the former to be the more effective method.[31] Consequences of repeated radiation dose are unclear, but are of concern. As there is little information available on the use of radiology as a mass-screening tool, compliance and willingness to return for repeated examinations are uncertain, and because it has not been formally tried in population screening, its use cannot be recommended.

Computed tomography (CT) colonography

CT colonography or 'virtual colonoscopy' provides a three-dimensional radiologic assessment of the colon using multi-slice X-ray technology. The debate around its place, usefulness now or in the future, and practicality, is vigorous, and several studies have generated much discussion.[32–35]

Sensitivity is variably reported as inferior, equivalent, or even better (for 'significant' neoplasia) to colonoscopy in practice-based settings.[33,34] A recent review that critically analyzed the most important studies[36] commented on the 'remarkable variability' in results between the studies and quoted sensitivities for colorectal neoplasia ranging from 55% to 94%. Obviously, the size of the lesion is important. Flat or small lesions are not well seen with a sensitivity of about 50% if <10 mm.[34] We can expect these results to improve and the variability to decrease as contrast media, subtraction methods, and better technology become more widely available.

Although true population participation studies are only just being commenced, an early study has shown a participation of 18%.[35] CT colonography presents the advantage of being less invasive than colonoscopy, is performed without sedation, and computer 'subtraction' of labeled stools might minimize the need for bowel preparation (Figure 8.9).

There are many uncertainties, some of which pose challenging barriers to the use of CT colonography in screening.

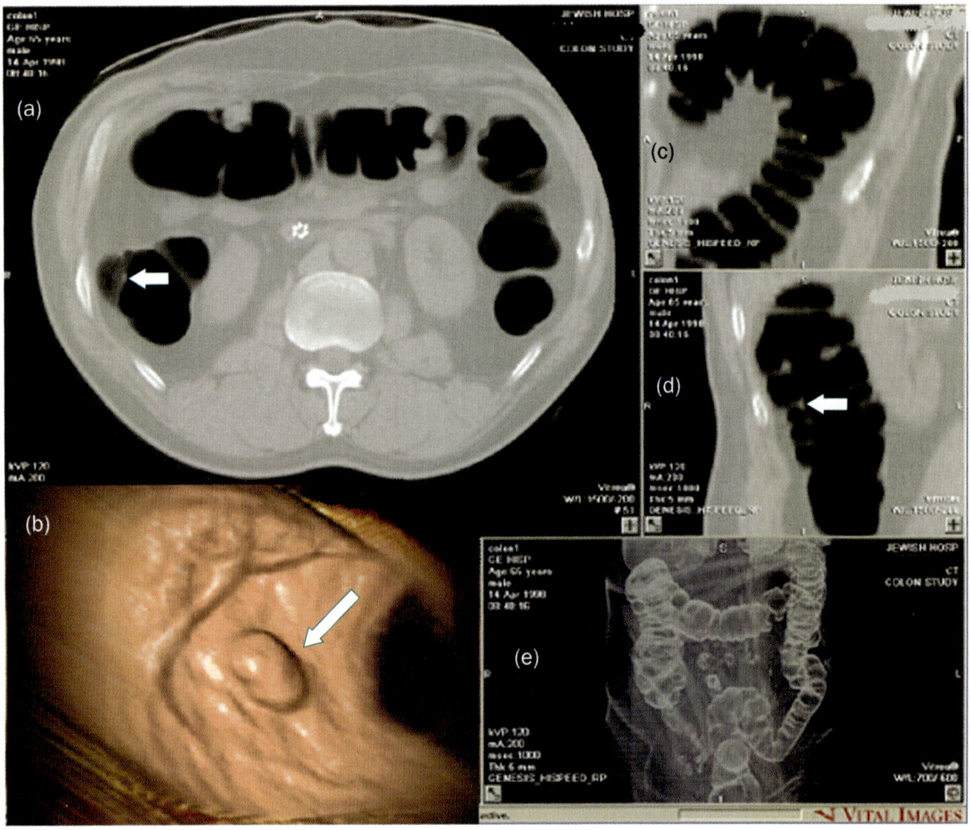

Figure 8.9 *CT colonography Photomontage of views generated by this technique (provided by the EZ-EM Company). (a) Top left, prone axial view of bowel and abdominal organs, with a filling defect indicated by arrow. (b) Bottom left, Computer-generated endoluminal three-dimensional appearance of a sessile polyp indicated by arrow. (c) and (d) Top and middle right—Magnified axial images illustrated a possible polyp protruding into the lumen indicated by arrow. (e) Bottom right—A computer generated overview of the colon.*

It is not therapeutic and, at least for the present, full bowel cleaning is necessary. The best radiologic equipment and imaging software are not widely available. The learning curve is long and the evaluation of images is time-consuming. False-positive results due to luminal content pose a problem, meaning that the colonoscopy follow-up rate is increased. Extracolonic lesions are found at a rate of up to 10% and 2–3% of these require procedural or therapeutic follow-up of uncertain longer-term benefit to the patient.[37] The radiation dose, although now lower, is not insignificant, especially with repeated procedures.

More studies are needed before the place of this procedure is established for screening. The use of magnetic resonance imaging (MRI) colonography is also being evaluated; it eliminates radiation, but is expensive.

CT colonography does have a definite benefit as a diagnostic test, by visualizing the bowel in case the colonoscopy examination was incomplete or was not performed because of patient refusal.

Endoscopic screening

There are significant differences between using a test for diagnostic purposes and for screening purposes, a distinction that is often overlooked. A diagnostic test is applied to an individual, often with symptoms, where the likelihood of disease is relatively high and test side effects are easily balanced against the benefit. A screening test is applied to a healthy individual with low likelihood of disease, where any level of complication could make it unacceptable. This distinction becomes critically important when considering endoscopic screening. On the other hand, endoscopic methods improve the chance of detecting smaller neoplastic lesions, especially adenomas, which can be removed or biopsied.

Rigid proctosigmoidoscopy

Rigid proctosigmoidoscopy examination is anatomically limited by its length and rectosigmoid angulations. Often, it will not pass through the rectosigmoid junction. In practice, it detects about 25–30% of colorectal cancers.[38] However, based on UK data on the distribution of cancers in the large bowel, 45% identification is theoretically possible if the rectosigmoid junction were always visualized (Figure 8.10).[39] It is far less comfortable than flexible sigmoidoscopy.

No special facilities are required, although training in technique and lesion recognition is essential. Because of the diagnostic limitations and discomfort associated with this examination, it is uncommonly used as a screening test.

Flexible sigmoidoscopy

The flexible sigmoidoscope achieves more comprehensive views of the rectum and sigmoid colon than does the rigid proctosigmoidoscope. Although 30 cm and 60 cm instruments are available, the former is rarely used. Its field of view is greater, with its length and flexibility allowing more comfortable insertion and manipulation around the rectosigmoid junction and sigmoid colon compared with the rigid sigmoidoscope (Figure 8.11). Significantly, more neoplastic lesions are identified than with rigid sigmoidoscopy, and one-half to two-thirds of neoplasms are within its reach with the 60 cm instrument.[40] This examination can be conducted without sedation and with only enema preparation, rather than taking an oral bowel preparation. But the facilities required for instrument maintenance and disinfection are the same as those for colonoscopy. Instruments with a removable sheath have been developed that do not need disinfecting (www.visionsciences.com).

A detailed comparison of the usage and efficacy of rigid and flexible sigmoidoscopy has been reported by the

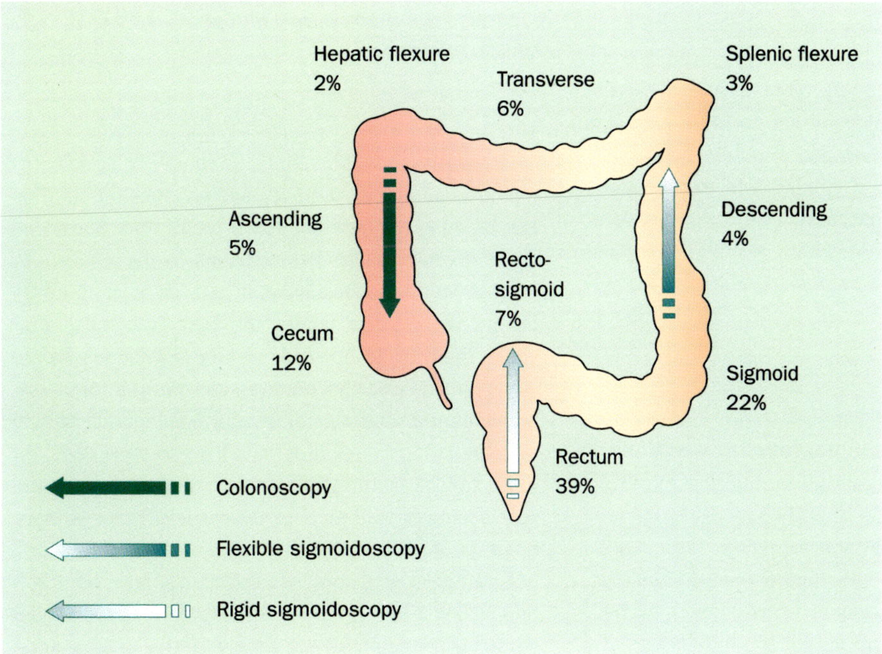

Figure 8.10 *Diagrammatic representation of the sensitivity of the various endoscopic methods according to reach around the colon and distribution of cancer.*[39,40]

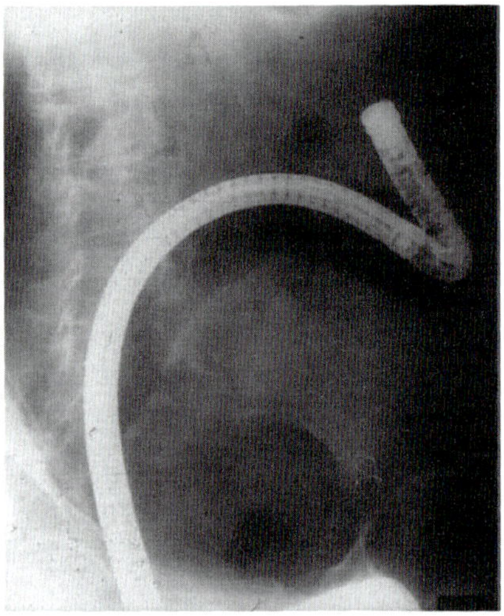

Figure 8.11 *X-ray of the abdomen during insertion of the flexible sigmoidoscopy through the sigmoid colon.*

American Medical Association.[41] Appropriate training and facilities are necessary and nurses can be trained to perform flexible sigmoidoscopy. The technique has been described in detail.[42,43] A DVD has been prepared describing all aspects of the procedure (contact MELZME@aol.com for details). To help training in its performance, simulator models have been developed to obtain initial experience before supervised and independent examinations (Figure 8.12) (www.simbionix.com). Due to the risk of explosion during cautery, polypectomy should not be performed during sigmoidoscopic screening unless full bowel preparation has been performed or CO_2 insufflation is available.

Organizing screening sigmoidoscopy sessions

This can be efficiently organized by utilizing existing endoscopy services outside clinical hours, or by devoting them to this purpose at specific times. The advantages are to not mix the apprehensive healthy screenees with clinical patients whose test may be prolonged, sometimes complicated, and require use of recovery facilities. After hours is frequently more convenient for the working screenee, whereas a dedicated morning session may be more convenient for those who work at home.

(a)

(b)

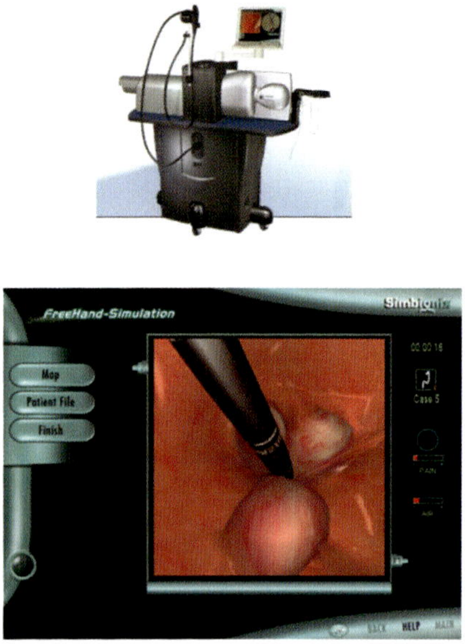

Figure 8.12 *Example of a simulator model for teaching endoscopy (a). Appearance of hemorrhoids on retroflexion (b). (Reproduced with permission of GI Monitor, Simbionix.)*

One of the main inhibitions to screening flexible sigmoidoscopy is the need for enema preparation. This can be done at home and many prefer that. Some prefer it done en-suite, i.e. adjacent to the endoscopy rooms. This is especially important for persons traveling some distance before the test or coming after work. There is no need for dietary restrictions before examination, and the enemas can be self- or nurse-administered. The sigmoidoscopy examination should take less than 10 minutes, and the screenee does not need special clothing other than being draped to prevent soiling of clothes or embarrassment; nor is there need for recovery facilities.

An efficient screening session should last about 2–3 hours, and allow for the examination of about 10–15 persons. The team should consist of the medical interviewer–receptionist, cleaning–reprocessing technician, one or two nursing assistants (one assisting in preparing for screening and another helping during screening), and physician or nurse–practitioner screener: if the latter, then a physician should be easily available. Equipment should be on-hand for biopsy and photography of lesions. Photographs are especially important when lesions are identified by nurse–practitioners. Videoendoscopy is advantageous for team observation and is often useful for promoting screenee cooperation and understanding. The conditions should be calm and sympathetic, so as to minimize the anxiety felt by the healthy screenee. These conditions will promote willingness for periodic recall examination and to persuade others to participate.

So as to minimize discomfort, it is important that an experienced endoscopist perform the test. The endoscopist can be a trained nurse–practitioner where this is allowed: they are not less efficient than specialist physician–endoscopists, who are often unwilling to spend their expensive time on such routine preventive examinations.

The most time-efficient session is to utilize several endoscopy rooms, so that the examiner can go quickly from one examination to another. This allows for at least 4 examinations to be performed in an hour. For efficiency, at least three endoscopic instruments should be available, allowing for cleaning and reprocessing of each endoscope, which takes at least 30 minutes.

The least-efficient is having sigmoidoscopy performed by the occasional endoscopist. There are endoscopy-training programs for primary care physicians.[43] However, skills are easily lost if not used frequently. The other major disadvantages are the need to invest in endoscopy instruments, having available skilled nursing help, and the need for quality-controlled cleaning and reprocessing of expensive equipment. Using an endoscope that has a disposable external sheaf can eliminate the need for cleaning and purchasing multiple instruments, but is more expensive.[44]

Colonoscopy

Colonoscopy is the most complete means for examining the colon. Combined with the ability to take biopsies and intervene therapeutically, it is the ideal diagnostic tool and for follow-up after polypectomies.[9,31] However, the need for vigorous bowel preparation and sedation of subjects, the time lost from employment, the need for trained personnel, limited availability in many countries, and the relatively high cost make it of questionable cost-effectiveness as the primary screening tool for the average-risk subject in many countries. As with flexible sigmoidoscopy, appropriate training is essential, special facilities are necessary, and training in sedation is essential.

Sensitivity and efficacy of colonoscopic screening are discussed later in this chapter.

Endoscopy technology summary

1. The proportions of colorectal cancers reached by rigid or flexible sigmoidoscopy or colonoscopy are determined by their reach into the colon and the adequacy of bowel preparation.
2. Whereas preparation for colonoscopy is complex, only an enema is required for flexible sigmoidoscopy.
3. The facilities required for the flexible endoscopic procedures are substantial.
4. Training is necessary for all procedures, but is most complex for colonoscopy.
5. Sedation is desirable for colonoscopy, but is not necessary for flexible sigmoidoscopy.

Follow-up of a positive screening test

A positive fecal occult blood test

Any positive FOBT sample warrants diagnostic evaluation, preferably by colonoscopy. In practice, primary care doctors have not adequately followed this directive, sometimes attributing the result to possible confounding factors such as hemorrhoids, lack of dietary compliance, participation in endurance sports, and menstruation. Even if a screenee should not have done the test (e.g. during menstruation) or did not follow the diet, colonoscopic follow-up should be carried out because it may be a true positive. Physician failure to encourage follow-up can adversely affect the value of screening and, if not documented, could be viewed as negligence.

A 'positive' sigmoidoscopy

The finding of an adenoma over 1 cm in diameter, a villous adenoma, or multiple adenomas at flexible sigmoidoscopy are definite indications for colonoscopic follow-up.[45]

Approximately 30% of cancers proximal to the splenic flexure have an index lesion situated more distally. Many argue on the potential sentinel status of a distal adenoma for proximal cancer or on the basis of the adenoma–cancer sequence, that colonoscopic follow-up is required for all adenomas, and it is common practice to do this in several countries such as the United States. As the follow-up colonoscopy rate in high-adenoma-prevalence countries could be as high as 25–35% with this recommendation, it would create a huge demand on resources. It also ignores the finding that in the UK, a small distal tubular adenoma, once removed, poses no future risk for cancer.[46] The current trial of flexible sigmoidoscopy in the UK should answer the question of what type of adenoma should trigger colonoscopic follow-up. This might not be applicable to other countries that have a lower prevalence of large, polypoid adenomas.

The principles of appropriate test follow-up are shown in Table 8.9.

Safety

Safety and adverse events

Safety is critically important when screening healthy people. Furthermore, the risks of screening are not just procedural but also relate to the anxiety that may be generated by increasing awareness of disease, by the delays between confirmation of potentially adverse findings, and by the relatively unseen adverse effects of missed cancers. Whichever screening tool is used, the mere process of public education and raised awareness of the possibility of disease in people who feel well has some consequences.[47]

Table 8.9 *Principles for follow-up of test results—positive means either the result of a fecal occult blood test or the finding of an adenoma at sigmoidoscopy*

- When offered screening, subjects should understand the **follow-up action** required for each test result.
  - **Negative** result: come back again for rescreening at the correct interval; report any symptoms in the interim
  - **Positive** result: total colorectal evaluation is required
- **Doctors** involved must understand and implement these actions
- **Resources** for prompt follow-up must be available

Safety of FOBTs

FOBTs in themselves are quite safe apart from the minor issue of hygiene. The consequences of testing create risks though. Following a positive test, there is a delay before colonoscopic follow-up that generates anxiety. If no neoplasia is found, then any anxiety experienced may be viewed as having been unnecessary. But given that a normal colonoscopy examination may indicate a very low risk for the next 5–10 years and probable lack of need for any screening during that time, the testing can be put in a positive light.

Following a negative test, a cancer may have been missed. However, it can be anticipated that if rescreening is undertaken annually, any missed neoplasm might be identified at a later time.[48] Repeated testing is inherent in the screening process. When screening is offered, it is important to indicate that the test is not a diagnostic test, but an aid to detection, and the screening test is a selection process for colonoscopy that directs colonoscopy to those more likely to have cancer. A one-time test might not lead to the detection of all cancers!

Safety of barium enema and CT colonography

The complication rate of these tests is very low, although when perforation occurs, the mortality due to barium peritonitis is high. There is an issue of increasing exposure to radiation if these methods are to be used repeatedly. As with FOBTs, any positive result must be followed up by colonoscopy to confirm the diagnosis of cancer by biopsy or to remove and evaluate the polyp. Hence, the same principles of anxiety in anticipation and missed lesions apply as for FOBT.

Safety of flexible sigmoidoscopy

Screening flexible sigmoidoscopy appears to be particularly safe, since endoscopic biopsy is safe: the perforation rate is less than 1 per 1000 procedures.[49] Sedation is not required for this procedure. Polypectomy should not be done unless the bowel has been prepared or CO_2 insufflation is available, and so significant bleeding or perforations are unlikely.

Safety of colonoscopy

The complication rate of screening colonoscopies under the carefully supervised and managed environment of a controlled trial is low: of 12 246 colonoscopies, there were 4 perforations and 11 episodes of serious bleeding, i.e. a rate of major complications of about 1 in 800.[48] Widespread use of colonoscopy by non-expert operators could result in an increased complication rate and an increased rate of incomplete examinations. Careful quality control will be needed.[50] Risk of perforation in less-expert settings is about 1 in 500, and increases in the presence of comorbidities.[49] Hemorrhage requiring transfusion is about twice as common as perforation. Overall, the risk of a significant instrument-related complication with colonoscopy is greater than 1 in 500, and possibly as high as 1 in 200. Complications related to sedation need to be added to this, but are not well documented.

Anxiety can be created by colonoscopy due to the delay between polypectomy and confirmation of histology. Also, the finding of an adenoma indicates increased risk, and hence a need for future colonoscopic surveillance.

Acceptability of screening tests

Acceptability of a test is critical to success of screening. If a targeted person will not do it, i.e. participate or comply with the offer, then no matter how good the test, it will not be effective. Participation rates do differ between screening tools and have to be considered in the context of a population-screening program.[51–54] Observed rates for the various screening methods are shown in Table 8.10.

Acceptance of FOBT

Occult blood testing requires manipulation of feces. Aversion to inspecting, sampling, and handling feces is common in many societies. Available sampling methods include making a smear of feces onto a test card with a stick, using a brush to sample feces from the bowl, scooping or inserting a probe into feces and placing it into a screw-capped jar, throw-in-the-bowl methods, and wiping the anus with a sampling pad. The latter method has poor clinical specificity. Throw-in-the-bowl, self-reporting tests are of concern with regard to accuracy of interpretation of color in the bowl, onus on follow-up action for a positive results rests with the screenee, and sensitivities lower than Hemoccult have been reported for a number of these tests.

Population screening studies have shown that despite the need for some dietary restriction, participation in G-FOBT screening can reach 55–70% (see Table 1.5).[48] In comparison with G-FOBT, FIT had significantly better participation.[51] This is explained by the fewer samples requested and the different collecting methods used for the FIT.[23,51] The collection of portions of stool in jars without protease enzyme inhibitors is to be discouraged, as it can lead to false-negative results because of enzymatic degradation of hemoglobin.[5]

Table 8.10 Observed participation rates for various methods of screening when applied to average-risk subjects or populations

Screening method	Participation rates
Fecal occult blood test	
• Done by physician	Unknown
• Provided as mass screening	25–78%,[48,54,Chapter 1—references 12,14,16] normally about 40–60%.
• G-FOBT vs FIT	23% vs 30% (spatula sampling) or 40% (brush sampling)[51]
Flexible sigmoidoscopy	
• Done by physician	Unknown
• Provided as mass screening	Normally 20–40%[52,53, Chapter 1—reference 29]
Colonoscopy	
• Done by physician	Unknown
• Provided as mass screening	6–10%[54, Chapter 1—reference 29] 30% (Italy, Dr Zappa pers comm)

Acceptance of sigmoidoscopy and colonoscopy

With screening by flexible sigmoidoscopy, participation rates in true mass population studies vary from 20 to 70%, with 30–40% seeming to be a usual rate in a typical Western population.[52,53] A rate of 65% has been achieved in population studies in Norway, which suggests that with education and encouragement, good rates are possible.[54] Flexible sigmoidoscopy is more invasive and inconvenient than FOBT, and hence one expects that compliance with the former will never be as good for mass screening when a physician or counselor is not included, but this remains to be fully explored.

With colonoscopy, there are only a few successful large-scale mass screening studies in an average-risk population: these include Germany and Poland (see Table 1.7).[3] In a US study, where screening colonoscopy was offered to physicians and dentists, participation was only 6%.[55] However, in a more recent US study of screening colonoscopy offered to Veterans (mainly men) at average and increased risk (family history of colorectal neoplasia), the acceptance was 69%.[56] In a recent trial in Tuscany, Italy, participation reached 30% (M Zappa, pers comm). This increased compliance in specific countries reflects the personal preferences of the treating physicians, the gastroenterology community, successful public education, and a compliant public.[7]

Effectiveness of screening tests

Outcomes and parameters of effectiveness

Various parameters are used to describe the performance of screening tests, and are similar to those used for diagnostic tests.[57] They include sensitivity, specificity, and predictive values (see Table 1.4). Whereas some are relatively theoretical, in the screening context each relates to a useful outcome or concept. Ultimately, it is important that the screening test leads to performance of sufficient colonoscopy examinations to detect enough curable cancers and removable adenomas so as to reduce mortality (and ideally incidence as well) at the population level.

With population screening, several practical outcomes need emphasis:

- To influence mortality, we must be able to detect curable cancers and/or adenomas; hence the overall detection rate or '*yield*' of cancers in a screening program is vital. This is a product of participation rate and sensitivity.
- To be cost-effective and practical at a resource level, it is important to know the number of follow-up colonoscopies that could be needed; hence, the test *positivity rate* is important.

Finally, in the two-step process of screening, the initial step (the screening test) serves to select out those who are at higher risk for neoplasia and who therefore get to colonoscopy. Thus, the *likelihood ratio* serves to emphasize this selection process.

Reduced mortality in FOBT screening

The value of FOBT-based screening is supported by the highest level of evidence—namely, four randomized, controlled trials of screening, which have allowed for participation rates, have included systematic, unbiased ascertainment of participants, and have used mortality as the endpoint. Results are summarized in Table 1.5. On an *intention-to-screen basis*, biennial screening with a G-FOBT (Hemoccult unrehydrated) reduces mortality by 15–20%, whereas annual screening (rehydrated Hemoccult) reduces mortality by 35–38%.[48]

On a *participatory* basis in the randomized population trials, i.e. those who actually perform the screening test, mortality is reduced by at least 40%. FOBT-based screening acts primarily by facilitating colonoscopic detection of curable cancers. Yet, 18 years after commencing screening with annual rehydrated Hemoccult, not only did community mortality fall but also incidence fell as well. Clearly, some adenomas are detected and removed as a result of detection of fecal occult blood, and this is not due to serendipitous detection at colonoscopy.[48] Recent studies have proved that adenomas bleed.[17]

These studies clearly demonstrate the benefit of FOBT as a means of reducing mortality at the population and individual level. Not only do they do it by detecting early-stage cancer but also, when using a more sensitive test, they lead to adenoma detection and removal, which results in a reduction in cancer incidence as well.[9,48]

They are also simple and easily performed in the convenience and privacy of one's home.

Cancer yield: a product of participation, sensitivity, and follow-up

Mortality reduction in the general population depends on cancer yield of the screening program; it is the product of participation rate, sensitivity of the test, and compliance with follow-up. As such, sensitivity and participation rate, together, are surrogate markers for impact on mortality—they should be considered jointly not separately. The interactive effect of participation and sensitivity is demonstrated in Table 8.11. It can be seen that even colonoscopy, with its excellent sensitivity, can be ineffective at the population level if participation is low.

Sensitivity of FOBTs

Despite the lower sensitivity of G-FOBTs, which varies from 50 to 90% depending on the type and frequency of screening, they come out well in this intention-to-screen analysis.[18] The sensitivity of a one-time FOBT actually compounds with repeated testing. For instance, if a cancer remains at a curable stage for 3 years, then there are three opportunities to detect it by annual testing. Assuming 50% sensitivity for any one-time test, this compounds to 87.5% over 3 years.

The sensitivity of Hemoccult can be increased with either hydration (which actually activates plant peroxidases, and is not to be recommended as the disadvantages of hydration outweigh the advantages) or with the enhanced reagents used for Hemoccult SENSA. However, specificity worsens with either if red meats or plant peroxidases are consumed, although the effect is not as great for Hemoccult SENSA.[18,20]

As far as tests types are concerned, FIT show better sensitivity than G-FOBT. HemeSelect had been shown to be better than Hemoccult II, without unacceptable worsening of specificity.[58] FlexSURE (now named Hemoccult-ICT) had similar sensitivity to Hemoccult SENSA, but with a better specificity.[21] More recently, early data for InSure show it to have superior sensitivity to Hemoccult II and Hemoccult SENSA.[17]

Participation rates with FOBT

This has been discussed above under 'Acceptability of screening tests'. It should be noted that the requirement for dietary restriction with G-FOBT is associated with a significant deterioration in population screening rates—of 15% in one study.[59]

Which FOBT should we use?

FITs show a number of major advantages over G-FOBTs. A more detailed description of FITs is provided elsewhere,[17] and Table 8.12 lists the type of FOBT that might be used in certain types of population settings.[18]

Table 8.11 *Interaction of* **participation** *in screening with the* **sensitivity** *of the initial test on yield (sensitivity × participation rate) of cancers in a screening program*[a]

Screening method[b]	Sensitivity (%)	Participation rate (%)	Cancer yield in program (%)
G-FOBT:			
Scenario 1	90[48]	78[48]	70
Scenario 2	55[see Table 1.5]	55 [see Table 1.5]	30
FIT:			
Scenario 1	78[57,58]	67[51,58,59]	52
Scenario 2	78	40[51]	31
Flex. Sig.:			
Scenario 1	75[40,60]	65[54]	49
Scenario 2	55[40,60]	23[52,61]	13
Colonoscopy:			
Scenario 1	95[30,55,56]	6[55]	6
Scenario 2	95[30,55,56]	69[56]	66

[a]For each test two combinations of sensitivity and participation are modeled on results from the literature. Specific values are either derived from publications cited or else estimated for purposes of modeling outcomes.
[b]G-FOBT, guaiac-based fecal occult blood test; FIT, fecal immunochemical test; Flex. Sig., flexible sigmoidoscopy.

Table 8.12 Matching the type of screening fecal occult blood test (FOBT) to available facilities for further evaluation (where colonoscopic or sigmoidoscopic screening is not feasible or accessible)[a]

Colonoscopy resources for follow-up	Population compliance with diet for guaiac tests (G-FOBT)	Suggested FOBT[b]
Unavailable		Do not screen
Limited	Generally good	High specificity G-FOBT, e.g. Hemoccult II
Limited	Poor or uncertain	FIT
Readily available	Generally good	A sensitive G-FOBT, e.g. Hemoccult SENSA
Readily available	Poor or uncertain	FIT
Readily available	Adenoma detection a priority	FIT

[a] Adapted from reference 10.
[b] G-FOBT, guaiac-based fecal occult blood test; FIT, fecal immunochemical test.

The major advantages of FITs are as follows:

- Results are unaffected by diet or drugs. This makes the testing process easier and reduces variability in specificity.
- They are selective for bleeding from the large bowel and are very insensitive for occult bleeding from the proximal gastrointestinal tract.
- They are more sensitive for cancer than the early G-FOBTs such as Hemoccult II.
- They are more specific than the sensitive G-FOBTs such as Hemoccult SENSA. This means that one can achieve better sensitivity without unacceptable specificity.
- They perform well when just two rather than three stools are sampled.
- They detect adenomas better than G-FOBTs.
- They often utilize more modern sampling methods that are more acceptable to people and hence lead to better participation.
- The test endpoint is usually more easily read, which increases likelihood of an accurate result and aids quality control.
- Endpoints can often be read objectively by an automated process, which reduces costs and increases reproducibility and quality control.
- Some of them can be used in a quantitative manner (MagStream-Bayer Detect, InSure, OC-Sensor, for example). This allows one to choose a suitable cutoff point for positivity.

FIT are more costly than G-FOBT but the many other advantages should overcome this.

Whichever FOBT is performed, it should be done so by the screenee away from the doctor's office. Digital rectal examination is an unsatisfactory way to collect samples.[15]

Sensitivity of sigmoidoscopic screening and impact on mortality

Case–control studies demonstrate an association between sigmoidoscopic examination of rectum or rectosigmoid and a reduction in chance from dying from CRC within reach of the endoscope.[38,61] A case–control study from the Oakland Kaiser-Permanente program examined the use of screening rigid sigmoidoscopy, and found that only 8.8% of the cancer patients had undergone screening sigmoidoscopy, compared with 24.2% of the controls, i.e. a risk reduction of 70% for *cancers within reach*.[38] The data suggested that screening sigmoidoscopy may provide risk reduction for as long as 10 years, although recent studies challenge this. Another case–control study found that a history of screening flexible sigmoidoscopy was present in 10% of those who died of CRC but in 30% of case controls, a reduction in a risk of death from CRC of 79%.[61] Population screening studies are now in progress.[44,53,62]

Because of the distribution of cancer in the large bowel, the sensitivity of sigmoidoscopy depends on the depth of insertion. The skill of the operator, the adequacy of the bowel preparation, and anatomy actually determine depth and adequacy of views. Figure 8.10 shows the distribution of cancer in the colon based on data of new cancer diagnoses during 1988 in the United Kingdom.[39] It can be seen that if flexible sigmoidoscopy were to reliably include the splenic flexure, then approximately 73% of CRCs would be detected directly. Experience with screening sigmoidoscopy has been reviewed by Neugut and Pita.[40] In practice, the sensitivity of flexible sigmoidoscopy for cancer and large adenomas within its potential reach is in the range 33–60%.

Using flexible sigmoidoscopy, 10–25% of screenees will have an index adenoma,[61] which means that the colonoscopic follow-up rate will be high. Given that approximately 30% of cancers proximal to the splenic flexure have an index lesion situated more distally, one-third of cancers not seen at sigmoidoscopy might be identified at subsequent colonoscopy, which would take the overall sensitivity of screening flexible sigmoidoscopy to 44–80%.[63] This is similar to but not better than the sensitivity of G-FOBT and FIT.

Some have argued against flexible sigmoidoscopy screening on the grounds that there is a shift towards more proximal cancers. This is not a universal observation even in North America; the actual rate of proximal cancers is not increasing in North America. In Italy, it is increasing at all sites. Clearly, the epidemiology of CRC distribution is variable and complex.[64–66]

Combining FOBT and sigmoidoscopy screening

The combination of FOBT with flexible sigmoidoscopy has intuitive merit because they have complementary benefits: one is capable of detecting cancer at any level, whereas the other adds more accurate adenoma and cancer detection within reach.[5] Adequate population trials have not been done to show the incremental benefit and, despite some calculations of cost-effectiveness suggesting it to be acceptable, the colonoscopic follow-up rate will be high. In practice, if this approach is used, the FOBT should be done first: if this is positive, proceed to colonoscopy, if negative, proceed to flexible sigmoidoscopy. Unfortunately, people often fail to see a need to proceed if the FOBT is negative. Also, they might avoid screening altogether if they have an aversion to preparing an FOBT. As a result, this combination of screening is not often used.

Sensitivity of colonoscopic screening on impact and mortality

If screening by FOBT or by flexible sigmoidoscopy is effective, then so must colonoscopic screening. However, the use of colonoscopy as a screening test for average-risk populations in some medical services is not supported by all data, recommendations, or cost-effectiveness analysis.[67] Funding bodies more frequently fund FOBT screening than colonoscopic screening because of the high initial costs, concerns about feasibility in terms of adequate resources to do large numbers of colonoscopies, and uncertain acceptability to a significant proportion of the target population.[68]

Some have proposed a single screening colonoscopy at around age 50–60 years. The rationale is based on the concept that those likely to develop CRC in the future are likely to have an adenoma by that age. This not supported by prospective data in representative populations. Others have proposed a screening colonoscopy at intervals of 10 years. But the evidence justifying this interval is only indirect.[69]

The use of surveillance colonoscopy in high-risk subjects, not to be confused with population screening of average-risk subjects, is generally accepted but not the subject of this chapter. Colonoscopy for post-polypectomy surveillance constitutes a huge potential effort that should be appropriately anticipated and managed.[69]

There have been several descriptive studies of the value of screening colonoscopy in specific target populations.[70–72] Further studies are ongoing to determine efficacy, feasibility, acceptance, cost-effectiveness, and safety. Preliminary studies on cost-effectiveness now support its use, although many of the assumptions used are estimates that require rigorous testing using data from true population studies.

Colonoscopy is not perfect and small adenomas and even proximal cancers may be missed in more than 5%.[73–75] The complication rate is also significant (see above) and trials have not yet been done of sufficient magnitude to determine the benefit–risk balance with certainty.

In spite of the above comments, screening colonoscopy is available in the United States through Medicare, every 10 years, similarly to the public health programs of Germany, Poland, and Italy (see Table 1.7).[3]

Colonoscopic screening overview

- Colonoscopic screening will be effective and will have the best impact on incidence of CRC through adenoma detection and removal. It should be included as an option where it is available.
- Initial costs as a mass screening tool are high and feasibility of resourcing it is uncertain in many countries.
- Acceptance of colonoscopic screening remains uncertain, and it will probably only be used for the minority, who will do it as the initial test and who can also afford access.
- Complications must not be underestimated and should be disclosed to potential screenees.
- There is still uncertainty about incremental cost–benefit over and above two-step screening with FOBT and/or flexible sigmoidoscopy, especially when acceptability and feasibility are considered.

Effectiveness summary

1. There is strong evidence that FOBT, flexible sigmoidoscopy, and colonoscopy reduce mortality from CRC, although the best-quality evidence and most convincing feasibility at the population level apply to FOBT.
2. Sensitivity of a screening method is critical to its impact on mortality, but must not be considered in isolation of the corresponding population participation rate.
3. Willingness to perform a test must be considered when predicting impact on mortality.
4. At present, participation with FOBT is better than demonstrated participation with sigmoidoscopic or colonoscopic screening.
5. FITs are superior to G-FOBTs and are the FOBT of choice.
6. FITs can aid the detection of adenomas but endoscopic methods are better.

Costs of screening

The initial costs of screening are largely due to the provision of the initial test plus the follow-up colonoscopies generated by positive tests (much the larger cost), where colonoscopy is not the first-line test.[76] The test positivity rate (TPR) is thus a critical parameter. TPR is the total of true positives plus false positives. Clearly, the initial cost is highest with colonoscopic screening.

FOBT positivity rates

FIT positivity rates are unaffected by diet. Positivity rates of the best studied tests (Immudia-HemSp and Heme-Select) are in the range 2–5%, a manageable rate for most Western populations.[57] More recent data suggest that the best advanced adenoma detection rates are seen with positivity rates of 8–9%.[77]

With G-FOBTs, additional problems arise. Confounding factors have been discussed in detail elsewhere and are summarized in Tables 8.5 and 8.6. Plant peroxidases can give false-positive results, whereas vitamin C can cause false-negative results. Iron probably does not cause positive reactions. It is critical that red meat consumption be restricted for the more sensitive G-FOBTs such as Hemoccult SENSA, and this is also desirable for the less sensitive G-FOBTs (e.g. Hemoccult), especially in populations where red meat consumption is high, e.g. United States, Canada, Australia, and New Zealand.

Positivity rates are reviewed in detail elsewhere.[5] For large studies using Hemoccult II, they have generally been in the range of 1–5%. Better sensitivities occur with the higher TPRs. For rehydrated Hemoccult, the sensitivity can be 8–13%. For Hemoccult SENSA, TPRs are intermediate between these values.[18]

It is now apparent that a better balance of TPR and sensitivity is achievable with FIT, but the latter are more expensive ($10–25 compared with $6–10 for three fecal samples). Costs of FIT will be less if it is shown that fewer samples provide the same sensitivity.

Sigmoidoscopy screening and implications for colonoscopy

Depending on the age group and national dietary lifestyle habits, 5–25% of screenees will have an index adenoma at flexible sigmoidoscopy, which means that the colonoscopic follow-up rate can be high after sigmoidoscopic screening. It should not be assumed that all polyps are adenomas. Not performing a pathologic examination of the polyps, prior to scheduling colonoscopic follow-up of a polyp, creates a major problem of specificity and should be discouraged. Up to 50% of polypoid lesions will be non-neoplastic, i.e. the observation of a polyp is 'false positive' for neoplasia half the time. Given the evidence that subjects with a small distal tubular adenoma, once removed, are not at increased risk of cancer, surveillance colonoscopy may be less effective in this group and so small adenomas, in some countries, present a possibly unnecessary burden.[46] A randomized trial confirming the value of adenoma removal according to type, size, and number is now in progress.[78]

Cost-effectiveness

For CRC screening to be acceptable as formal public health policy, its cost-effectiveness must be of the same order as that of other cancer screening programs that are already in place. A number of modeling studies in the United States, the UK and Europe, and Australia, have shown that the cost per life-year saved by FOBT screening is in the range \$10 000–40 000 and is similar or less than that of breast cancer screening.[76,79]

The costs of endoscopic screening will be considerable, due to the cost of the initial screening test and the competition for other healthcare resources. Nonetheless, calculations of cost-effectiveness of endoscopic screening provided so far are promising, even though they are largely theoretical and suffer from the lack of real outcome data such as that used to calculate cost-effectiveness for FOBT screening.[79] Formal trials are clearly indicated to clarify cost-effectiveness of colonoscopic screening (see also Chapter 10).

Identifying those who will have the target lesion

The detection of blood is not intended to be the definitive diagnostic procedure, but rather to identify those more likely to have colorectal neoplasia at the present moment in time. This concept is embodied in the pre-test/post-test likelihood ratio, i.e. the chance of having CRC when one returns an abnormal test result.[5] It is simply the sensitivity of a test divided by its false-positive rate. It provides a robust way of describing the utility of a test because it is not affected by prevalence of cancer in the target population. Based on the sensitivity and specificity data, using hydrated Hemoccult from the Minnesota controlled trial of screening (90.4% and 92.2%, respectively), the likelihood ratio is 12. Using an approximation of sensitivity (50%) and specificity (99%) from the Danish controlled trial of screening with standard Hemoccult, the likelihood ratio is 50 (see Table 1.5). Such predictors of likelihood for cancer are obviously higher than any other, including age and family history, and perhaps even visible blood! These points are summarized in Table 8.13.

In other words, screening by FOBT ensures that colonoscopy is targeted at those more likely to have a neoplasm.

Endoscopic screening, where selection is based on age, is random compared with FOBT-based screening, and many more procedures will be done on people without neoplasia. With G-FOBT, the predictive value of a positive test for cancer is 5–10% (see Table 1.5).[48] Random colonoscopy in a population over 50 years old would detect about 3 cancers per 1000. This is a predictive value of 0.3%, or one-tenth to one-twentieth that of FOBT.

When screening for colorectal cancer, the target lesions are curable cancers and removable adenomas—especially those persons who have multiple adenomas, an adenoma >1 cm, an adenoma containing villous changes, or high-grade dysplasia. FOBTs largely target detection of curable cancer, although the Minnesota study shows a further reduction in incidence due to adenoma removal (see

Table 8.13 *Factors that influence an individual's likelihood for having colorectal cancer in effect, these serve as risk predictors*

- **Age:** exponential rise beyond 45–50 years of age (see Figure 2.5)
- **Personal** history of adenoma or cancer: increases risk by a 3- to 7- fold increment
- **Family** history: increases risk by a 2- to 6-fold increment (even higher in the dominantly inherited syndromes)
- **Fecal occult blood test:** a positive result increases chance 11- to 45-fold relative to a negative test

Figure 8.1).[48] Visualization by endoscopy obviously improves adenoma detection, although how reliable it is remains to be seen, as some studies indicate that flat adenomas and 'de novo' cancers are more significant than previously accepted.[80] The sensitivity of colonoscopy for smaller lesions has now been well studied and is of the order of 70–80%.[75] How much value adenoma removal adds to the benefit of FOBT-based screening at the population level, where compliance will be different between the two modalities, remains to be demonstrated.

Rescreening

The complete screening program, where it is a two-step process, requires ongoing participation, biennially or annually for FOBT and every 5 years for sigmoidoscopy. The many possible outcomes of the initial screen and the subsequent process (see Table 8.1) are outlined below. It is desirable that the screening process checks subjects for symptoms, personal history and/or family history of colorectal neoplasia, and ascertains the presence of multisystem or serious disease where CRC screening would not be a priority. The outcomes that might occur are thus:

1. Unwell—exclude from screening.
2. Symptomatic—send for diagnostic testing.
3. Personal history—provide colonoscopic surveillance at the correct interval.
4. Family history—profile actual risk and design a personalized surveillance program.
5. Flexible sigmoidoscopy negative—repeat in 5 years with intervening annual FOBT.
6. Flexible sigmoidoscopy shows neoplasia—for cancer, operate; for adenoma, perform colonoscopic polypectomy and plan ongoing surveillance at correct interval.
7. FOBT negative—repeat at 1-year (preferable) or 2-year intervals, advise need to report symptoms occurring in intervals between tests.
8. FOBT positive—full diagnostic evaluation of colon; in the absence of symptoms and iron deficiency, upper gastrointestinal endoscopy is not indicated if colonoscopy is negative.

Rescreening is important for all outcomes except the first situation. It is especially important after a negative FOBT, since a cancer might have been missed and repeated screening increases the chance of detecting this while it is still curable.

Some argue that this process of needing to repeat screening is cumbersome, costly, and not ideal for participants! It is argued that colonoscopic screening is more accurate, needs to be done only once, or every decade, and provides a simpler process. There is some appeal with this argument. Unfortunately, in practice, the sensitivity of colonoscopic screening is not ideal.[73,74] We need formal trials to resolve this uncertainty.

As pointed out, the risk for CRC increases exponentially with age, and in the United States, with the aging population, there is some evidence of more cancers, especially in women, occurring in the right colon.[64,65] The possibility of changing screening methodology with aging is being examined.[3]

Individual choice and responsibility to the public in screening

For the individual seeking care (case-finding), rather than being offered screening as part of a population mass screening program, the key difference is motivation and willingness to undertake the test and ability of the healthcare system to provide the test that is agreed upon. For the population, doing something is better than doing nothing. For the individual, doing what is best is the issue, but cost and safety have to be considered.

Screenee-initiated screening and physician-initiated screening are the two mains forms of case-finding. Involvement of healthcare practitioners (e.g. primary care physicians) has advantages in that there should be better motivation of the subject, symptomatic subjects are redirected from screening to appropriate diagnostic investigations, the screenee's risk status can be assessed prior to choice of the screening tool, and those at low risk because of age are excluded. Furthermore, the ongoing screening program can be tailored to the nature and degree of risk of the individual. The process is the same as in Table 8.1, but is highly personalized and augmented by the encouragement from the physician involved.

Counseling about screening must include explanations of the following:

- there are options for those ≥50 years old (FOBT and/or flexible sigmoidoscopy, or colonoscopy, etc.)
- there is proven value for the participant in repeated annual FOBT screening (mortality reduction of 40% or more to those who do it)
- FOBT screening acts as a selection process for those most likely to have neoplasia and so most likely to benefit from colonoscopy
- negative tests should not give false reassurance and ongoing participation and early response to new symptoms are essential, as cancer can be missed
- a positive test requires diagnostic follow-up in a two-step screening process
- the risk of major complication from colonoscopy is not trivial and is probably at least 1 in 500
- colonoscopic screening can also miss lesions
- informed consent is based on consideration of the above facts.

Relevant screening documentation and medical responsibility

It is essential that a medical interviewer or the physician obtain and document minimal medical information before initiating screening. This includes family history of neoplasia and past medical history of important gastrointestinal or other diseases or symptoms that could change screening methodology or even remove screening as a priority for that person. Before initiating screening, it should be made clear to the screenee that neither FOBT nor sigmoidoscopy, nor even both screening tests together, are absolute, and even within a screening program (usually a 5-year cycle) do not identify all colorectal neoplasia. So, screenees should be warned that if symptoms appear, they need to be investigated promptly. These points would ideally appear on the informed consent form.

Records may be computerized and at the end of the session provide a report for the screenee and primary care physician and allow for recall or follow-up to be arranged according to the established protocol. The importance of routine recall for tests should be emphasized. In the case of a positive finding at flexible sigmoidoscopy or a positive FOBT, the screenee must be notified personally and this is recorded in the medical file. Failure to appear at a follow-up test should be recorded, including the attempts to contact the patient personally.

When providing a final report, it is often beneficial to combine it with general preventive health recommendations. These relate to diet, tobacco smoking and alcohol consumption, weight control, mammography screening, routine gynecologic examinations, and measurement of blood pressure, blood sugar, and lipids. These recommendations can be given by the examining physician, or in a busy practice by a nurse–practitioner or trained medical interviewer. Advice is usually well appreciated, and can be followed-up by the primary care physician (see Chapter 10).[81]

National recommendations

National bodies throughout the world are now reaching the conclusion that population colorectal screening is justified (see Table 1.7).[3] For an organized healthcare system, there are two key questions: should it allow reimbursement for individual screening and/or should it implement a comprehensive population policy where it organizes and offers screening from a central national register either free, subsidized, or at cost? In either case, there needs to be defined criteria of performance, quality control, and promotion.[7]

Japan has a population screening policy based on FIT that is effective, whereas Germany's policy has been of limited acceptance for G-FOBT but is now more actively promoting colonoscopic screening.[3] The United States has approved reimbursement through Medicare, and some HMOs for screening tests of all types, but does not have a national population-based strategy for implementation (see Chapters 1 and 10). Excellent guidelines have been made available in the United States and in many other countries such as Australia.[8–10] In Israel, FOBT screening is available upon request to every person over 50 years old. Endoscopic screening is available for all persons at increased risk because of the family history or personal past history of premalignant disease. In the UK and Australia, they have completed pilot population trials of FOBT and are highly likely to implement widespread national programs.[82]

Given that FOBT screening has been shown to be of proven efficacy by the highest level of evidence, and that endoscopic screening also has a strong evidence base, screening should at least be accessible to the individual, even if formal population programs are not funded.[3]

Conclusions

Screening for CRC is effective. Randomized trials of two-step screening indicate that mortality from CRC can be reduced using annual FOBT as the first step; they show a 15–38% reduction on an intention-to-screen basis at the population level, or at least a 40% reduction at the individual level when participation occurs. Although there have been no randomized population trials of one-step endoscopic screening, the observational and case–control studies reported are persuasive, and two-step screening only works because it leads to colonoscopy. Endoscopic screening will provide improved adenoma detection, but it costs more to initiate, is less acceptable to the general population, and results in colonoscopy being done on a higher proportion of people without neoplasia.

Professional bodies around the world recommend that screening for colorectal cancer in average-risk persons begin at 50 years of age. Although there is some variation between the national guidelines, all support annual or biennial FOBT-based screening with or without flexible sigmoidoscopy every 5 years. There is full support for colonoscopic screening for those at increased risk, whereas only partial support for nationally funded colonoscopy screening programs in average-risk people. Radiologic methods for screening are not widely supported, as the evidence base for CT colonography is considered inadequate, although with technologic advances being made, this might be added to the list of options in the near future. Advances are being made in stool molecular tests and, within the next decade, it is expected that this innovative technology will eventually lead to more specific and simple tests that provide an effective first test in a two-step screening process. When it comes to choice of an FOBT, FITs are superior to G-FOBTs and should replace them. Ideally, quantifiable FITs that enable control of test performance characteristics, and which use technology to reliably read test endpoints, should be used for mass screening.

In practice, where there is face-to-face interaction between the doctor and the potential screenee, the options of FOBT with or without flexible sigmoidoscopy, flexible sigmoidoscopy alone, or colonoscopy should be discussed where they are available and fundable. However, the risks should also be carefully explained as well as the benefits, and the imperative to do no harm must be carefully applied when screening the asymptomatic average-risk person. Individual preferences should be considered, because without participation there is no detection. The ultimate success of screening is not dependent so much on the test itself but rather on the fact that a proven test is done.

References (*Reviews and general articles)

1. Watson JMG, Junger G, Principles and Practice of Screening for Disease. WHO Public Health Papers No. 34, 1968.
2. Greegor DH, Diagnosis of large-bowel cancer in the asymptomatic patient. JAMA 1967; 201: 943–5.
3. *Rozen P, Winawer SJ, Report of the OMED Colorectal Cancer Screening Committee Meeting, New Orleans, 2004—in collaboration with the IDCA. Eur J Cancer Prev 2004; 13: 461–4.
4. Weller D, Hiller J, Beilby J et al, Screening for colorectal cancer. Knowledge, attitudes and practices of South Australian GPs. Med J Aust 1994; 160: 620–4.
5. *Young GP, Macrae FA, St John DJB, Clinical methods of early detection: basis, use and evaluation. In: Prevention and Early Detection of Colorectal Cancer (Young GP, Rozen P, Levin B, eds). London: WB Saunders, 1996: 241–70.
6. Allison JE, Screening for colorectal cancer 2003: Is there still a role for the FOBT? Gastrointest Endosc 2003; 5: 127–33.
7. *Rozen P, Blanchard J, Campbell D et al, Implementing Colorectal Cancer Screening: Group 2 report. ESGE/UEGF Colorectal Cancer—Public Awareness Campaign. The Public/Professional Interface Workshop: Oslo, Norway, June 20–22, 2003. Endoscopy 2004; 36: 354–8.
8. Summaries for patients. Screening for colorectal cancer: recommendations from the United States Preventive Services Task Force. Ann Intern Med 2002; 137: I38.
9. *Winawer S, Fletcher R, Rex D et al, Colorectal cancer screening and surveillance: clinical guidelines and rationale—update based on new evidence. Gastroenterology 2003; 124: 544–60.
10. Guidelines for the Prevention, Early Detection and Management of Colorectal Cancer. Canberra, Australia: National Health and

Medical Research Council, 1999: 23–32.
11. *Young GP, Screening for colorectal cancer: an introduction. In: Prevention and Early Detection of Colorectal Cancer (Young GP, Rozen P, Levin B, eds). London: WB Saunders, 1996: 271–4.
12. *Austoker J, Gaining informed consent for screening. BMJ 1999; 319: 722–3.
13. Molina L, Carlos RC, Fendrick AM et al, Completion of colorectal cancer screening in women attending screening mammography. Acad Radiol 2004; 11: 1237–41.
14. Bini EJ, Rajapaksa RC, Weinshel EH, The findings and impact of nonrehydrated guaiac examination of the rectum (FINGER) study: a comparison of 2 methods of screening for colorectal cancer in asymptomatic average-risk patients. Arch Intern Med 1999; 159: 2022–6.
15. Zhang B, Nakama H, Fattah AS et al, Lower specificity of occult-blood test on stool collected by digital rectal examination. Hepatogastroenterology 2002; 49: 165–7
16. Collins JF, Lieberman DA, Durbin TE et al, Accuracy of screening for fecal occult blood on a single stool sample obtained by digital rectal examination: a comparison with recommended sampling practice. Ann Intern Med 2005; 142: 81–5.
17. Young GP, Fecal immunochemical tests (FIT) vs office-based guaiac fecal occult blood test (FOBT). Pract Gastroenterol 2004; 28: 46–56 (www.practicalgastro.com).
18. *Young GP, St John DJB, Winawer SJ et al, Choice of fecal occult blood tests for colorectal cancer screening: recommendations based on performance characteristics in population studies. Am J Gastroenterol 2002; 97: 2499–507.
19. Selinger RR, Norman S, Dominitz JA, Failure of health care professionals to interpret fecal occult blood tests accurately. Am J Med 2003; 114: 64–7.
20. Sinatra M, St John DJB, Young GP, Interference of plant peroxidases with guaiac-based fecal occult blood tests is avoidable. Clin Chem 1999; 45: 123–6.
21. Rozen P, Knaani J, Samuel Z, Comparative screening with a sensitive guaiac and specific immunochemical occult blood test within an endoscopy study. Cancer 2000; 89: 46–52.
22. Saito H, Yoshida Y, Mass screening: Japanese perspective. In: Prevention and Early Detection of Colorectal Cancer (Young GP, Rozen P, Levin B, eds). London: WB Saunders, 1996: 301–11.
23. Crotta S, Castiglione G, Grazzini G et al, Feasibility study of colorectal cancer screening by immunochemical faecal occult blood testing: results in a northern Italian community. Eur J Gastroenterol Hepatol 2004; 16: 33–7.
24. Pierson RN, Holt PR, Watson RM et al, Aspirin and gastrointestinal bleeding. Am J Med 1961; 31: 259–65.
25. Macrae FA, St. John DJB, Relationship between patterns of bleeding and Hemoccult sensitivity in patients with colorectal cancers or adenomas. Gastroenterology 1982; 82: 891–8.
26. Young GP, St John DJ, Cole SR et al, Prescreening evaluation of a brush-based faecal immunochemical test for hemoglobin. J Med Screen 2003; 10: 123–8.
27. Osborn NK, Ahlquist DA, Stool screening for colorectal cancer: molecular approaches. Gastroenterology 2005; 128: 1–22.
28. Imperiale TF, Ransohoff DF, Itzkowitz SH et al, Fecal DNA versus fecal occult blood for colorectal-cancer screening in an average-risk population. N Engl J Med 2004; 351: 2704–14.
29. Ferrucci JT, Screening for colon cancer: programs of the American College of Radiology. AJR Am J Roentgenol 1993; 160: 999–1003.
30. Bampton PA, Young GP, Screening for colorectal cancer: use of colonoscopy or barium enema. Semin Colon Rectal Surg 2000; 11: 9–15.
31. Winawer SJ, Stewart ET, Zauber AG et al, A comparison of colonoscopy and double-contrast barium enema for surveillance after polypectomy. N Engl J Med 2000; 342: 1766–72.
32. Morrin MM, LaMont JT, Screening virtual colonoscopy—ready for prime time? N Engl J Med 2003; 349: 2261–4.
33. Cotton PB, Durkalski VL, Pineau BC et al, Computed tomographic colonography (virtual colonoscopy): a multicenter comparison with standard colonoscopy for detection of colorectal neoplasia JAMA 2004; 291: 1713–19.
34. *Van Gelder RE, Nio CY, Florie J et al, Computed tomographic colonography compared with colonoscopy in patients at increased risk for colorectal cancer. Gastroenterology 2004; 127: 41–8.
35. Scott RG, Edwards JT, Fritschi L et al, Community-based screening by colonoscopy or computed tomographic colonography in asymptomatic average-risk subjects. Am J Gastroenterol 2004; 99: 1145–51.
36. van Gelder RE, Florie J, Stoker J, Colorectal cancer screening and surveillance with CT colonography: current controversies and obstacles. Abdom Imaging 2005; 30: 5–12.
37. Rajapaksa RC, Macari M, Bini EJ, Prevalence and impact of extracolonic findings in patients undergoing CT colonograph. J Clin Gastroenterol 2004; 38: 767–71.
38. Selby JV, Friedman GD, Quesenberry CP Jr et al, A case-control study of screening sigmoidoscopy and mortality from colorectal cancer. N Engl J Med 1992; 326: 653–7.
39. Austoker J, Cancer prevention: setting the scene. BMJ 1994; 308: 1415–20.
40. Neugut AI, Pita S, Role of sigmoidoscopy in screening for colorectal cancer: a critical review. Gastroenterology 1988; 95: 492–9.
41. Diagnostic and therapeutic technology assessment. Rigid and flexible sigmoidoscopies. JAMA 1990; 264: 89–92.
42. *Schapiro M, Lehman GA, Flexible Sigmoidoscopy: Techniques and Utilization. Baltimore: Williams & Wilkins, 1990.

43. American Society for Gastrointestinal Endoscopy, Guidelines for training non-specialists in screening flexible sigmoidoscopy. Gastrointest Endosc 2000; 51: 783–5.
44. Bretthauer M, Hoff G, Thiis-Evensen E, Use of a disposable sheath system for flexible sigmoidoscopy in decentralized colorectal cancer screening. Endoscopy 2002; 34: 814–18.
45. *Rex DK, Johnson DA, Lieberman DA et al, Colorectal cancer prevention 2000: screening recommendations of the American College of Gastroenterology. Am J Gastroenterol 2000; 95: 868–77.
46. Atkin WS, Morson BC, Cuzick J, Long-term risk of colorectal cancer after excision of rectosigmoid adenomas. N Engl J Med 1992; 326: 658–62.
47. Irwig L, Glasziou P, Informed consent for screening by community sampling. Eff Clin Pract 2000; 3: 47–50.
48. *Mandel JS, Church TR, Ederer F et al, Colorectal cancer mortality: effectiveness of biennial screening for fecal occult blood. J Natl Cancer Inst 1999; 91: 434–7.
49. Gatto NM, Frucht H, Sundararajan V et al, Risk of perforation after colonoscopy and sigmoidoscopy: a population-based study. J Natl Cancer Inst 2003; 95: 230–6.
50. Macrae FA, Tan KG, Williams CB, Towards safer colonoscopy: a report on the complications of 5000 diagnostic or therapeutic colonoscopies. Gut 1983; 24: 376–83.
51. *Cole SR, Young GP, Esterman A et al, A randomised trial of the impact of new faecal haemoglobin test technologies on population participation in screening for colorectal cancer. J Med Screen 2003; 10: 117–22.
52. Olynyk JK, Aquilia S, Fletcher DR et al, Flexible sigmoidoscopy screening for colorectal cancer in average risk subjects: a community-based pilot project. Med J Aust 1996; 165: 74–6.
53. Atkin WS, Hart A, Edwards R et al, Uptake, yield of neoplasia, and adverse effects of flexible sigmoidoscopy screening. Gut 1998; 42: 560–5.
54. Gondal G, Grotmol T, Hofstad B et al, The Norwegian Colorectal Cancer Prevention (NORCCAP) screening study: baseline findings and implementations for clinical work-up in age groups 50–64 years. Scand J Gastroenterol 2003; 38: 635–42.
55. Rex DK, Lehman GA, Hawes RH, et al, Screening colonoscopy in asymptomatic average-risk persons with negative fecal occult blood tests. Gastroenterology 1991; 100: 64–7.
56. Lieberman DA, Weiss DG, Bond JH et al, Use of colonoscopy to screen asymptomatic adults for colorectal cancer. N Engl J Med 2000; 343: 162–8.
57. Young GP, Screening for colorectal cancer: alternative fecal occult blood tests. Eur J Gastroenterol Hepatol 1998; 10: 205–12.
58. Allison JE, Tekewa JS, Ransom LJ et al, A comparison of fecal occult blood tests for colorectal cancer screening. N Engl J Med 1996: 334: 144–59.
59. Cole SR, Young GP, Participation in faecal occult blood test-based screening for colorectal cancer is reduced by dietary restriction. Med J Aust 2001; 175: 195–8.
60. Levin TR, Flexible sigmoidoscopy for colorectal cancer screening: valid approach or short-sighted? Gastroenterol Clin North Am 2002; 31: 1015–29.
61. Newcomb PA, Norfleet RG, Storer BE et al, Screening sigmoidoscopy and colorectal cancer mortality. J Natl Cancer Inst 1992; 84: 1572–5.
62. Schoen RE, Pinsky PF, Weissfeld JL et al, Results of repeat sigmoidoscopy 3 years after a negative examination. JAMA 2003; 290: 41–8.
63. Selby JV, Targeting colonoscopy. Gastroenterology 1994; 106: 1702–5.
64. Rabeneck L, Davila JA, El-Serag HB, Is there a true 'shift' to the right colon in the incidence of colorectal cancer? Am J Gastroenterol 2003; 98: 1400–9.
65. Cucino C, Buchner AM, Sonnenberg A, Continued rightward shift of colorectal cancer. Dis Colon Rectum 2002; 45: 1035–40.
66. Ponz de Leon M, Marino M, Benatti P et al, Trend of incidence, subsite distribution and staging of colorectal neoplasms in the 15-year experience of a specialised cancer registry. Ann Oncol 2004; 15: 940–6.
67. Ransohoff DF, Screening colonoscopy in balance. Issues of implementation. Gastroenterol Clin North Am 2002; 31: 1031–44.
68. Klabunde CN, Riley GF, Mandelson MT et al, Health plan policies and programs for colorectal cancer screening: a national profile. Am J Manag Care 2004; 10: 273–9.
69. Schoen RE, Surveillance after positive and negative colonoscopy examinations: issues, yields, and use. Am J Gastroenterol 2003; 98: 1237–46.
70. Rex DK, Rationale for colonoscopy screening and estimated effectiveness in clinical practice. Gastrointest Endosc Clin N Am 2002; 12: 65–75.
71. Harewood GC, Lieberman DA, Prevalence of advanced neoplasia at screening colonoscopy in men in private practice versus academic and Veterans Affairs medical centers. Am J Gastroenterol 2003; 98: 2312–16.
72. *Lieberman DA, Weiss DG, Bond JH et al, Use of colonoscopy to screen asymptomatic adults for colorectal cancer. Veterans Affairs Cooperative Study Group 380. N Engl J Med 2000; 343: 162–8.
73. Postic G, Lewin D, Bickerstaff C et al, Colonoscopic miss rates determined by direct comparison of colonoscopy with colon resection specimens. Am J Gastroenterol 2002; 97: 3182–5.
74. *Bressler B, Paszat LF, Vinden C et al, Colonoscopic miss rates for right-sided colon cancer: a population-based analysis. Gastroenterology 2004; 127: 452–6.

75. Villavicencio RT, Rex DK, Colonic adenomas: prevalence and incidence rates, growth rates, and miss rates at colonoscopy. Semin Gastrointest Dis 2000; 11: 185–93.
76. Salkeld S, Young G, Irwig L et al, Cost-effectiveness analysis of screening by faecal occult blood testing for colorectal cancer in Australia. Aust J Pub Health 1996; 20: 138–43.
77. Young GP, Smith A, Cole S, How many colonoscopies are needed to detect advanced neoplasia in population screening using immunochemical fecal occult blood tests? J Gastroenterol Hepatol, in press.
78. Taylor T, Williamson S, Wardle J et al, Acceptability of flexible sigmoidoscopy screening in older adults in the United Kingdom. J Med Screen 2000; 7: 38–45.
79. *Wagner JL, Tunis S, Brown M et al, The cost-effectiveness of colorectal cancer screening in average-risk adults. In: Prevention and Early Detection of Colorectal Cancer (Young GP, Rozen P, Levin B, eds). London: WB Saunders, 1996: 321–56.
80. Chen C-D, Yen M-F, Wang W-M et al, A case-cohort study for the disease natural history of adenoma-carcinoma and de novo carcinoma and surveillance of colon and rectum after polypectomy: implication for efficacy of colonoscopy. Br J Cancer 2003; 88: 1866–73.
81. *Smith RA, Wender RC, Cancer screening and the periodic health examination. Cancer 2004; 100: 1553–7.
82. UK Colorectal Cancer Screening Pilot Group, Results of the first round of a demonstration pilot of screening or colorectal cancer in the United Kingdom. BMJ 2004; 329: 133. doi:10.1136/bmj.38153,491187,7C.

9 When colorectal cancer is detected, what to do next?

Bernard Levin, John Skibber, Paul Rozen, Graeme P Young

Primary treatment of colorectal cancer

Whereas the primary treatment of colorectal carcinoma must rely heavily on expert surgical resection, the comprehensive care of the patient with colorectal neoplasia requires a multidisciplinary approach.[1] The need for adjuvant systemic chemotherapy, with or without concurrent radiation therapy, depends on tumor location (colon vs rectum) and stage of disease. Systemic chemotherapy may also be indicated in those with metastatic colorectal cancer. Other supportive medical and nursing services are often required.

Surgical principles of management

Adenomas containing high-grade dysplasia or adenocarcinoma

Since adenomatous polyps represent a spectrum of abnormalities between normal mucosa and invasive colorectal carcinoma, it is important to accurately determine the presence of tumor invasion in a colorectal adenoma containing high-grade dysplasia/adenocarcinoma. Invasion through the muscularis mucosae and into the submucosa indicates the ability to spread through lymphatics and blood vessels.

Lesions in which high-grade dysplasia cells extend through the muscularis mucosae require complete excision and accurate assessment of the histology. The depth of invasion, degree of differentiation, adequacy of excision margins, and presence or absence of lymphatic or vascular invasion are all important characteristics that need to be assessed in an adenoma containing adenocarcinoma. Adenomatous polyps may be either sessile or pedunculated. Invasive cancer occurs in about 10% of sessile polyps and 4.5% of pedunculated polyps, and overall about 3–5% of colorectal polyps contain invasive cancer.[2,3] Sessile polyps that have been removed in a piecemeal fashion usually cannot be properly staged. In the case of pedunculated polyps, when invasion does not extend into the base of the stalk, endoscopic removal is adequate treatment. Haggitt et al[4] studied a series of patients in whom colorectal cancers arose in adenomatous polyps with only minimal invasion of the colonic wall (Figure 9.1). They created a staging system for the depth of penetration into the stalk or base of the polyp that was correlated with outcomes. Polyps treated by piecemeal excision or those inadequately oriented are difficult to assess using this system. Level 1 tumors invade into the muscularis mucosae but are limited to the head of the polyp; level 2 carcinomas invade into the neck of the adenoma; level 3 lesions invade into the stalk; and level 4 indicates invasion into the submucosa of the bowel wall below the polyp but above the muscularis propria. Any invasion below the muscularis mucosae in sessile lesions represents level 4 invasion, whereas invasive carcinoma in a pedunculated adenoma must traverse a greater distance before reaching the submucosa. Level 4 invasion signifies a T1 carcinoma. In 65 patients, in their study, with only carcinoma in situ, there were no recurrences or carcinoma in lymph nodes at the time of colectomy. The group with pedunculated polyps where the carcinoma invaded only into the head of the polyp also had no adverse outcomes after endoscopic polypectomy (Table 9.1). These criteria have been confirmed in other series.[3,5] Recently, there have been more studies correlating the microscopic features with prognosis. The width of submucosal invasion (>4 mm) and presence of tumor 'budding' were associated with lymph node metastases. Moreover, a 1 mm or more margin outside of the coagulated area was found adequate to exclude residual tumor.[6]

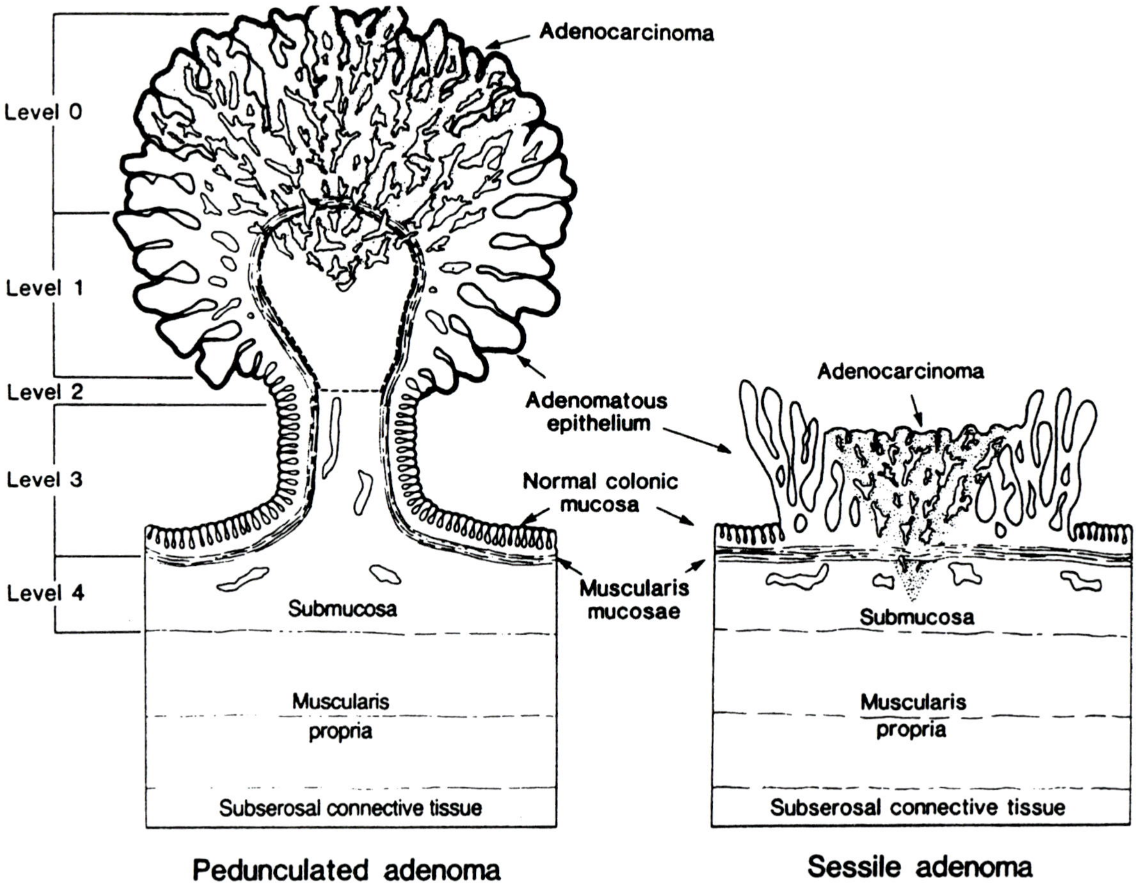

Figure 9.1 *Grading of neoplasia arising in an adenomatous polyp. (From reference 4, with permission.)*

Ultimately, the decision to undertake a surgical resection in a patient with an adenoma containing adenocarcinoma must consider the gross and histologic pathology, the location of the lesion, the presence of comorbid disease, and the patient's wishes for treatment. The management of polyps is summarized in Table 9.2.

Endoscopic mucosal resection of rectal lesions

Endoscopic mucosal resection (EMR), a technique developed by Japanese endoscopists, refers to the removal of sessile or flat neoplasms confined to the mucosa. EMR is an alternative to surgical resection for the management of sessile colorectal villous adenomas, adenomas with carci-

Table 9.1 *Risk factors for adverse outcome in patients with an adenoma containing adenocarcinoma*[4,6]

	Low risk	High risk
Polypectomy margin	Clear or >1 mm	Involved by cancer
Invasion of submucosal bowel wall	Absent	Present
Width of submucosal invasion		<4 mm
Degree of differentiation	Well or moderate	Poor
Tumor 'budding'	Absent	Present
Venous or lymphatic invasion	Absent	Present

Table 9.2 *Malignant colorectal adenomatous polyps that should have a curative cancer operation*[a]

A. Lesions in colon:
   a. Pedunculated polyp with invasion into outer third of submucosa or pedunculated lesions with lymphovascular invasion
   b. Sessile lesions removed with margin <1 mm
   c. Sessile lesions removed piecemeal
   d. Sessile lesions with depth of invasion into outer third of submucosa
   e. Sessile lesions with lymphovascular invasion

B. Lesions in middle third and upper third of rectum identical to A above.

C. Lesions in distal third of rectum:
   a. Pedunculated with invasion into outer third of submucosa or pedunculated lesions with lymphovascular invasion.
   b. All sessile lesions (see endoscopic mucosal resection in text)

[a] Modified with permission from Nivatvongs S, Surgical management of malignant colorectal polyps. Surg Clin N Am 2002; 82: 959–66.

noma in situ and some T1 lesions. This technique can provide a complete specimen for histopathologic assessment that can be contrasted with endoscopic polypectomy, in which the sessile polyp is provided to the pathologist in a piecemeal fashion. Submucosal injection is used to elevate the lesion to be resected on to a cushion of injectate, thus creating a pseudostalk. A snare is placed over the base of the raised area and the lesion is resected with electrocautery. Determination of the depth of invasion of the lesion and the presence or absence of lymph node metastases is of paramount importance in the selection of patients for EMR, and is accomplished by endoscopic ultrasound.[7] The main complications of EMR are bleeding, perforation, and transmural burn syndrome. EMR is useful in the hand of experts who are able to minimize the risk of serious complications.

Relationship between stage of cancer and survival

The principles of staging of colorectal cancer are important, since there is a correlation between stage at diagnosis and survival.

In Table 9.3, the TNM classification used by the American Joint Committee on Cancer (AJCC) and the Union Internationale Contre le Cancer (UICC) is shown, together with a graphical demonstration of the T classification in Figure 9.2.[8] The relationship of stage to survival is indicated in Table 9.4.

Table 9.3 *The TNM classification according to the American Joint Committee on Cancer (AJCC) and the Union Internationale Contre le Cancer (UICC)*[a]

Tx	Minimum requirements to assess the primary tumor cannot be met
T0	No evidence of primary tumor
Tis	In situ carcinoma
T1	Tumor extends into the submucosa
T2	Tumor extends into the muscularis propria
T3	Tumor extends through the muscularis propria into the subserosa or into the non-peritonealized pericolic or perirectal tissues
T4	Tumor extends directly into other organs or tissues, or tumor perforates the visceral peritoneum of the specimen
Nx	Minimum requirements to assess the regional lymph nodes cannot be met
N0	No lymph node metastasis
N1	Metastatic tumor in one to three pericolic or perirectal lymph nodes
N2	Metastatic tumor in four or more pericolic or perirectal lymph nodes
N3	Metastatic to any lymph node along the course of a major named vascular trunk
Mx	Minimum requirements to assess distant metastasis cannot be met
M0	No distant metastasis
M1	Distant metastasis present

[a] Reproduced from reference 8, with permission from McGraw-Hill.

Colon cancer resection: principles

The preoperative *evaluation* for resection of colon carcinoma includes an assessment of the patient's fitness for surgery and of the extent of spread of the tumor. Evaluation for synchronous colonic neoplasia by colonoscopy is important due to a 3–5% risk of having another large bowel cancer and in many westernized countries of having a 30–40% incidence of adenomatous polyps. However, one cannot perform a preoperative evaluation of the entire colon in patients with obstructive lesions or in those who must have emergency surgery (e.g. for perforation), and postoperative colonoscopy is advisable in such patients.

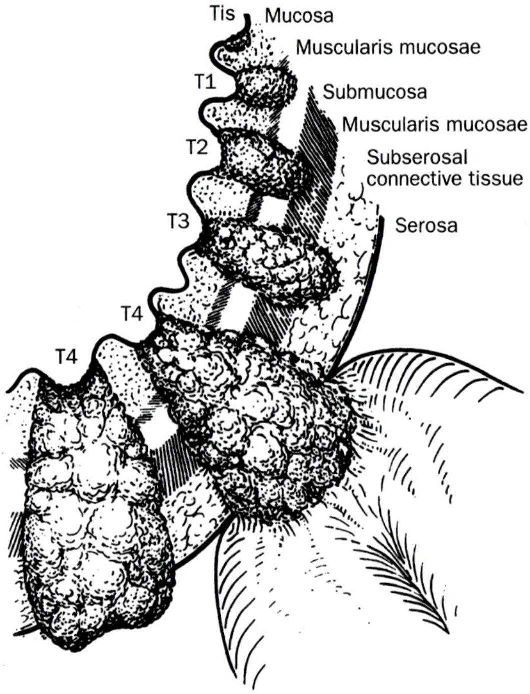

Figure 9.2 *Schematic demonstration of TNM classification. (Reproduced from reference 8 with permission from McGraw-Hill.)*

Table 9.4 *Classification of large-bowel cancer by its degree of spread (stage; TNM features) and its correlation with survival*[a]

Stage groupings	TNM classification	5-year survival rate (%)
Stage 0	Tis, N0, M0	100
Stage I	T1, N0, M0 T2, N0, M0	100 85
Stage II	T3, N0, M0 T4, N0, M0	70 30
Stage III	Any T, N1, M0 Any T, N2, M0 Any T, N3, M0	60 30
Stage IV	Any T, any N, M1	3

[a] Reproduced from reference 8, with permission from McGraw-Hill.

Surgical *resection* with an anastomosis is the treatment of choice in >85% of patients with colon cancer. The majority of resections carried out for colon carcinoma are done with curative intent, even though some patients may have microscopic metastases that are undetectable at the time of laparotomy. During the surgical procedure, information is gained about the presence of visceral metastases and lymph node involvement. In performing a curative resection, the segment of colon bearing the primary tumor is first resected with adequate margins of normal-appearing tissue together with its major vascular pedicle and parallel lymphatic drainage, and an anastomosis is then performed (Figure 9.3).

For patients undergoing curative resection for colon cancer, overall survival rates vary between 55% and 75%, with

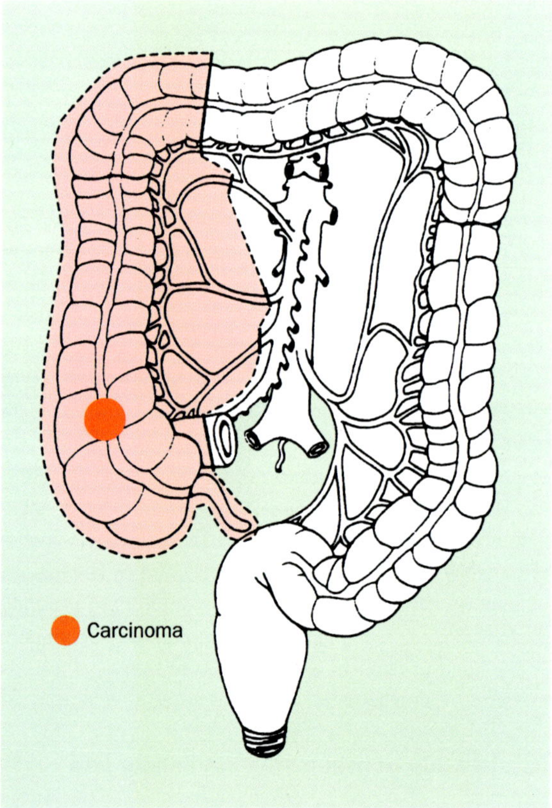

Figure 9.3 *Demonstrating principles of resection for colon cancer: (1) resection with wide luminal margins; (2) lymphadenectomy by mesenteric resection to include the major arterial vessels supplying the affected segment; (3) reconstruction by primary anastomosis.*

most recurrences seen in the first 2 years of follow-up. Survival after curative resection is markedly affected by the presence of nodal metastases. For node-negative patients, survival with surgery alone varies between 75% and 90%. Even in these cancers, such factors as depth of penetration, contiguous organ involvement, differentiation, lymphatic, vascular and perineural invasion, as well as molecular and cellular characteristics, will affect survival. An emergency presentation (obstruction, gross bleeding, or perforation) is associated with worse outcome. In one series, overall survival at 5 years was 57.5% after elective surgery and 39.1% after emergency curative surgery ($p<0.001$).[9]

Important issues in surgically resected, apparently node-negative colon cancer are the methods of lymph node evaluation and the detection of occult metastatic disease. Studies have indicated that 13 or more nodes need to be examined to indicate true nodal negativity.[10] Standardizing node evaluation and using immunohistochemical techniques can identify occult nodal metastases in up to 26% of those whose nodes are negative for the presence of metastasis by routine techniques.[11] The clinical significance of this finding has not been confirmed and it is not routinely performed. The likelihood is high that standard post-surgical dissection methods by the pathologist will identify node-negative patients if an adequate number of nodes is examined.[12]

Various biologic tests on the neoplastic tissue have been evaluated for their usefulness for suggesting response to chemotherapy and/or prognosis. Microsatellite instability, also associated with hereditary nonpolyposis colon cancer, has been shown to be associated with survival independent of tumor stage and 5-fluorouracil (5-FU) therapy.[13] The presence of cyclooxygenase-2 (COX-2) but not cyclooxygenase-1 (COX-1) expression suggests adverse prognosis.[14] Other molecular markers include DNA synthesis-related genes (thymidylate synthase), growth factor receptor genes (epidermal growth factor receptor; *EGFR*), angiogenesis-related genes (vascular endothelial growth factor; *VEGF*), proliferation indices (e.g. Ki-67), and tumor suppressor genes and oncogenes. To date, these have not become routine tests, even though they could influence therapy and assessment of prognosis.

For *palliative* purposes, to relieve the symptoms of obstruction or bleeding, a more limited resection may be performed. In certain select circumstances, such as advanced carcinomatosis, or in the presence of extensive tumors that invade the retroperitoneum or adjacent organs, simple diversion and colostomy, or bypass surgery, may be an alternative. By managing bleeding, obstruction, fistula formation, and perforation, surgical resection provides palliation.

In carcinoma of the *proximal half of the colon*, the distal 10–15 cm of ileum is resected together with the right half of the colon. This includes the related blood vessels and lymph nodes up to the base of the ileocolic artery. After transection of the distal ileum and the midtransverse colon, an anastomosis is then created (see Figure 9.3). In tumors of the *transverse colon*, essentially the same operation can be performed with an extension of the resection margin to the left of the middle colic arcade and inclusion of this arcade with the specimen. For lesions in the *left colon*, left colectomy involves a resection of the bowel supplied by the inferior mesenteric artery, and anastomosis is done between the distal transverse colon and rectum. In carcinomas of the *sigmoid colon*, a similar operation is performed to that for left colon carcinoma. When an *obstructing* lesion or *synchronous lesions* are present in the left colon, a total abdominal colectomy may be performed, with an anastomosis between the terminal ileum and the rectum. Most commonly, *perforated tumors* adhere to adjacent organs and should be resected en bloc with any adherent organs. Free perforation causes peritonitis, and should be managed urgently by resection of the perforated segment.

Postoperatively, the most troublesome complications are bleeding and anastomotic leaks. Whereas bleeding manifests itself during or immediately after the operation, anastomotic leaks usually occur 3–7 days after surgery. Fever, leukocytosis, abdominal pain, and prolonged ileus may occur as a result, and signs of systemic sepsis may supervene. In leaks that are walled off, a fistula may develop. A computed tomography (CT) scan is often helpful in identifying abscesses due to anastomotic leaks. Percutaneous drainage may occasionally be useful in managing this complication, but most patients require reoperation.

Laparoscopic colectomy

Laparoscopic techniques have become widely used in the management of benign and malignant colorectal conditions.[15] These techniques can be carried out safely and successfully, in the hands of an experienced laparoscopic surgeon. Even assessment of the liver is carried out by laparoscopic intraoperative ultrasonography.[16] With laparoscopic colectomies, there is a theoretical advantage of a shortened hospital stay and a more rapid recovery. The shortened stay associated with laparoscopic colectomy, attributable to early postoperative feeding, has also resulted in a change in the management of colon resection patients who are treated by open techniques.[17]

In a large randomized trial of laparoscopic and open colectomy in the United States, the overall complications of laparoscopic colorectal surgery were comparable to those of open resection.[18] However, the intra-abdominal complications attributable to laparoscopic surgery may be somewhat different from those seen with open surgery, and include cauterization injury to the bowel, hypercapnia, ureteric injury, and development of hernia at the port site.[19] The risk of an anastomotic leak from a colonic anastomosis in a laparoscopically assisted procedure is similar to the leak rate seen after open resection and anastomosis. A unique problem of laparoscopic resection can be the inability to localize a small mucosal lesion due to loss of ability to palpate the bowel. This may be avoided by tattooing small lesions during colonoscopy, or using endoscopically placed clips near the lesion in question.[20]

Available data on the extent of lymphadenectomy and resection margins suggest that oncologic laparoscopic resection is comparable to open colectomy for cancer.[21] Among candidates for a curative resection, approximately 10% will have malignant cells after peritoneal lavage. If positive cytologic findings persist on postoperative peritoneal lavage, the risk of locoregional failure is high.[22] Although there is experimental evidence of an increase in trocar-site implantation of colorectal cancer cells by pneumoperitoneum, the clinical importance of this is not clear.[23] Studies have documented estimated recurrence rates in port sites of 1.08–3.8% after laparoscopic resection. These recurrence rates are similar to those associated with laparotomy wounds in patients treated by open resection.[18]

Laparoscopic vs open resection for colon cancer

Two prospective, randomized trials have been done to compare the efficacy of laparoscopic colectomy with open colectomy for carcinoma.[24,25] The COST (Clinical Outcomes of Surgical Therapy) study involved patients with right, left, or sigmoid colon adenocarcinoma, and patients were randomly assigned to laparoscopically assisted or open colectomy. The primary endpoints of the study were disease-free and overall survival. The secondary endpoints were examinations of morbidity, cost-effectiveness, and quality of life.

The COST trial demonstrated, in a multi-institutional trial, that rates of recurrence and overall survival rates were equivalent for open and laparoscopic colectomy.[24] Wound recurrence rates were less than 1% in both groups. Laparoscopic resection was found to be associated with lower use of narcotics and a shorter hospital stay. Complication rates were similar in both groups. It is important to recognize that this trial excluded rectal cancer and transverse colon cancer. The authors also imposed strict controls over the quality of the surgery and the experience of the surgeons prior to enrolling patients in the study.

In the study by Lacy et al,[25] although the criteria for entry were similar, it was conducted in a single hospital unit. This study favors laparoscopic resection in terms of survival and recurrence rates. Lower rates of wound infection and ileus were noted in the laparoscopic resection group and were responsible for an overall lower morbidity rate for this group. The probability of cancer-free survival was significantly higher in the laparoscopic resection group.

Rectal cancer resection: principles

In rectal cancer, treatment decisions are based on accurate preoperative clinical and radiologic staging. The extent of tumor spread locally and distantly greatly affects treatment planning. Endorectal ultrasound is a useful and accurate technique for determining the depth of penetration of the bowel wall by primary rectal tumors (Figure 9.4). It can also provide aspiration biopsy of suspected lymph node metastases.

The principles of resection for rectal cancer involve removal of the tumor with normal tissue margins, the assessment of lymph node involvement, and the restoration of function. Due to the anatomic location of the rectum in the pelvis and the tendency for lateral spread of these tumors, local recurrence rates are higher than in colon cancer. In addition, the presence of a low rectal cancer may limit the ability to excise a lesion while preserving the anus, thus making a colostomy likely.

Local excision for rectal cancer

Transrectal full-thickness local excision is an effective treatment of selected early low rectal cancers. Local excision is used as curative therapy for patients who have a

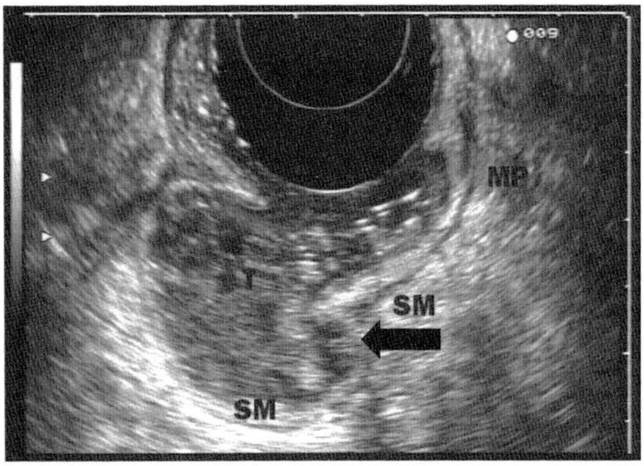

Figure 9.4 *Endoscopic ultrasonogram of a T2 rectal adenocarcinoma, demonstrating depth of tumor invasion: SM, submucosa; MP, muscularis propria; arrow, tumor invading submucosa. (Figure provided by Dr M Santo, Tel Aviv.)*

superficial tumor and as alternative therapy in medically compromised patients and those who refuse standard therapy.

The intent of local excision is to obtain a negative-margin full-thickness excision in a patient with a low risk of lymph node metastases. Physical assessment, CT, and endorectal ultrasound with aspiration biopsy of suspected metastatic lesions are helpful in the preoperative evaluation of rectal cancer patients. Imaging findings can be used to select patients for local excision procedures by determining the depth of tumor penetration into the rectal wall and the absence of enlarged and involved lymph nodes. Most patients with rectal cancer do not meet the criteria for treatment by local excision alone due to the size or extent of the tumor spread. Curative surgical treatment for rectal cancer entails tumor excision with margins of normal tissue and resection of locoregional lymph nodes, whereas local excision alone achieves a negative-margin excision without resection of the mesorectal lymph nodes.

The incidence of lymph node metastases in patients with T1 tumors approximates the recurrence rate for T1 cancers treated by local excision, which is a 3–10% rate of local recurrence.[26] Survival rates in patients with T1 rectal carcinomas treated by local excision or radical resection are 90–100%. Local excision is a reasonable treatment for T1 carcinoma of the rectum if favorable criteria are present. Poor differentiation, perineural, blood vessel, or lymphatic invasions are significant predictors of lymph node involvement and poor survival. In such cases, standard surgical therapy should be used. If the patient refuses or cannot tolerate standard surgical therapy, the use of adjuvant therapy after local excision should be considered.

The risk of lymph node metastasis is 10–30% in patients with T2 rectal carcinoma.[27] Studies show higher local recurrence rates for tumors involving the muscularis propria treated by local excision, because of the failure to treat lymphatic metastases. Recurrence rates are 17–24% in patients with T2 tumors, and survival rates are 78–82% in those treated by local excision. In patients with T2 carcinomas of the rectum, the risk of lymph node metastasis in the mesorectum must be addressed by resection of the mesorectum during proctectomy or, if a local excision is done, by the addition of chemotherapy and radiation therapy to reduce the incidence of pelvic recurrence. Excellent disease control rates are possible for patients with selected T1 and T2 rectal cancers treated by local excision and postoperative adjuvant radiotherapy (Table 9.5).[28] In contrast, local excision cannot be recommended for T3 rectal cancer.

Locoregional resection and multimodality treatment for rectal cancer

About 60–80% of patients with rectal cancer have stage II or stage III lesions that are frequently large and biologically aggressive. Patients are at higher risk of local and systemic recurrence after treatment. The risk of spread to local lymph nodes and of local recurrence increases as tumor penetration of the rectal wall deepens. This has led to the development of surgical procedures, such as abdominoperineal resection, that can achieve tumor-free proximal and distal tissue margins and remove the proximal pathways of lymphatic spread from rectal cancer. A distal margin of 2 cm from the edge of the tumor has been shown to be adequate. However, the work of Quirke and colleagues has demonstrated the importance of lateral tumor spread in influencing local recurrence of rectal cancer after resection.

The bony sidewalls of the pelvis confine the rectum together with major blood vessels and nerves, and the pelvis contains viscera that are important to functional well-being. These anatomic characteristics do not facilitate obtaining wide margins of normal tissue around a transmural rectal tumor. Tumor involvement at the

Table 9.5 Patterns of failure by AJCC[a] tumor (T) stage of disease after local excision and adjuvant therapy for rectal cancer[b]

	T1 (*n* =16)	T2 (*n* =15)	T3 (*n* =15)	Total (*n* =46)
Local recurrence only	0	0	2	2 (4%)
Distant recurrence only	0	0	4	4 (7%)
Combined recurrence	0	1	1	2 (4%)

[a] AJCC = American Joint Commission on Cancer
[b] Derived from reference 28 with permission from WB Saunders.

circumferential margin of resection is associated with local recurrence in 85% of cases, with a resulting poor prognosis (Figure 9.5).[29] Whereas distal margins are measured in centimeters, circumferential margins are measured in millimeters; controlled sharp dissection must be performed with close attention to these margins. Involvement of the circumferential margins can be due to direct spread, mesenteric implants, vascular or lymphatic invasion, or cancer-bearing lymph nodes.[29] Tumor involvement of the circumferential margins of resection is frequently due to spread in the mesorectum distal to the primary tumor.[29] The mesorectum is the extension of the large-bowel mesentery along the posterior wall of the rectum. This blood vessel and lymph node-bearing structure is enveloped by the fascia propria of the rectum. Total mesorectal excision has been demonstrated to be effective in the surgical management of rectal cancer. Consequently, there is much interest in the use of surgery alone for node-negative T2 and T3 rectal cancer when optimal surgical techniques such as total mesorectal excision and sharp dissection are used.[30]

For rectal cancer patients, a major component of quality of life is sphincter preservation. This is simple to accomplish in middle and upper-third rectal cancers, for which low anterior resection allows adequate removal of the tumor and surrounding lymphatics and an end-to-end anastomosis. In patients with low rectal cancers that do not involve the levator muscles or sphincters, the anus may

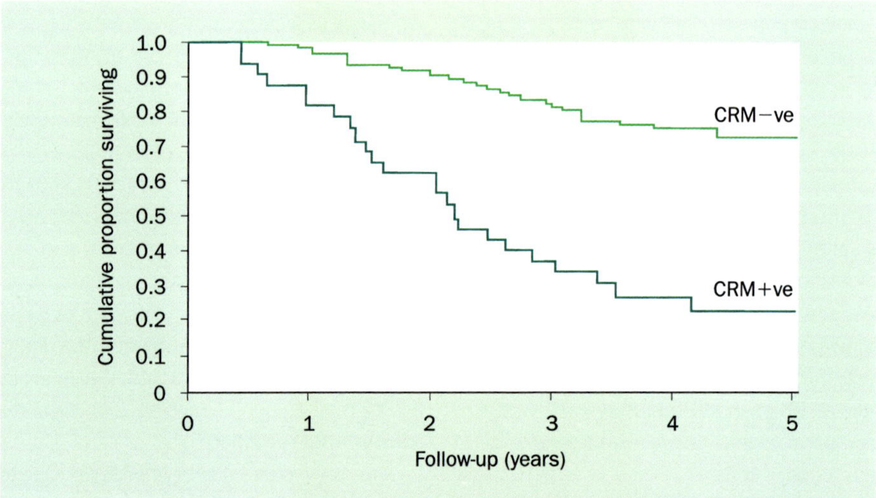

Figure 9.5 *Survival comparing presence or absence of tumour at the circumferential resection margin (CRM) in patients who underwent potentially curative resection. (Derived from Adam IJ, Mohamdee MO, Martin I et al, Role of circumferential involvement in the local recurrence of rectal cancer. Lancet 1994; 344: 707–11, with permission from The Lancet.)*

still be spared by proctectomy and coloanal anastomosis. Preoperative chemoradiation may facilitate this goal. However, patients with levator ani or sphincter involvement are best managed by abdominoperineal resection and permanent colostomy.

Proctectomy and coloanal anastomosis can be useful in patients with low rectal cancer, as demonstrated in a study in which the median distance of the tumor from the anal verge was 6–7 cm.[31] The operation required complete mobilization of the rectum to the levators, transanal transection of the rectum, complete mobilization of the left colon, and endoanal anastomosis. The effectiveness of the procedure was demonstrated by a relatively low local recurrence rate of 7%. Fecal continence was satisfactory in 78% of patients, and overall bowel function appeared to be improved in patients who had a colonic J-pouch reservoir created with a coloanal anastomosis (Figure 9.6). Early and late complications were related to anastomotic leakage (10%) and stricture formation. Major long-term postoperative complaints are related to diminished rectal capacity. This function gradually improves over an approximately 9-month period after closure of the temporary stoma.

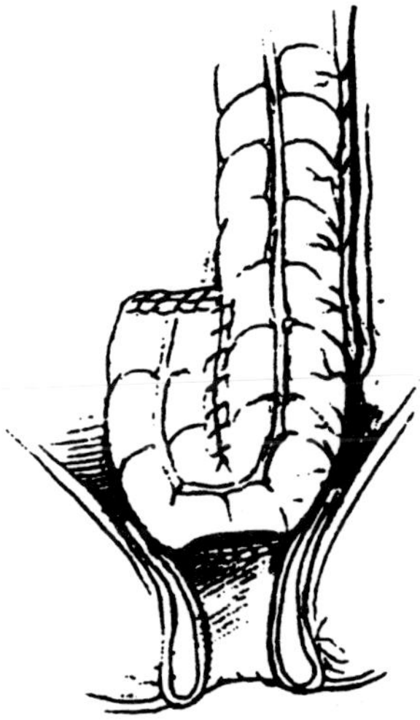

Figure 9.6 *Coloanal anastomosis is defined as a method of restoring bowel continuity by uniting the descending colon to the anal canal. It is in wide use in the management of cancers of the middle and lower thirds of the rectum. A detailed anal continence history and physical examination by an experienced surgeon are very important in predicting the postoperative outcome. Impaired functional results of a 'straight' coloanal anastomosis, especially increased bowel movement frequency, have led to the preference for use of a coloanal J-pouch. This has the functional consequence of creating a reservoir for fecal contents.*

Preoperative radiation or chemoradiation

Considerable tumor shrinkage can occur after neoadjuvant (preoperative) radiation or chemoradiation. With radiation alone, the complete pathologic response rate of lesions that have infiltrated through the bowel wall and/or have involved local lymph nodes is reported to be 10–17%. With preoperative chemoradiation, complete response can be increased to 20–30%.[32–34] The role of neoadjuvant chemoradiation has evolved from its use solely in those with T4 lesions, to its application in stage II and III patients with two objectives, better local tumor control and lower morbidity.[35] A German trial compared preoperative with postoperative long-term chemoradiation (50.4 Gy/5-FU) in those with resectable cancer (T3/4, N positive); 5-year local recurrence rates were 6% vs 13%, respectively ($p = 0.006$). However, distant-recurrence rates and survival were similar in both patient groups. Preoperative treatment was better tolerated than postoperative treatment. Of the patients considered by the surgeon to need abdominoperineal resection before randomization within the two treatment groups, 19% underwent a sphincter-preserving procedure in the postoperative period compared with 39% in the preoperative treatment group ($p = 0.004$).[35] Current approaches include the addition of new chemotherapeutic agents such as oxaliplatin, and capecitabine, to radiotherapy regimens.

In a patient with a *locally advanced* primary rectal cancer or in the presence of pelvic recurrence, an extensive surgical procedure is often needed to provide clear margins. Preoperative chemoradiation is frequently used for such tumors, especially if they appear fixed.[32] Increased resectability rate can be achieved without increasing morbidity. Perineal reconstructive procedures are often required to manage the pelvic defect. The majority of *local recurrences* from rectal cancer are unresectable due to a variety of factors, and palliative measures including stent placement or laser photoablation of the luminal tumor may be indicated. Rectal cancer in the *elderly* (>65 years of age) should be treated as usual, unless the patient cannot tolerate a major operation and/or has poor sphincter function.[36]

Surgical management of hepatic metastases

Fifteen percent of patients will have liver metastases at the time of presentation with the primary tumor. Failure of curative treatment for colorectal cancer will be frequently manifested by the occurrence of hepatic metastases, and in about 30% of patients, the liver will be the only site of metastatic disease at the time of death from colorectal cancer.

Untreated, hepatic metastases will generally result in a median survival of <2 years.[37] The length of survival is influenced by the extent of hepatic disease, the presence of extrahepatic metastases or an unresected primary, and the severity of comorbid disease. About 60% of patients who present with a solitary liver metastasis will survive over 1 year even if untreated, whereas only 5% of patients with widespread disease will survive more than 1 year. Although unresected hepatic metastases will cause death in almost all patients within 5 years of diagnosis, it has been demonstrated that hepatic resection in appropriately selected patients can result in survival of approximately 25–30% at 5 years, with median survival of 28–35 months.[37]

The majority of patients found to have liver metastases during follow-up after curative therapy will have these discovered by a CT scan, whose performance was prompted by a rising carcinoembryonic antigen (CEA) level, abdominal pain, or jaundice (Figure 9.7). About 80% of patients with hepatic metastases will have elevated CEA levels. A multiphase helical abdominal CT scan can determine the extent of hepatic metastases, and identify extrahepatic metastases. Abdominal ultrasound is less sensitive and is not useful for determining resectability. Additional procedures to determine the extent of disease in patients found to have hepatic metastases are chest CT scan and/or PET (positron emission tomography)—CT scan (Figure 9.8) and colonoscopy. The exclusion of extrahepatic disease is critical to the selection of patients for hepatic resection. More effective systemic chemotherapy regimens are enhancing the likelihood that a greater portion of hepatic metastases can become resectable.[38]

Hepatic resection: principles

To be successful, hepatic resection must accomplish the complete removal of the tumor with adequate margins of normal tissue. Usually, margins of approximately 1 cm are obtained. The major limitation to wider resection margins, within the liver, is the relationship of the tumor to major vascular structures within or adjacent to the liver, including the vena cava or hepatic veins, the portal vein, or the hepatic arteries. Recognition of intrahepatic structures can be greatly enhanced by intraoperative ultrasound, and tumors as small as 5 mm can be identified. At times, ultrasound techniques can be also useful in guiding fine-needle aspiration biopsies of suspicious lesions. At the time of laparotomy, the surgeon performs a thorough exploration for extrahepatic spread before attempting hepatic tumor resection.

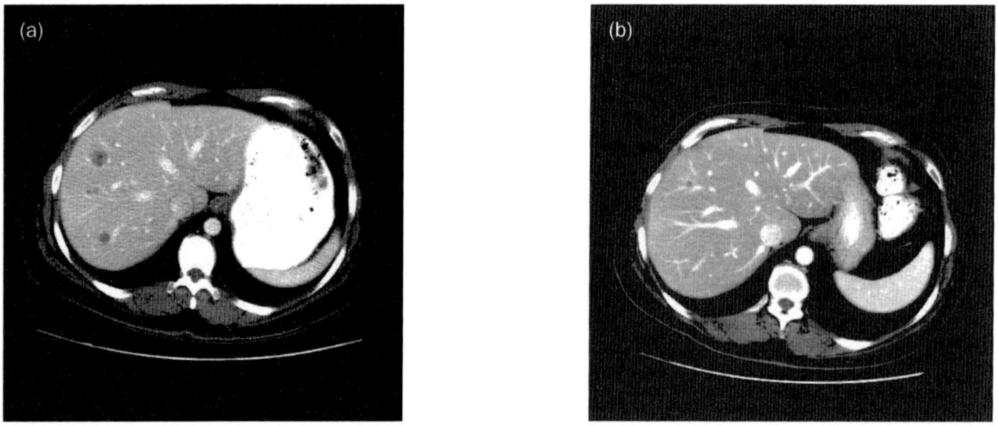

Figure 9.7 *(a) Pretreatment computed tomography (CT) scan, demonstrating multiple hepatic metastases. (b) Post-chemotherapy CT scan after 3 months of combination therapy with an oxaliplatin-based regimen in combination with bevacizumab demonstrated significant shrinkage of the metastatic disease (Figure provided by Dr R DuBrow, Houston, Texas.)*

Hepatic resections are broadly defined as either anatomic or non-anatomic. Non-anatomic resections are also known as segmental resections. Anatomic resections are usually termed right and left lobectomy, lateral segmentectomy, and trisegmentectomy. Anatomic resection is not necessary for small lesions in a favorable location. The benefit of non-anatomic resection is that it limits the amount of functional hepatic parenchyma that is removed, thereby diminishing postoperative hepatic insufficiency. Non-anatomic resections have also been shown to decrease blood loss and shorten operating room times and hospital stays. For larger tumors and those located adjacent to major portal or hepatic vein branches, anatomic resection is usually preferable. Mortality associated with liver resection for colorectal metastases is ≤5%, with the majority of deaths occurring due to hemorrhage, infection, liver failure, or biliary leaks. Among those whose cancer recurs, the liver is the most likely site of recurrence.

Because the majority of patients with liver metastases are not candidates for hepatic resection, other regional treatment measures include cryoablation of the hepatic tumor with a margin of surrounding hepatic parenchyma. Percutaneous or laparoscopic radiofrequency ablation can produce a response rate of 67% with a high degree of safety. There are, however, no prospective randomized trials that show any therapeutic advantage of these ablative techniques over chemotherapy alone in non-resectable metastatic disease confined to the liver. Such trials are in progress in Europe.[37] Another type of treatment is hepatic arterial chemotherapy that is based not only on the selective vascular supply of hepatic metastases from the arterial blood flow but also on the high hepatic extraction of certain chemotherapeutic agents such as floxuridine. Whereas hepatic arterial pump placement may be associated with many complications such as arterial thrombosis and cholangitis, intra-arterial therapy does provide a high degree of tumor shrinkage in the liver. A major drawback to this treatment, however, is that metastatic disease may develop at extrahepatic sites during treatment. The overall impact on patient survival is modest, and use of this approach has declined with the advent of more effective systemic therapy.[39]

Lung metastasis

The management of lung metastases follows similar principles of management to those for liver metastasis. In the absence of other sites of metastatic disease, several lung metastases may be resected with reasonable results in a significant number of patients.[40] The size of the metastases and the completeness of resection have been identified as independent prognostic factors. However, the majority of patients have extensive recurrence that is more appropriately treated with systemic chemotherapy.

Patterns of failure

As a basis for selecting additional therapy, it is important to understand where colorectal cancer spreads after attempted curative resection. Approximately 75% of all patients with colorectal cancer will present at a stage when all gross carcinoma can be surgically resected. The natural history and patterns of failure (local recurrence or distal spread) following apparently 'curative' resection differ for colon and rectal cancer. Locoregional failure, as the only or major site of recurrence, is more common in rectal cancer, although pulmonary metastases are well described. The rationale for a locally effective therapy in rectal cancer, such as pre- or postoperative pelvic irradiation, is based on this natural history. Colon cancer frequently spreads to the liver, peritoneum, and other distant sites, and is associated with a lower rate of local failure.

Colon cancer: adjuvant therapy

Despite an apparently high rate of surgical resectability, about half of all patients with colorectal cancer die from metastatic disease. In particular, those with locally advanced tumors (transmucosal spread or with lymph node involvement) may have subclinical micrometastases. Viable tumor cells may have metastasized prior to primary tumor resection. They may be in the adjacent lymph nodes or bone marrow but not detectable except by highly specialized histologic, molecular, or imaging techniques. This realization has led to the use of adjuvant cytotoxic therapy administered with intent to cure. The target of such therapy is the pool of rapidly cycling cancer cells that may be circulating. The aim is to eradicate them before they become established and relatively refractory to treatment. Postoperative adjuvant therapy after surgery is advised for most patients with stage III colon cancer, and this is based on the recommendations of the 1990 US National Institutes of Health (NIH) consensus statement as well as subsequent trials.[41] Recently, an expert panel concluded

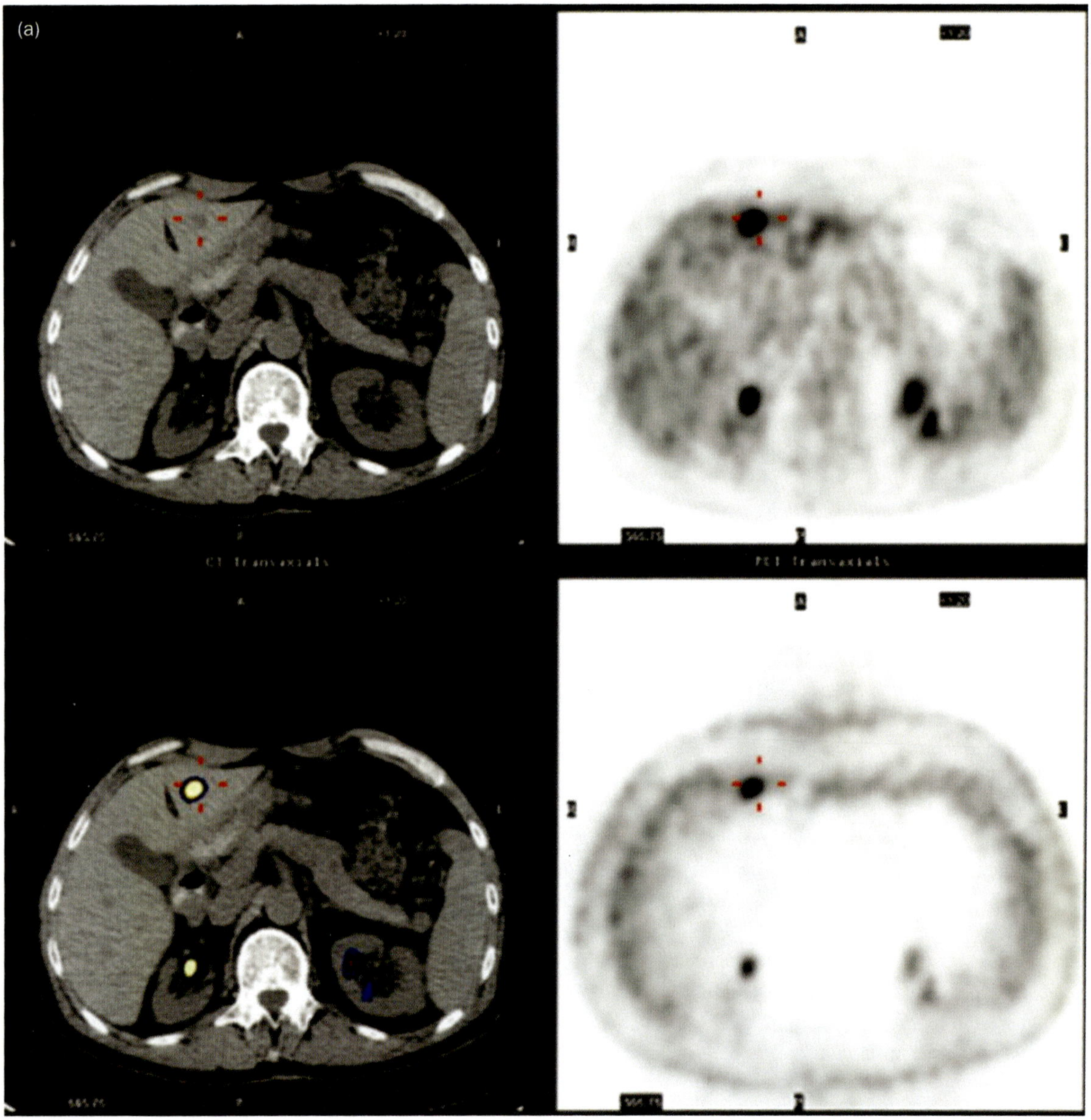

Figure 9.8 *F-18 fluorodeoxyglucose (FDG) positron emission tomography (PET) image of the liver in a patient known to have colorectal cancer and hepatic angiomas. (Figures provided by Drs Even-Sapir and Metser, Tel Aviv, Israel). (a) Top left is a transaxial computed tomography (CT) image, top right is the corresponding attenuation—corrected PET image, and bottom left is the fused PET-CT image. Uptake (blue) in the urinary tract is a normal finding. Increased FDG uptake was detected in one of the hypodense liver lesions, including coexisting liver metastasis (marked red) in addition of the hemangiomas. (b) Right upper and lower PET transaxial figures illustrating areas of increased FDG uptake. Left upper and lower CT figures illustrating normal CT appearing and sized retroperitoneal lymph nodes. However, in the fused PET-CT image there was also increased FDG update in these nodes (marked red), indicating metastasis.*

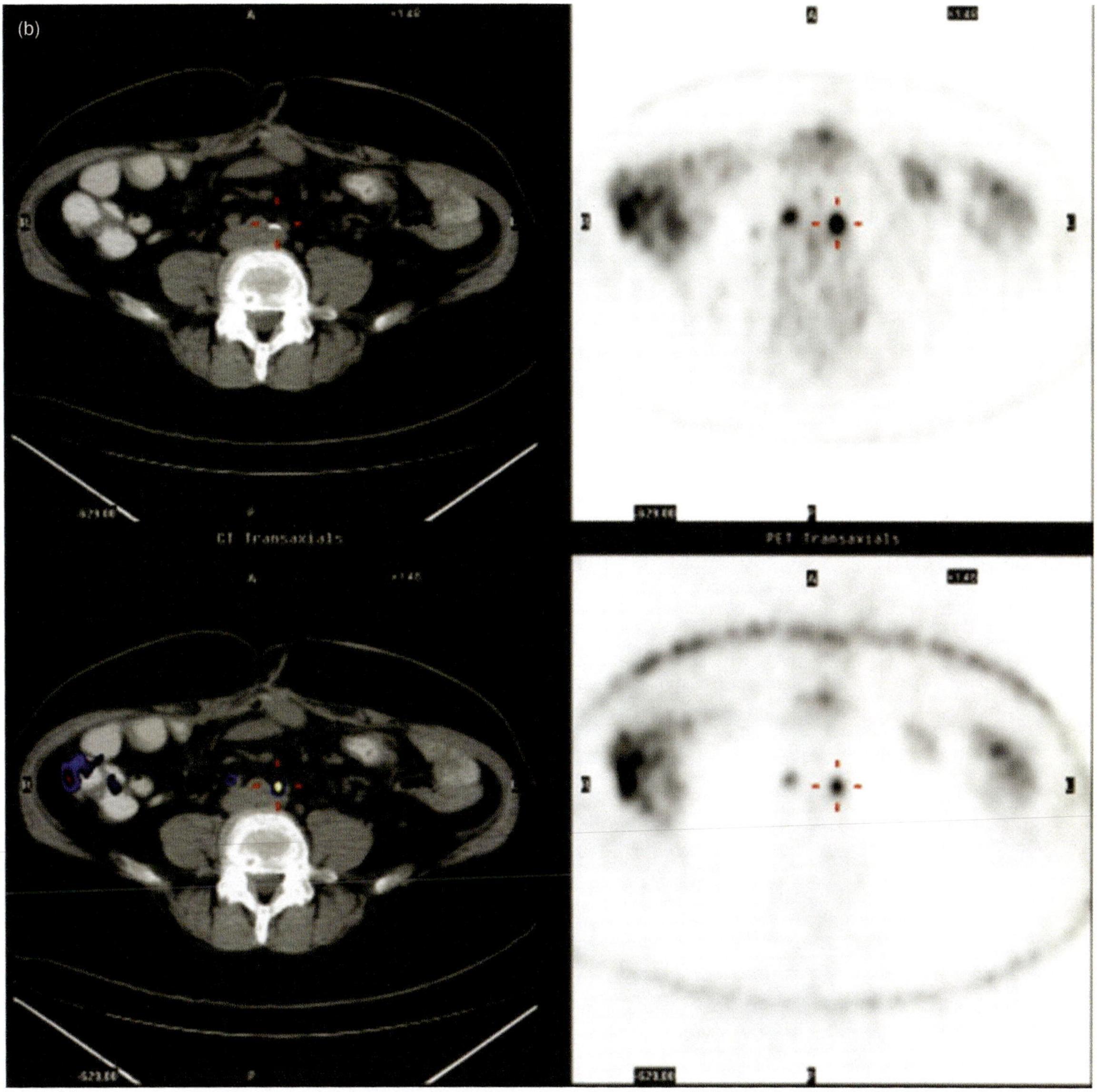

that systemic adjuvant chemotherapy is not indicated for stage II colon cancer patients who have undergone successful surgical resection. Extenuating circumstances favoring therapy in stage II patients may include an inadequate number of lymph nodes analyzed after surgery (e.g. less than 13), the presence of an adverse prognostic lesion such as perforation, peritumoral lymphovascular involvement, or poorly differentiated histology. Assessment of comorbidities and anticipated life expectancy must also be considered in making the decision to offer adjuvant therapy.[42]

For approximately 40 years, the only drug to show reproducible therapeutic activity in colorectal cancer was five flourouracil (5-FU), which is believed to act mainly by intracellular conversion to the corresponding deoxyriboside monophosphate, 5-fluorodeoxyuridine monophosphate. This compound binds to and inhibits the enzyme thymidylate synthase, which is the rate-limiting step in the de-novo synthesis of thymidine nucleotides required for DNA synthesis. When compared with 5-FU alone, the compound calcium leucovorin modulates the activity of 5-FU, thereby enhancing therapeutic response rates. In the IMPACT analysis of three studies, mortality was reduced by 22%.[43] In an intergroup study in the United States, mortality was reduced by 16%.[44]

As a result of a recent multicenter, international trial of oxaliplatin, fluorouracil, and leucovorin as adjuvant therapy for colorectal cancer, this regimen has been approved in the United States as adjuvant therapy in the management of stage III colon cancer. The rate of disease-free survival at 3 years in the group receiving the three drugs was 78.2% (95% CI 75.6–80.7) and 72.9% (95% CI 70.2–75.7) in the group who received fluorouracil plus leucovorin. Side effects such as febrile neutropenia and sensory neuropathy were higher in the group receiving oxaliplatin.[45] The oral fluoropyrimidine, capecitabine, may also be used because of its convenience, and under some circumstances (e.g. presence of comorbid conditions), 5-FU plus leucovorin may still be appropriate. It may be combined with other chemotherapeutic agents such as irinotecan.[41]

Molecular genetic changes and chemotherapy

Tumor-related factors with relevance to chemotherapy response include loss of heterozygosity (chromosomal instability) and microsatellite instability (MSI). A survival benefit from 5-FU chemotherapy was reported if heterozygosity was retained at chromosome 17p or 18q sites.[46]

Fluorouracil-based adjuvant chemotherapy benefits patients with stage II or stage III colon cancers with microsatellite-stable tumors or tumors exhibiting low-frequency MSI but not those with tumors exhibiting high-frequency MSI.[47] Immunohistochemical demonstration of MSI by staining for MSH2 and MLH1 in sporadic colorectal cancer (about 17% exhibit MSI) has been shown to be associated with an excellent prognosis in T3N0M0 colon cancer, thereby obviating a need for adjuvant therapy.[48,49] However, to date, few oncologic centers have implemented MSI evaluation as routine before deciding on therapy.

Adjuvant therapy of rectal cancer

As surgical advances have reduced the need for abdominoperineal resection in the management of carcinoma of the rectum, adjuvant therapy has been shown to be valuable in reducing local and distant tumor recurrences. Local recurrence in the pelvis is often painful because of the involvement of contiguous organs and soft and bony tissues. Presenting symptoms vary from vague pelvic fullness to difficulty in voiding and sciatica. The effectiveness of postoperative irradiation and 5-FU-based chemotherapy as adjuvant therapy for resected high-risk rectal cancer (stage II or III disease) was established by prospective randomized trials during the 1980s and 1990s.

Management of advanced colorectal cancer

The patient with advanced colorectal cancer may present with local recurrence and/or widespread metastases. Characteristic sites of spread include the pelvis, retroperitoneum, liver and lungs. The prognosis may vary considerably in each individual, depending on the extent of the disease and the presence of comorbid illnesses. A decision to offer chemotherapy or other treatment will depend upon the patient's general level of fitness (performance status), the extent of metastatic spread, and the wishes of the patient. Increasingly, because of access to and use of the Internet, patients and their family members have more information concerning available treatment alternatives.

The management of advanced colorectal cancer requires appropriate integration of palliative measures such as chemotherapy and radiation therapy, as well as control of anorexia, fatigue, pain and nausea. Mechanical bowel obstruction may require surgical decompression. Occasionally, depression and anxiety may be severe enough to warrant pharmacologic therapy. The support of the medical oncologist and primary care physician is especially crucial during this phase of the patient's illness. Palliative care services may also offer additional benefit under some circumstances.

Systemic chemotherapy

Early randomized studies explored the best possible doses and schedules of 5-FU and its modulators such as leucovorin with respect to efficacy and site effects. The development of oral fluoropyrimidines, in particular capecitabine, has been an important advance. Capecitabine is a rationally designed prodrug intended to mimic the continuous infusion of 5-FU while avoiding the complications of intravenous drug administration. On the basis of two large phase III studies, capecitabine has been approved as a first-line alternative to intravenous 5-FU in advanced metastatic colorectal cancer.[50]

In the past 7 years, several new drugs have appeared (Table 9.6). Irinotecan, an inhibitor of the nuclear enzyme topoisomerase I, when combined with 5-FU, has been shown to produce tumor response rates as high as 36% in those who had never received prior treatment. In addition, quality of life and survival were enhanced.[51] Currently, this drug is used largely in combination with cetuximab because of toxicity considerations.

Table 9.6 *Common chemotherapy drugs used for therapy of colorectal cancer*

Class	Generic drug name
Antimetabolite	5-fluorouracil (5-FU)
Antimetabolite	Capecitabine
Biomodulator	Leucovorin
Topoisomerase inhibitor	Irinotecan
Alkylating agent	Oxaliplatin
Monoclonal antibody	Cetuximab (anti-EGFR)[a]
Monoclonal antibody	Bevacizumab (anti-VEGF)[b]

[a] EGFR, epidermal growth factor.
[b] Vascular endothelial growth factor.

Oxaliplatin is a third-generation platinum analogue that is less toxic than cisplatin. In randomized phase III trials of combinations of infusional 5-FU plus oxaliplatin (FOLFOX), significant improvements in response rate and progression-free survival have been reported when compared with infusional 5-FU alone or oxaliplatin alone in patients whose cancers had become resistant to irinotecan.[52]

Targeted therapies in advanced disease: use of monoclonal antibodies

Cetuximab

Cetuximab is a chimeric monoclonal antibody that binds to the external domain of the epidermal growth factor receptor (EGFR). In patients with tumors that express EGFR and who no longer responded to treatment with irinotecan alone or in combination with other chemotherapy, the combination of cetuximab and irinotecan shrank tumors in 23% of patients and delayed tumor progression by approximately 4 months. For patients who received cetuximab alone, the tumor response rate was 10.8%, and tumor growth was delayed by 1.5 months. The most common adverse side effects were acneiform rash, malaise, and diarrhea.[53]

Bevacizumab

Bevacizumab is a human chimeric antibody to vascular endothelial growth factor (VEGF), which is a powerful

Table 9.7 *Historical comparisons and estimates of the impact of palliative chemotherapy on colorectal cancer patient survival*[a]

Therapy[b]	Survival		
	Median (months)	1 year (%)	2 years (%)
BSC	6	42	14
BSC with 5-FU	12–14	50–60	20
BSC with 5-FU and irinotecan	15–17	60–70	25–30
BSC with 5-FU, irinotecan, and oxaliplatin in various singleton or doublet sequences	21	75	40
BSC with 5-FU and irinotecan and bevacizumab	21	75	40
BSC with 5-FU or capecitabine, irinotecan, oxaliplatin, and bevacizumab in various combinations	24?	80–85?	45–50?

[a] Modified from reference 38 with permission.
[b] BSC, best supportive care; 5-FU, 5-fluorouracil.

stimulant of angiogenesis. New blood vessel formation is critical for tumor growth, invasion, and metastasis. Bevacizumab prevents ligand–receptor interaction and thereby inhibits signal transduction. Following phase I and phase II trials, a recent phase III trial was performed in patients with advanced colorectal cancer.[54] Half of the 80 patients received irinotecan, 5-FU and leucovorin, whereas the other half received bevacizumab every 2 weeks in addition. Overall, those receiving the combination lived about 5 months longer (20 months), and the average time before tumors started regrowing or new tumors appeared was 4 months longer than in patients receiving the three-drug combination alone. The overall response rate to the treatment was 45%, compared with 35% for the control arm. Serious but uncommon side effects included gastrointestinal perforation, impaired wound healing, and pulmonary hemorrhage.

Combinations of chemotherapy and the two monoclonal antibodies cetuximab and bevacizumab are under further study as well as their use in combination with radiation therapy.

Estimates of the impact of the newer therapies now available on patient survival are illustrated in Table 9.7. The common toxicities associated with current therapy are summarized in Table 9.8.

Surveillance after colorectal cancer resection

The major aims of postoperative follow-up are the following:

- discover metastatic tumor at an early enough stage to permit definitive therapy
- assess the results of surgical therapy and identify disease that requires further treatment
- monitor patients for metachronous tumor development in the large bowel.

The value of such follow-up has been challenged because an estimated 17–61% of cancers may recur between scheduled return appointments and also because great expense is incurred by the use of radiologic and laboratory tests, including CEA determinations.[55,56] In addition, one must consider the psychologic distress caused by false-positive results, the possible failure of early detection, the discovery of asymptomatic, incurable recurrences, and the morbidity related to exploratory laparotomy done as a result of true-positive or false-positive results. However, survival is significantly improved

Table 9.8 Toxicity of currently available agents used in metastatic colorectal cancer[a]

Agent[b]	Common toxicities	Uncommon toxicities
Fluoropyrimidines		
5-FU (bolus)	Mucositis, diarrhea, neutropenia, photosensitivity, conjunctivitis	Coronary spasm, cognitive dysfunction, cerebellar ataxia
5-FU (infusion), capecitabine (oral)	Hand and foot syndrome, diarrhea	Myelosuppression, nausea, vomiting
Camptothecins		
Irinotecan	Early-onset diarrhea, late-onset diarrhea, neutropenia, alopecia, nausea, vomiting, mucositis	Pulmonary syndrome (fever, dyspnea, eosinophilia, reticulonodular infiltrates)
Platinum analogues		
Oxaliplatin	Early peripheral neuropathy (cold), late peripheral neuropathy, neutropenia, nausea, vomiting, mucositis	Anaphylaxis, hemolytic anaemia

[a] Derived from reference 38 with permission.
[b] 5-FU, 5-fluorouracil.

if surgically resectable recurrent disease is detected during surveillance, as compared to disease found during interval visits.[57]

The most important time for follow-up is during the first 3 years after primary tumor resection. During this time, 85% of recurrences usually occur. Although controversy still reigns about the most appropriate schedule of follow-up procedures, the following represents the practice of some physicians for relatively fit patients with stages I–III disease in whom further surgical or other therapies would be appropriate if recurrence were demonstrated.

For successfully treated patients who have no known residual disease, a history is obtained and a physical examination is performed every 3 months for the first 3 years, then every 6 months for the next 2 years.

For those with T2 or greater lesions, a CEA test is performed at baseline and every 3 months for 2 years, and then every 6 months for the next 3 years. Colonoscopy is indicated within 1 year of resection, and is performed thereafter every 3 years if no abnormalities have been found or more often if adenomas are discovered. Flexible proctosigmoidoscopy is performed at 6- to 12-month intervals for the first 3 years in patients who have undergone a low anterior resection. It is worth noting that curable anastomotic recurrence is infrequent.

When an elevated CEA is detected in a patient in whom it was normal postoperatively, the test should be repeated for confirmation. After confirmation, further evaluations may include imaging studies (CT or magnetic resonance imaging (MRI)) of the abdomen, chest X-ray, and colonoscopy. PET–CT may then be useful to see if isolated, surgically resectable, metastases can be demonstrated, especially if the other imaging tests are equivocal (see Figure 9.8). It is also useful for monitoring response to treatment, as it can usually differentiate between viable tumor and fibrosis.

Multidisciplinary approach to management

The optimal management of the patient with colorectal cancer requires a comprehensive and multidisciplinary approach that involves the primary care physician, surgeon, gastroenterologist, medical oncologist, radiation oncologist, pathologist, diagnostic radiologist, specialized nurses (e.g. enterostomal therapist), as well as other support personnel.

Conclusions

The best outcome in the management of patients with colorectal neoplasia is achieved by detection of colorectal neoplasms at the earliest possible stage. The importance of screening and early detection cannot be overemphasized. The modern, largely successful management of patients with stages I and II colorectal cancer rests heavily on the expertise of the surgeon, pathologist, and gastroenterologist. For patients with stage III and especially stage IV colorectal cancer, more effective management techniques are needed, although the recent introduction of novel therapeutic agents is reason for some optimism regarding future directions and improved outcomes.

References (*Reviews and general articles)

1. *Weitz J, Koch M, Hohler T et al, Colorectal cancer. Lancet 2005; 365: 153–65.
2. Wolff WI, Shinya H, A new approach to colonic polyps. Ann Surg 1973; 178: 367–76.
3. *Hamilton SR, Pathology and biology of colorectal neoplasia: In: Prevention and Early Detection of Colorectal Cancer (Young GP, Rozen P, Levin B, eds). London: WB Saunders, 1996: 3–21.
4. Haggitt RC, Glotzbach RE, Soffer EE et al, Prognostic factors in colorectal carcinomas arising in adenomas: implications for lesions removed by endoscopic polypectomy. Gastroenterology 1985; 89: 328–36.
5. Volk EE, Goldblum JR, Petras RE et al, Management and outcome of patients with invasive carcinoma arising in colorectal polyps. Gastroenterology 1995; 109: 1801–7.
6. *Ueno H, Mochizuki H, Hashiguchi Y et al, Risk factors for an adverse outcome in early invasive colorectal carcinoma. Gastroenterology 2004; 127: 385–94.
7. Ahmad VA, Kochman ML, Ginsberg GC, Endoscopic ultrasound and endoscopic mucosal resection for rectal cancers and villous adenomas. Hematol Oncol Clin North Am 2002; 16: 897–906.

8. *Fielding LP. Staging systems. In: Cancer of the Colon, Rectum and Anus (Cohen AM, Winawer SJ, Friedman MA et al, eds). New York: McGraw-Hill, 1995: 207–15.
9. McArdle CS, Hole DJ, Emergency presentation of colorectal cancer is associated with poor 5-year survival. Br J Surg 2004; 91: 605–9.
10. Joseph NE, Sigurdson ER, Hanlon AL et al, Accuracy of determining nodal negativity in colorectal cancer on the basis of the number of nodes retrieved on resection. Ann Surg Oncol 2003; 10: 213–18.
11. Mainprize KS, Kulacoglu H, Hewavisinthe J et al, How many lymph nodes to stage colorectal carcinoma? J Clin Pathol 1998; 51: 165–6.
12. Brown HG, Luckasevic TM, Medich DS, Efficacy of manual dissection of lymph nodes in colon cancer resections. Mod Pathol 2004; 17: 402–6.
13. Gryfe R, Kim H, Hsieh HT et al, Tumor microsatellite instability and clinical outcome of patients with colorectal cancer. N Engl J Med 2000; 42: 69–77.
14. Soumaoro LT, Uetake H, Higuchi T et al, Cyclooxygenase-2 expression: a significant prognostic indicator for patients with colorectal cancer. Clin Cancer Res 2004; 10: 8465–71.
15. *Delaney CP, Kiran RP, Senagofe AJ et al, Case-matched comparison of clinical and financial outcome after laparoscopic or open colorectal surgery. Ann Surg 2003; 238: 67–72.
16. Foley EF, Kolecki RV, Schirmer BD, The accuracy of laparoscopic ultrasound in the detection of colorectal cancer liver metastases. Am J Surg 1998; 176: 262–4.
17. Khalili TM, Fleshner PR, Hiatt JR et al, Colorectal cancer: comparison of laparoscopic with open approaches. Dis Colon Rectum 1998; 41: 832–8.
18. Fleshman JW, Nelson H, Peters WR et al, Early results of laparoscopic surgery for colorectal cancer. Retrospective analysis of 372 patients treated by Clinical Outcomes of Surgical Therapy (COST) Study Group. Dis Colon Rectum 1996; 39: S53–8.
19. Bokey EL, Moore JW, Keating JP, Laparoscopic resection of the colon and rectum for cancer. Br J Surg 1997; 84: 822–5.
20. Feingold DL, Addona T, Forde KA et al, Safety and reliability of tattooing colorectal neoplasms prior to laparoscopic resection. J Gastrointest Surg 2004; 8: 543–6.
21. Kockerling F, Reymond MA, Schneider C et al, Prospective multicenter study of the quality of oncologic resections in patients undergoing laparoscopic colorectal surgery for cancer. The Laparoscopic Colorectal Surgery Study Group. Dis Colon Rectum 1998; 41: 963–70.
22. Hase K, Ueno H, Kuranaga N et al, Intraperitoneal exfoliated cancer cells in patients with colorectal cancer. Dis Colon Rectum 1998; 41: 1134–40.
23. Kim SH, Milsom JW, Gramlich TL et al, Does laparoscopic vs. conventional surgery increase exfoliated cancer cells in the peritoneal cavity during resection of colorectal cancer? Dis Colon Rectum 1998; 41: 971–8.
24. The Clinical Outcomes of Surgical Therapy Study Group, A comparison of laparoscopically assisted and open colectomy for colon cancer. N Engl J Med 2004; 350: 2050–9.
25. Lacy AM, Garcia-Valdecasas JC, Delgado S et al, Laparoscopy-assisted colectomy versus open colectomy for treatment of non-metastatic colon cancer: a randomised trial. Lancet 2002; 359: 2224–9.
26. Graham RA, Gainsey L, Jessup JM, Local excision of rectal carcinoma. Am J Surg 1990; 160: 306–12.
27. Minsky BD, Rich TA, Recht A et al, Selection criteria for local excision with or without adjuvant radiation therapy for rectal cancer. Cancer 1989; 63: I42I–9.
28. Ota DM, Skibber JM, Rich TA, M.D. Anderson Cancer Center experience with local excision and multimodality therapy for rectal cancer. Surg Clin North Am 1992; 1: 147–53.
29. *Quirke P, Scott N, The pathologist's role in the assessment of local recurrence in rectal carcinoma. Surg Oncol Clin North Am 1992; 1: 1–17.
30. Kapiteijn E, van de Velde CJ, The role of total mesorectal excision in the management of rectal cancer. Surg Clin North Am 2002; 82: 995–1007.
31. Cavaliere F, Pemberton JH, Cosimelli M et al, Coloanal anastomosis for rectal cancer: long-term results at the Mayo and Cleveland Clinics. Dis Colon Rectum 1995; 38: 807–12.
32. Rich TA, Skibber JM, Ajani JA et al, Preoperative infusional chemoradiation for stage T3 rectal cancer. Int J Radiat Oncol Biol Phys 1995; 32: 1025–9.
33. Chan S, Tyler DS, Anscher MS et al, Preoperative radiation and chemotherapy in the treatment of adenocarcinoma of the rectum. Ann Surg 1995; 221: 779–87.
34. Gunderson LL, Haddock MG, Schild SE, Rectal cancer: preoperative versus postoperative irradiation as a component of adjuvant treatment. Semin Radiat Oncol 2003; 13: 419–32.
35. *Sauer R, Becker H, Hohenberger W, Preoperative versus postoperative chemoradiotherapy for rectal cancer. N Engl J Med 2004; 351: 1731–40.
36. *Abir F, Alva S, Longo WE, The management of rectal cancer in the elderly. Surg Oncol 2004; 13: 223–34.
37. *Poston GJ, Surgical strategies for colorectal liver metastases. Surg Oncol 2004; 13: 125–36.
38. *Damjanovic D, Thompson P, Findley MP, Evidence-based update of chemotherapy options for metastatic colorectal cancer. ANZ J Surg 2004; 74: 781–7.
39. Meta-Analysis Group in Cancer, Re-appraisal of hepatic arterial infusion in the treatment of nonresectable liver metastases from colorectal cancer. J Natl Cancer Inst 1996; 88: 252–8.
40. Vogelsand H, Haas S, Hierholzer C et al, Factors influencing survival after resection of pulmonary

metastases from colorectal cancer. Br J Surg 2004; 91: 1066–71.
41. *Meyerhardt JA, Mayer RJ, Systemic therapy for colorectal cancer. N Engl J Med 2005; 325: 476–87.
42. *Benson AB, Schrag D, Somerfield MR et al, American Society of Clinical Oncology recommendations on adjuvant chemotherapy for stage-2 colon cancer. J Clin Oncol 2004; 16: 3408–19.
43. IMPACT Trial, Efficacy of adjuvant fluorouracil and folinic acid in colon cancer. Lancet 1995; 345: 939–44.
44. O'Connell M, Maillard J, MacDonald J et al, Controlled trial of fluorouracil and low-dose leucovorin given for six months as post-operative adjuvant therapy for colon cancer. J Clin Oncol 1997; 15: 246–50.
45. Andre T, Boni C, Moundedji-Boudiaf L et al, Oxaliplatin, fluorouracil, and leucovorin as adjuvant treatment for colorectal cancer. N Engl J Med 2004; 350: 2343–51.
46. Barrett PL, Seymour MT, Stenning SP et al, DNA markers predicting benefit from adjuvant fluorouracil in patients with colon cancer: a molecular study. Lancet 2002; 360: 1381–91.
47. Ribic CM, Sargent DJ, Moore MJ et al, Tumor microsatellite-instability status as a predictor of benefit from fluorouracil-based adjuvant chemotherapy for colon cancer. N Engl J Med 2003; 349: 247–57.
48. Carethers JM, Smith EJ, Behling CA et al, Use of 5–fluorouracil and survival in patients with microsatellite-unstable colorectal cancer. Gastroenterology 2004; 2: 394–401.
49. *Parc Y, Gueroult S, Mourra N et al, Prognostic significance of microsatellite instability determined by immunohistochemical staging of MSH2 and MLH1 in sporadic T3N0M0 colon cancer. Gut 2004; 53: 371–5.
50. Hoff PM, Ausari R, Batist G et al, Comparison of oral capecitabine versus intravenous fluorouracil and leucovorin as first-line treatment in 605 patients with metastatic colorectal cancer: results of a randomized phase III study. J Clin Oncol 2001; 19: 2282–92.
51. Douillard JY, Cunningham D, Roth AD et al, Irinotecan combined with fluorouracil compared with fluorouracil alone as first-line treatment for metastatic colorectal cancer: a multicentre randomised trial. Lancet 2000; 355: 1041–7.
52. Rothenberg ML, Oza AM, Bigelow RH et al, Superiority of oxaliplatin and fluorouracil-leucovorin compared with either therapy alone in patients with progressive colorectal cancer after irinotecan and fluorouracil-leucovorin: interim results of a phase III trial. J Clin Oncol 2003; 21: 2059–69.
53. Cunningham D, Humblet Y, Siena A et al, Cetuximab monotherapy and cetuximab plus irinotecan in irinotecan-refactory metastatic colorectal cancer. N Engl J Med 2004; 351: 337–45.
54. Hurwitz H, Fehrenbacher L, Novotny W et al, Bevacizumab plus irinotecan, fluorouracil and leucovorin for metastatic colorectal cancer. N Engl J Med 2004; 350: 2335–42.
55. Berman JM, Chenng RJ, Weinberg DS, Surveillance after colorectal cancer resection. Lancet 2000; 355: 395–9.
56 *Renehan AG, Egger M, Saunders MP et al, Impact on survival of intensive follow-up after curative resection for colorectal cancer: systemic review and meta-analysis of randomised trials. BMJ 2002; 324: 813.
57. Bonthuis DC, Landheer MLEA, Bilgen EJS et al, Small but significant survival benefit in patients who undergo routine follow-up after colorectal cancer surgery. Eur J Surg Oncol 2004; 30: 1093–7.

10 The pros and cons of population-based colorectal cancer preventive strategies

Stephen J Spann, Paul Rozen, Bernard Levin, Graeme P Young

Primary prevention: can we prevent colorectal cancer?

The primary prevention of disease is the ultimate goal of any clinician. Is this feasible for colorectal cancer? The answer must logically be yes. Why? Because it is a condition that is occurring with a rapidly rising incidence in countries that have adopted both the negative as well as the positive features of the lifestyle and diet of the industrialized (westernized) world. Preventing these negative aspects from happening and even reversing this trend is the first goal. This is true especially in those areas of Asia, the Mediterranean countries, and Europe where colorectal cancer was not a public health problem until recently (see Chapters 2 and 4).[1]

What about the situation today in countries where habits are so established and seemingly impervious to change, such as the United States, Australia, and South America? The situation is not so immutable. We have examples from the United States, where some years ago cardiovascular disease was occurring in epidemic proportions. Risk factors were identified: these included lack of physical activity, overeating saturated fats of meat origin, and not detecting and treating hypertension and hyperlipemia. Within a few years, a concerted public health campaign dramatically reduced the mortality from coronary artery disease. We have also seen the successful results of governmental policy to reduce tobacco smoking in some Western countries, especially the United States, and can look forward to a reduction in tobacco-related diseases there.

What about colorectal cancer? As pointed out in Chapters 2 and 3, its etiology is multifactorial and seemingly nebulous. There is no single major preventable risk factor, but it is the total lifestyle that seems important. A healthy lifestyle is largely applicable to the prevention of many disorders—cardiovascular, hypertension, diabetes, and some common cancers. A step in this direction has been, at least, a trend in reduction of meat consumption in Australia and the United States.

As pointed out in Chapter 4, the maintenance of an ideal body weight, the promotion of physical activity, the reduced consumption of animal fats, and the increased consumption of fruits and vegetables have salutary effects beyond the primary prevention of colorectal cancer. However, lifestyle modifications do not come easily to individuals, and interventions to promote these have certain costs. Tosteson and colleagues evaluated the cost-effectiveness of promoting a cholesterol-lowering diet at a community level; the marginal cost-effectiveness ratio of lowering the average serum cholesterol by 2% was estimated to be \$3200–\$38 500 per year of life added, well within the acceptable threshold.[2]

Chemoprevention

What is the place of chemoprevention for colon cancer, as a public health or individual's health policy (see Chapter 5)? Low-dosage aspirin is used to prevent the onset and/or the recurrence of coronary artery disease. Aspirin also reduces some of the risk for colorectal cancer, but there are no recommendations for its use, or for the dosage needed because of the side effects that occur. This may change with the development of newer and safer medications. In the meantime, we have an armamentarium of naturally occurring and safer products, including olive oil, fish, tea, and calcium, which experimentally and epidemiologically have been associated with a reduction in colorectal cancer incidence (see Chapter 5).

Secondary prevention: screening for colorectal cancer

What are the potential benefits?

Colorectal cancer is one of the most commonly diagnosed cancers, and a leading cause of cancer deaths, worldwide. The International Agency for Research on Cancer (IARC) estimates that in 2002 there were 1 023 000 new cases of colon cancer diagnosed, and 529 000 colorectal cancer deaths worldwide.[3] Lieberman has estimated the impact of screening for colorectal cancer in the United States over a 10-year period using various screening methods (Table 10.1).[4] For example, he estimated that a screening program consisting of a yearly guaiac fecal occult blood test (FOBT), combined with every 3–5 year flexible sigmoidoscopy in individuals 50–70 years of age, would prevent 50% of cancers and reduce colorectal cancer mortality by 66%, assuming 100% compliance with the screening program. Thus, if a universal screening program were instituted using these tests, the worldwide incidence of colorectal cancer could potentially be reduced to 511 500 new cases per year, and worldwide mortality reduced to 179 900 deaths per year. The reduction in the number of cancers, and the detection of cancers in earlier stages, would result in a significant reduction in disease and treatment morbidity, as well (see also Chapter 8 for a discussion on the different and improved FOBTs).

A recent comparison of the costs of prediagnosis evaluation (3 months prior to diagnosis) and treatment (12 months following diagnosis) of colorectal cancer in patients screened with FOBT vs not screened in the Group Health Cooperative, a large health maintenance organization (HMO) in the state of Washington in the United States, found that screening produced significant cost savings. Prediagnosis evaluation costs were significantly lower for patients in the screened population ($7 346) vs those who had not been screened ($10 042). Treatment costs during the first 12 months after diagnosis were also lower in the screen-detected group ($22 369) vs the symptom-detected group ($29 471).[5] The reduction in cancer mortality and increase in life expectancy, as well as the ultimate reduction in cancer incidence due to adenomatous polyp detection and removal, will necessarily lead to increased economic productivity in the screened population. From an individual's point of view, early polyp identification and removal, as well as early cancer detection and treatment, should result in decreased colorectal cancer morbidity and mortality and increased quality of life and life expectancy.

Is population screening feasible?

If we take the example of mammographic screening for breast cancer, this has been implemented successfully as a national policy in many high-risk countries. This required

Table 10.1 Modeling of impact of screening over a 10-year period on prevention, using various initial screening tools[a]

Screening test[b]	Compliance (%)	Cancers prevented (%)	Deaths prevented (%)
FOB testing alone (annual)	100	22	48
	50	11	24
FS alone (every 3–5 years)	100	38	52
	50	20	30
FS (every 3 years) plus guaiac FOBT (annual)	100	50	66
	50	25	33
Barium enema (every 5 years)	100	38	57
	50	19	29
Colonoscopy (every 10 years)	100	70	80
	50	35	40

[a]Adapted from reference 4.
[b]FS, flexible sigmoidoscopy; FOBT, guaiac fecal occult blood test.

a concerted proactive policy of health authorities and cancer societies. With consistent reinforcement in some countries, population compliance has improved to include the majority of women at risk, with a significant reduction in breast cancer mortality. Its cost has been accepted as feasible for national health care, and a similar benefit, but at an even lower cost, has been established for colorectal cancer screening.[6,7]

What are the potential risks of screening for colorectal cancer?

Any healthcare intervention that offers potential benefits also has associated potential risks (see Chapter 8). The risks associated with screening for colorectal cancer include the risks of false-negative and false-positive tests, the risks of complications of the tests per se, and the risks associated with the treatment of disease identified through the screening process. No screening test is perfectly accurate; any screening test can potentially yield false-negative and false-positive results. False-negative test results are harmful because they offer false reassurance to the screened individual, while resulting in a delay in the diagnosis and treatment of the disease which is being screened for. False-positive test results are harmful because they typically lead to additional diagnostic tests, with their costs and own associated risks, or to unnecessary treatment of a supposed disease which isn't really present, with the risks associated with that treatment. Telling an individual that she has a positive screening test may result in significant psychologic distress, as well.

Consider the case of FOBT screening for colorectal adenomas and cancer. The one-time sensitivity of unrehydrated Hemoccult II slides for the detection of adenomas has been reported to range from 3% to 14% and for the detection of cancer from 18% to 24%.[7] Thus, a patient with adenomatous polyps would have a probability even as high as 97% of having a false-negative test, and being falsely reassured. The specificity of unrehydrated Hemoccult II slides for FOBT has been estimated to be 98%.[7] Thus, a patient without adenoma or colorectal cancer would have a 2% probability of a having a false-positive test. For a 50-year-old American with an average 30% risk of having large-bowel adenomatous polyps, the negative predictive value of a one-time FOBT would be approximately 73%, while the positive predictive value would be around 75%. A negative FOBT alone does not add much reassurance that the patient is free from colorectal adenomas; a positive FOBT substantially increases an individual's probability of having adenomatous polyps. Table 10.2 displays the average sensitivity and specificity of the different screening tests for detecting colorectal adenomas, as well as the positive and negative predictive

Table 10.2 The predictive values of various screening tests for colorectal adenomatous polyps in a 50-year-old American at average risk[a]

Test[b]	Sensitivity (%)	Specificity (%)	Negative predictive value (%)	Positive predictive value (%)
FOBT	14	98	73	75
FS	45	98	81	91
FOBT/FS combination (both tests negative)[c]			83	
DCBE	70	90	88	75
FS/DCBE combination (both tests negative)[c]			93	
Colonoscopy	90	100	96	100

[a]Adapted from reference 7.
[b]FOBT, guaiac fecal occult blood test; FS, flexible sigmoidoscopy; DCBE, double-contrast barium enema.
[c]Assumes that 50% of colorectal adenomas will be within the reach of the 60 cm flexible sigmoidoscope.

values of these tests in a 50-year-old American at average (30%) risk for such neoplasia.

The most significant risk of flexible sigmoidoscopy, double-contrast barium enema, and colonoscopy is colonic perforation. The risk of perforation from flexible sigmoidoscopy has been reported to vary between 1 in 5000 and 1 in 25 000; the risk from barium enema is reported to be as high as 1 in 25 000. The risk of perforation during diagnostic colonoscopy is reported to be between 0.029% and 0.61%; the risk during therapeutic colonoscopy is reported to be between 0.07% and 0.72%. The mortality rate for complications of screening colonoscopy is estimated to be 1 per 20 000.[8] These risks must be weighed against the almost 1 in 2 chances of dying from clinically diagnosed colorectal cancer.

It should be noted that the above-described modeling calculations are based on using the least-sensitive guaiac FOBT. Also, in contrast to periodic endoscopic screening, FOBT needs to be repeated annually to obtain cumulative program sensitivity (see Chapter 8).

What is patient compliance with colorectal cancer screening recommendations?

Despite the evidence regarding the efficacy of screening tests in reducing colorectal cancer mortality in many communities, at present compliance with screening recommendations is moderate, at best. Vernon[9] performed an extensive literature review of participation in colorectal cancer screening. Rates of patient adherence to FOBT screening varied widely according to the location of the screening program (physician practice, community, or work site), whether or not the study tested the impact of a specific intervention on screening adherence, and the country in which the study was performed; the median adherence rate among studies was 40–50%. Rescreening rates were found to be less variable, and ranged between 60% and 90%. Rates of patient adherence to sigmoidoscopy were lower, and less variable, as well.[9] In the United States, an analysis of the 2001 Behavior Risk Surveillance System conducted by the Centers for Disease Control and Prevention showed that only 23.5% of the population surveyed reported receiving an FOBT within the previous 12 months; 38.7% had received lower endoscopy within the past 5 years and 43.4% within the past 10 years; 53.1% had received FOBT within the previous 12 months and/or lower endoscopy within 10 years.[10] During the same period of time, the results of a similar survey from California were superior, indicating the importance of both population and provider awareness.[11]

In the Minnesota colon cancer control study, the compliance with annual FOBT in the screened group (11 screening opportunities over the length of the study) was 75%; the compliance with biennial FOBT (6 screening opportunities) was 78%.[12] Blom et al[13] reported on acceptance of an invitation for screening sigmoidoscopy in a population of 60 year olds in Uppsala and Lund, Sweden. Compliance was 47% in Uppsala and 30% in Lund; there was no difference in compliance between male and female invitees.

Subramanian et al[14] reviewed some 50 studies to evaluate factors impacting patient adherence with colorectal cancer screening in the United States. Age was found to be a significant factor, impacting adherence in 11 of 14 studies, with older individuals proving more compliant than younger ones. Higher education was correlated with undergoing recommended screening tests in the majority of studies. Gender, race, and marital status tended to be non-significant factors, while medical insurance was significantly correlated with adherence, and membership in an HMO was related to higher levels of adherence. Income did not appear to have a consistently significant impact on adherence to colorectal cancer screening recommendations. Acknowledging that cancer is preventable and curable positively impacted on screening behaviors, whereas fear of cancer and pessimism was reported as a barrier to screening, with fatalism being a strong negative predictor of non-adherence in patients. Family history of colorectal cancer was positively related to cancer screening tests. Physician recommendation was found to be strongly related to patient adherence, so that patients with a usual source of care and patients having regular doctor visits were more likely to be more compliant, as well.

Lieberman[4] demonstrated the potential impact of compliance on reducing colorectal cancer mortality through a 10-year screening program. He estimated that a program combining annual FOBT with triennial flexible sigmoidoscopy with 100% compliance by the population would reduce colorectal cancer deaths by 66%; with a population compliance of 50%, colorectal cancer mortality would be reduced by 33%; and with a population compliance of 25%, the colorectal cancer mortality would be reduced by only 21%.

How can compliance with colorectal cancer screening recommendations be increased?

Cancer screening can be offered in an opportunistic or an organized manner.[15–17] Opportunistic screening depends on individuals to request screening, or on their health care providers to recommend screening. Cancer screening in the United States typically takes place opportunistically: patients request or are offered cancer screening tests during a health maintenance visit, or their healthcare provider offers a screening test during a visit for care of an acute or chronic health problem. Organized screening programs are planned and are usually based on a public health approach to health care; they consist of elements which form a coherent structure offering a standardized system of care, with national guidelines that define who should be invited, how frequently they should be screened, and how detected abnormalities should be followed up and treated. Invitations are issued from centralized population registries. The quality of the overall program and component parts are monitored through quality assurance, including setting and monitoring key targets for various performance parameters such as population uptake rates, cancer detection rates, and false-positive and false-negative rates. Opportunistic screening involves fewer formal decisions regarding whether to screen, whom to screen, and at what interval. Quality assurance may be more variable, and few opportunities are available to monitor the achievements and failures of the program as a whole. The existence of high screening rates in the United States for several cancers, such as cervix and breast, shows that opportunistic screening can achieve a high level of population coverage, matching or exceeding that of the best organized systems.[17] Miles et al have identified a number of lessons learned from countries that use organized screening programs:

1. Organized screening has greater potential to reduce cancer incidence and mortality due to higher achievable levels of population coverage, follow-up and quality compared with opportunistic screening.
2. Organized programs aim to achieve a population-level benefit and a balance of benefits and harms; as a result, they may not provide screening that offers maximum individual protection, but do offer greater protection from harms.
3. Equality of access is often a key principle of healthcare provision in countries with organized screening programs.
4. In organized programs, the opportunity to be screened is determined by health policy and the adequacy of the call–recall system; in opportunistic screening, the opportunity is determined more by individual factors, such as patient and provider knowledge and behavior, insurance coverage, and the patient's pattern of healthcare encounters.
5. The cost of screening as a barrier is largely remedied by organized programs, but some limitations to access remain.
6. Organized programs do not totally eliminate socioeconomic and ethnic disparities in screening uptake, and each model faces challenges related to informed consent.
7. Introducing an organized screening program presents many challenges related to infrastructure, resources, vested interest, and public and provider acceptance of centralized health care.[17]

There are a number of interventions available at the patient and provider level to enhance compliance with recommendations for colorectal cancer screening. Individual participant (or patient) compliance can be enhanced through a number of interventions. Improved knowledge about the disease and the benefits of screening can improve compliance. Studies have shown that people are poorly informed concerning colorectal cancer risk factors and colorectal cancer screening; they don't appear to understand the differences between tests or their relative benefits and limitations. The public can be educated about the importance of screening through the use of mass communications media, such as newspapers, television, and billboards. Well-known personalities who have experienced the disease, such as politicians and actors, can be powerful spokespersons for screening.[18,19] National activities such as designation of a month for 'colon cancer awareness' and national cancer societies' concerted actions have spread from the United States to many countries. Actions of voluntary organizations such as the Cancer Research and Prevention Foundation in the United States and their 'colossal colon' engage public attention have been copied internationally. The receipt of written educational materials and a written or telephone invitation or reminder to participate in a screening intervention can increase individual compliance.[20]

Physician and practice compliance with screening programs can also be improved through a number of interventions. The existence of a specific screening guideline motivates physicians to carry out screening interventions. Improving the physician's knowledge of the efficacy and effectiveness of the screening intervention enhances physician compliance, as well.[20] This can be achieved through continuing medical education programs and academic detailing. The costs for any test have to be adequate to compensate for physician effort. If not, then there is little incentive to promote screening.[21] The German National FOBT Screening Program has exemplified this, where there had been poor physician compliance until recent improvement in physician compensation. Payment for the intervention, by third-party insurers, is also a positive incentive.[18]

Systems to help remind the physician when specific preventive interventions are due help improve compliance with screening.[18,20,21] A health maintenance flow sheet, which shows when specific interventions are due and allows a place to record their completion, is useful (Figure 10.1).[18] Colored stickers placed on the patient's chart can serve as a reminder to obtain certain screening tests at defined intervals. Physician reminders about preventive interventions becoming due can be generated by computer, at each visit, to enhance compliance with screening guidelines.[22] Either a computerized billing system or a computerized medical record system can be programmed to accomplish this task. Patient-recall systems are also helpful for reminding patients when it is time for specific screening tests. These can be as simple as a card-based reminder file system, or as sophisticated as a computerized system based on a practice billing system or computerized medical record. A card-based reminder file can be developed by completing a reminder postcard with the patient's mailing address, which is then placed in a box which has dividers organized according to future dates. If Mr Smith is on a once-yearly FOBT screening protocol and completes the test in June 2005, then a reminder postcard is completed and placed in the reminder file box behind the divider for June 2006. On June 1, 2006 all cards behind that divider will be removed and mailed, and Mr Smith will receive his reminder that he is due for his yearly FOBT. Practices can develop continuous quality-improvement programs, involving measurements of physician compliance with specific prevention guidelines. Practices involved with such programs typically strive to show continuous improvement in their performance. The use of physician practice pattern audits against certain external quality markers, developed and carried out by external agencies, also serve as an incentive to enhance physician compliance with screening interventions. One

	Age																									
Preventive intervention	**50**	**51**	**52**	**53**	**54**	**55**	**56**	**57**	**58**	**59**	**60**	**61**	**62**	**63**	**64**	**65**	**66**	**67**	**68**	**69**	**70**	**71**	**72**	**73**	**74**	**75**
Weight	*	*	*	*	*	*	*	*	*	*	*	*	*	*	*	*	*	*	*	*	*	*	*	*	*	*
Blood pressure	*	*	*	*	*	*	*	*	*	*	*	*	*	*	*	*	*	*	*	*	*	*	*	*	*	*
Tetanus–diphtheria booster	*										*										*					
Influenza vaccine	*	*	*	*	*	*	*	*	*	*	*	*	*	*	*	*	*	*	*	*	*	*	*	*	*	*
Pneumococcal vaccine																*										
Pap smear	*			*			*			*			*			*			*			*			*	
Clinical breast examination	*	*	*	*	*	*	*	*	*	*	*	*	*	*	*	*	*	*	*	*	*	*	*	*	*	*
Mammograms	*	*	*	*	*	*	*	*	*	*	*	*	*	*	*	*	*	*	*	*	*	*	*	*	*	*
FOBT	*	*	*	*	*	*	*	*	*	*	*	*	*	*	*	*	*	*	*	*	*	*	*	*	*	*
Flexible sigmoidoscopy	*					*					*					*					*					*
Discuss DRE and PSA	*	*	*	*	*	*		*	*	*	*	*	*	*	*	*	*	*	*	*	*	*	*	*	*	*
Serum cholesterol	*					*					*					*					*					*

Figure 10.1 *Flow chart of preventive medical examinations that a family physician needs to perform. FOBT, fecal occult blood test; DRE, digital rectal examination; PSA, prostate-specific antigen.*

example is the Health Plan Employer Data and Information Set (HEDIS) criteria established by the National Committee on Quality Assurance (NCQA); these are used by US managed care organizations seeking NCQA accreditation, in the audit of provider physician practices.[23] Current HEDIS criteria include screening for breast and cervical cancer.

Involving non-physician office personnel in managing a screening program through protocols has also been shown to increase compliance with cancer screening.[24] To some extent, these preventive measures can be delegated to nurse–practitioners, but the physician has a crucial role in initiating discussion of the topic, including a warm recommendation to follow through with implementation. In some medical systems, there is centralized managed preventive care for promoting and organizing mammographic screening. If there is, it would seem more cost-efficient to also add colorectal cancer screening to this framework.[25] This is important not only to utilize the existing administrative organization but also to impress on women that large-bowel screening is an integral part of their preventive health evaluation. In addition, they are then more likely to influence their husbands to undergo screening. In summary, there are a number of methods which can be utilized to enhance compliance with cancer screening recommendations; these are summarized in Table 10.3.

What are patient attitudes and preferences for colorectal cancer screening tests?

Several studies have evaluated patient attitudes and preferences for the different colorectal cancer screening tests. Leard and colleagues[26] asked 100 patients aged 50–75 years old from three primary care practices in San Diego, California which of five different colorectal cancer screening options they would choose, how likely they would be to undergo each of the options, and whether or not they would undergo the test if recommended. Colonoscopy was the screening test which most patients (38%) selected as their first choice. FOBT (guaiac) was the test, which most patients ranked as highly likely that they would undergo, and which the most patients would undergo if the test was recommended. Patients who had previously undergone colonoscopy were most likely to choose this test as their preferred screening option (Table 10.4).[26]

Pignone and colleagues[27] evaluated patient preferences for four different colorectal cancer screening strategies in 146 adults in a university adult internal medicine practice in North Carolina. Patient preferences were measured at three points: after descriptive information about colon cancer and screening options; after information about test performance but with no out-of-pocket costs; and finally with hypothetical out-of-pocket costs. After receiving descriptive information about testing procedures, most

Table 10.3 Methods to enhance compliance with cancer screening

Target	Method
Individual participant (patient)	• Improve knowledge through public education • Provide written educational materials, written and/or telephone invitation/reminder to participate • Involve the patient in the decision to screen
Physician/ practice	• Provide specific screening guidelines • Cover cost of intervention through health insurance • Educate the physician about the efficacy and effectiveness of screening • Reminder systems: health maintenance flow sheets, chart stickers, computer-generated reminders • Patient-recall systems: card-based reminder file, computer-generated • Continuous quality-improvement program • External audits • Involve non-physician office personnel through protocols

Table 10.4 Patient ($n = 100$) preferences of test options, as assessed by three different approaches[a]

	No. screening	Fecal occult blood test (FOBT)	Flexible sigmoidoscopy	Barium enema	Colonoscopy
Percentage of patients who selected test as first preference[b]	4	31	13	14	38
Mean likelihood of patients undergoing test (1 = highly unlikely, 5 = highly likely)[c]	1.6	4.4	3.4	3.4	3.4
Percentage of patients who would undergo test if recommended[d]	N/A	96	82	92	86
Percentage of patients who have had this test and who prefer this screening test[e]	14	36	17	15	71

[a]Adapted from reference 26.
[b]Colonoscopy vs FOBT, $p = 0.40$; colonoscopy vs barium enema, $p = 0.0007$; FOBT vs barium enema, $p = 0.01$.
[c]FOBT vs colonoscopy, $p < 0.0001$.
[d]FOBT vs colonoscopy, $p = 0.01$.
[e]Colonoscopy vs FOBT, $p < 0.0001$.

patients (45%) chose the FOBT (guaiac) alone option. Following receipt of information on test performance, most patients preferred the FOBT plus flexible sigmoidoscopy option. After receiving the out-of-pocket cost information, most preferred the FOBT alone strategy (Table 10.5).[27] Dominitz and Provenzale[28] used the time trade-off method to measure patient preferences for flexible sigmoidoscopy and colonoscopy, each to be performed every 5 years for

Table 10.5 Preferences of subjects ($n = 146$) for colon cancer screening[a]

Specific strategy[b]	Descriptive information on testing procedure (%)	Test performance information, no out-of-pocket costs (%)	Test performance information, with out-of-pocket costs (%)
FOBT alone	45	36	53
FS alone	13	12	8
FOBT and FS	38	47[c]	31[d]
Colonoscopy	1	1	2
Neither	3	3	5
Unable to answer	1	1	1

[a]Table reprinted by permission of Blackwell Science, Inc., from the *Journal of General Internal Medicine* 1999; 14: 434 (reference 27).
[b]FOBT, fecal occult blood test; FS, flexible sigmoidoscopy.
[c]$p = 0.12$.
[d]$p < 0.001$.

20 years. Four different groups of patients aged 50–75 years old were identified at the Veterans Administration Hospital in Durham, North Carolina: unscreened patients who had never undergone colorectal cancer screening; screened patients who were undergoing flexible sigmoidoscopy; 'cooperative study' patients who were enrolled in a multicenter prospective study of risk factors for large adenomas of the colon and were about to undergo colonoscopy; and colorectal cancer patients who had previously been diagnosed with and treated for colorectal cancer. Unscreened patients were willing to give up significantly more time (life expectancy) to avoid screening sigmoidoscopy and colonoscopy (median 91 days and 183 days, respectively) than were patients undergoing screening sigmoidoscopy (median 0 days and 7 days, respectively), screening colonoscopy (median 0 days and 0 days, respectively), or patients with colorectal cancer (median 0 days and 0 days, respectively). Ling and colleagues[29] used a patient decision aid to evaluate patient preferences for five alternative colorectal cancer screening methods at the Boston Medical Center. Most patients preferred annual FOBT (43%) or colonoscopy once every 10 years (40%). There was much less interest in combining annual FOBT with flexible sigmoidoscopy every 5 years (12%), or double-contrast barium enema every 5–10 years (3%), or flexible sigmoidoscopy every 5 years (2%).

These studies suggest that patients are most likely to choose, and comply with, FOBT screening over more invasive screening procedures. On the other hand, patients who have already decided to undergo, or have previously experienced invasive tests, are much less reticent to have these performed.

Patients often find that invasive screening procedures are not as embarrassing, uncomfortable, or painful as they have feared they would be. McCarthy and Moskowitz[30] found that 41.1% of individuals undergoing screening flexible sigmoidoscopy expected to experience moderate to extreme embarrassment, but only 27.4% actually did; 55.5% expected to experience moderate to extreme discomfort, but only 41.7% did; and 40.8% expected to experience moderate to extreme pain, but only 30.9% did. When asked about their willingness to have screening sigmoidoscopy again, 25.7% said they probably would, and 63.5% said they definitely would.[30] In Melbourne, Australia, Cockburn and colleagues[31] evaluated the acceptance of screening flexible sigmoidoscopy in 187 general practice patients, aged 50–60 years old. Forty-nine percent of patients received the recommended sigmoidoscopy: 65% experienced either no or mild discomfort; while 15% experienced moderate or severe pain. Eighty percent experienced a bloated feeling, but only 36% felt moderate or extreme bloating. Sixty-four percent experienced no embarrassment, although 9% reported moderate to extreme embarrassment. There are no large published population studies, but in initial studies the method of preparing an FOBT and the number of samples requested do influence compliance (see Chapter 8). Similarly, although there is the public impression that CT (computed tomography) colonography is a less invasive test, there are no large-scale screening and follow-up studies to assess compliance.

Involving patients in the decision to screen

There is an increasing call for patients to understand the risks, benefits, and alternatives for screening tests, and to make informed decisions about them. This is consistent with the concept that high-quality health care should be patient-centered—respectful of and responsive to patient preferences, needs, and values, ensuring that patient's values guide all clinical decisions. 'Informed decision-making' is said to occur when an individual understands the disease or condition being addressed, what the clinical service involves, as well as the benefits, risks, limitations, alternatives, and uncertainties of the same. Steps in the informed decision-making process include: (1) understanding the screening test, its risks, benefits, and alternatives; (2) understanding personal values and preferences; (3) weighing the pros and cons of the test; (4) clarifying decisional preferences; (5) finding additional information, if needed; and (6) deciding on an action plan. 'Shared decision-making' connotes a process in which physicians and patients share in the decision-making process, which is conducted through one or more face-to-face encounters. Shared decision-making is a subset of informed decision-making.[32] Although the evidence for colorectal cancer screening is strong, individuals typically face options for screening test selection; each test has its own level of accuracy, discomfort, potential risk, and cost. To be able to make an informed decision regarding screening test choice, the individual should be well informed about these issues. Decision aids are interventions designed to help individuals make specific and deliberative choices among options by providing information on the options and outcomes relevant to an individual's health status. They include information on the disease or condition, probabilities (benefits and harms) of outcomes for each option (preferably tailored to personal risk factors), some type of values clarification exercise, and guidance in the process of decision-making. Rimer and colleagues[32] list 7 lessons learned regarding informed decision-making and its role in cancer screening (Table 10.6).[32]

A few studies have examined the impact of informed decision-making in colorectal cancer screening. Pignone and colleagues[33] tested whether or not a decision aid consisting of an educational video, a patient education brochure based on the patient's readiness to be screened, and a marker for the patient's change signifying that readiness increased the performance of colorectal cancer screening with FOBT or flexible sigmoidoscopy in primary care practices in a randomized controlled trial. Patients in the intervention group were more likely to have colorectal screening tests ordered (47.2% vs 26.4%) and completed (36.8% vs 22.6%) than patients in the control group. The decision aid used in this study can be viewed on the Internet.[34] Dolan and Frisina[35] conducted a randomized controlled trial comparing a patient decision aid based on multicriteria decision-making theory with a simple educational intervention in 96 patients at average risk for colorectal cancer seen in an internal medicine practice in Rochester, New York to evaluate the patient decision-making process and the decision outcome. Patients who used the decision aid had lower decisional conflict regarding screening decisions due to increased knowledge, better clarity of values, and higher ratings of the quality of the decisions they made. There was no difference between the experimental and control groups in completion of planned screening tests (49% vs 52%). Wolf and Schorling[36] evaluated, in a randomized controlled trial conducted in four general internal medicine practices, the impact of two informational interventions (one describing colorectal cancer mortality reduction in relative terms, the other in absolute terms) vs a simple description of FOBT and flexible sigmoidoscopy screening on the intent of elderly patients to begin or continue those screening tests. There was no difference in screening interest between the control group and the two information groups; the majority of patients (63%) intended to begin or continue screening. Informed patients were able to gauge more accurately the positive predictive value of screening. Control patients rated the efficacy of screening higher than did patients receiving relative risk reduction information, who rated it higher than did patients receiving absolute risk reduction information.[36]

It has been shown that recommendation by the family or treating physician is crucial in initiating a particular screening test.[14] This has been demonstrated successfully in the UK and Norway, where they have had an overall 40% agreement to participate and a 70% compliance for a sigmoidoscopy screening program that included tens of thousands of persons in defined geographic areas of both countries (see Chapter 8 references 53 and 54). However, in other countries, national prejudices in the average risk population would inhibit cooperation with such an invasive screening procedure (Dr M Crespi, Rome, pers comm).

Table 10.6 *Lessons learned regarding informed decision-making (IDM): what is its role in cancer screening?*[a]

1. IDM interventions increase short-term improvements in knowledge, beliefs, and accuracy of cancer risk perceptions
2. There is insufficient evidence to conclude whether or not IDM interventions result in decisions that are consistent with a patient's preferences
3. The impact of IDM interventions on screening is modest. These generally have resulted in small decreases in prostate cancer testing and small increases in testing for breast and cervical cancers
4. IDM interventions are needed, especially for those cancer screening tests for which the evidence is uncertain or is very sensitive to patients' preferences
5. Numerous patient, provider, and system factors pose challenges to the optimal integration of IDM into healthcare decision-making
6. In the short run, participation in IDM should be facilitated for those patients who want it. Greater numbers of individuals should be encouraged to participate more fully in their health care
7. Decision-making information can be provided to individuals outside clinical encounters. This may not only attenuate health disparities but may also enhance the efficiency of patient–physician interactions.

[a]Adapted from reference 32.

What are the economics of screening for colorectal cancer?

In every country, healthcare resources are limited, while healthcare needs are limitless.[1] Rationing decisions about allocation of healthcare resources are inevitable. With advances in modern medical technology, there are a growing number of healthcare interventions that have been proven to be efficacious and effective. The problem is that no society can afford to implement all of them. Some interventions are cost-saving: they save more in downstream healthcare expenditures than they cost. Most interventions, however, are not cost saving: their implementation would add incremental healthcare costs to society, while yielding incremental (improvement in) health. Since policymakers are frequently forced to choose among several potentially effective healthcare interventions for implementation, they need a methodology to help them make rationing decisions. Cost-effectiveness analysis is a methodology that allows policymakers to compare healthcare interventions by evaluating the relative cost per unit of outcome achieved by a given intervention. Costs are typically expressed in monetary units: dollars, pounds, euros, etc. Outcomes may be expressed in a number of ways: cancers diagnosed, deaths prevented, years of life saved, etc. Since a year of life with cancer is not equal to a year of life with heart disease, life-expectancy outcomes are typically normalized (quality-adjusted) to a state of perfect health, and expressed as quality-adjusted life-years (QALYs). Individuals value different health states according to their personal preferences or 'utilities'; utilities are typically expressed as a value between 1 (perfect health) and 0 (death). Quality-adjusted life expectancy (QALYs) is obtained by multiplying the life expectancy in a given health state by the individual's utility for that health state.[37] Thus, if an individual has been diagnosed with a Dukes' C stage colon cancer and has a life expectancy of 5 years, and has a utility of 0.95 for his post-treatment health state, then his quality-adjusted life expectancy is 4.75 QALYs. A cost-effectiveness analysis that expresses outcomes in terms of quality-adjusted life expectancy is called a 'cost-utility' analysis. A marginal cost-effectiveness (or cost-utility) analysis compares the relative costs and outcomes of two interventions:

$$\text{Marginal cost-effectiveness ratio} = \frac{C_2 - C_1}{E_2 - E_1}$$

C_2 is the cost of intervention 2, C_1 is the cost of intervention 1, E_2 is the effectiveness of intervention 2, and E_1 is the effectiveness of intervention 1.[37]

Marginal cost-effectiveness analyses can be utilized to compare various intervention strategies designed to achieve the same outcome; for example, as seen below, Wagner and colleagues[7] have performed an analysis comparing the marginal cost-effectiveness of various strategies for colorectal cancer screening. This type of analysis may also be used to decide whether the cost-effectiveness of a given intervention is comparable to that of other healthcare interventions that have already been accepted and implemented. This requires a 'threshold' range of acceptability. In the United States, for example, a healthcare intervention is currently considered to be cost-effective if its marginal cost-effectiveness ratio is under \$50 000 per QALY saved.[38]

Cost-effectiveness analysis typically involves the development of a statistical model, or decision tree, which seeks to represent the various interventions that are being considered, along with the various potential outcomes for each intervention, and the probability of each one of those outcomes. The cost and the health outcomes are then estimated for each intervention. Cost-effectiveness analysis modeling is a complicated exercise, and must take into account all of the variables that affect the outcomes of the intervention.[37]

A number of studies have been published that evaluate the cost-effectiveness of various testing strategies screening for colorectal cancer. Most of these are based on modeling exercises, and because different models utilize different assumptions, results differ between models. Pignone and colleagues[39] performed a systematic review of the medical literature on the cost-effectiveness of colorectal cancer screening, identifying 7 unique studies satisfying strict inclusion criteria. Five of these evaluated more than one screening strategy.[7,40–43] In most base-case analyses, strategies had average cost-effectiveness ratios ranging from \$10 000 to \$25 000 (US dollars in year 2000) per year of life saved, not adjusted for quality. Alternative sensitivity analyses that assumed 'worst-case' scenarios about the biologic behavior of neoplasms and effectiveness of treatment generally produced cost-effectiveness ratios of less than \$100 000 per year of life saved. Table 10.7 summarizes the findings from these studies.[39] With regard to the most effective strategy in terms of greatest average number of years of life saved,

Table 10.7 *Cost-effectiveness ratios of various screening tests or combination for colorectal cancer compared with no screening*[a]

Test	Study, year (reference)				
	Wagner et al, 1996[7]	**Frazier et al, 2000**[40]	**Khandker et al, 2000**[41]	**Sonnenberg et al, 2000**[42]	**Vijan et al, 2001**[43]
Annual FOBT, $	11 725	17 805	13 656	10 463	5 691
FS every 5 years, $	12 477	15 630	12 804	39 359	19 068
Annual FOBT + FS every 5 years, $	13 792	22 518	18 693		17 942
DCBE every 5 years, $	11 168	21 712	25 624		
Colonoscopy every 10 years, $	10 933	21 889	22 012	11 840	9 038

[a]Reproduced from reference 39, with permission of the Annals of Internal Medicine.
[b]All costs are updated to US dollars ($) in 2000. DCBE, double-contrast barium enema; FOBT, guaiac-based fecal occult blood test; FS, flexible sigmoidoscopy.

three of the studies found annual FOBT plus sigmoidoscopy every 5 years to be most effective, and two of the studies found colonoscopy every 10 years to be most effective.[39] The most 'cost-effective' strategy depends on the cost threshold beyond which no one wishes to 'pay' for additional years of life saved. Table 10.8 shows the preferred strategy at different thresholds of 'acceptable' costs per life-year saved.[39]

Patient utilities for the different health outcome states were not included in these analyses. However, Whynes and colleagues[44] chose patients diagnosed with colorectal cancer in the Nottingham FOBT screening trial to evaluate their quality of life following surgery for colorectal cancer, and to compare the quality of life between patients whose cancer was detected by screening with that of patients whose cancer presented symptomatically. The mode of entry to diagnosis and treatment (screening vs no screening) did not appear to affect post-intervention quality of life. The stage of cancer progression was not closely related to outcome quality of life, either. A quality of life adjustment coefficient for surviving patients was estimated to lie within the range of 0.95–0.98. When the life-expectancy outcomes in the above models are quality-adjusted, utilizing a coefficient of 0.95, the marginal cost-utility ratios still fall well within the range of what is typically considered to be cost-effective.

Whynes[45] has published a cost-effectiveness analysis using actual data from the Nottingham FOBT screening trial. For individuals aged 45–74 years old undergoing biennial FOBT screening, the estimated marginal cost-effectiveness ratio is £1584 per year of life saved (at 2002 prices). Gyrd-Hansen and colleagues[46] utilized actual data from the Funen screening trial in Denmark to evaluate the cost-effectiveness of colorectal cancer screening using FOBT, modeling a number of different screening intervals, as well as age groups targeted for the program. Marginal cost-effectiveness ratios ranged from DKK 17 000 (Danish kroner) per life-year added for screening individuals 65–74 years old biennially to 42 500 DKK per life-year added for screening individuals 50–74 years old every year (DKK 1 = US$ 0.17).

How does the cost-effectiveness of colorectal cancer screening compare to that of screening for other cancers? Lindfors and Rosenquist[6] evaluated breast cancer screening using effectiveness estimates derived from a variety of sources, including trials conducted in the UK, Sweden, and the United States. The marginal cost-effectiveness ratios varied, depending on the frequency of screening and the age group screened. For women aged 50–79 years old, the ratio for annual mammography was estimated at $31 000 per year of life added; this fell to $19 000 per year of life added for biennial screening programs. Eddy[47] estimated that the marginal cost-effectiveness ratio for cervical cancer screening, in women aged 20–75 years old with Pap smears every 4 years, to be $14 000 per year of life added. The cost-effectiveness of colorectal cancer screening compares favorably to both that of breast cancer and cervical cancer screening.

Table 10.8 Preferred screening test(s) strategy at different levels of 'acceptable' costs per life-year saved[a]

Study, year (reference)	Most effective strategy[b]	Preferred strategy if willing to pay[c]			
		<$20 000 per life-year saved	$20 000–30 000 per life-year saved	$30 000–$50 000 per life-year saved	$50 000–$100 000 per life-year saved
Wagner et al, 1996[7] (alternatives)[d]	FOBT + FS	Colonoscopy every 10 years	Colonoscopy every 10 years	FOBT + FS	FOBT + FS
Frazier et al, 2000[40]	FOBT + FS	Annual FOBT	Annual FOBT	FOBT + FS	FOBT + FS
Khandker et al, 2000[41]	Colonoscopy every 10 years	FS every 5 years	FS every 5 years	Annual FOBT	Colonoscopy every 10 years
Sonnenberg et al, 2000[42]	Colonoscopy every 10 years	Colonoscopy every 10 years	Colonoscopy every 10 years	Colonoscopy every 10 years	Colonoscopy every 10 years
Vijan et al, 2001[43]	FOBT + FS	Annual FOBT	Annual FOBT	Colonoscopy at 55 and 65 years of age only	Colonoscopy at 55 and 65 years of age only

[a]Reproduced from reference 39, with permission of the Annals of Internal Medicine.
[b]Most effective strategy = largest number of life-years saved among 5 main stratgegies. FOBT, guaiac-based fecal occult blood test; FS, flexible sigmoidoscopy.
[c]All costs are updated to US dollars in 2000.
[d]Using sensitivity of 50% for double-contrast barium enema, rather than 70% used in base case.

The cost-effectiveness of other preventive interventions has also been estimated. Edelson and colleagues[48] estimated the marginal cost-effectiveness ratio for treating hypertension with hydrochlorothiazide to be $16 400 per year of life added. Goldman and colleagues[49] estimated the cost-effectiveness of primary prevention of coronary artery disease by treating individuals with hypercholesterolemia with lovastatin; the cost-effectiveness ratios varied according to individual risk status. For males aged 45–54 years old who were smokers, moderately hypertensive, ≥130% of ideal body weight, with a serum cholesterol level ≥300 mg/dl (7.76 mmol/L), the cost-effectiveness ratio was estimated to be $22 000 per year of life added. The cost-effectiveness of colorectal cancer screening compares favorably to that of all of these preventive interventions.

The above calculations refer mainly to the United States and some European countries, where medical costs are relatively high. Other countries, having managed medical care and lower costs for diagnostic procedures, find that it is markedly cost-effective to screen the average-risk population with any one of the recognized screening methods.[50]

All these calculations referred to the average-risk population whose lifelong colorectal cancer risk is about 5–6%, i.e. 1:20. Where there is a familial risk for colorectal cancer, the individual's risk rises dramatically to 1:5–10 or even 1:2 (see Chapter 6). The economic evidence strongly supports screening those family members at risk for colorectal cancer.[51]

Colorectal cancer screening and national health policies

Given that colorectal cancer screening has been shown to be efficacious, acceptable to individuals, and cost-effective, one would anticipate that routine periodic screening for this disease would be common health policy in most countries. This, in fact, is not the case, but it is changing. The World Health Organization (WHO) recommends yearly FOBT and digital rectal examination and flexible sigmoidoscopy every 3–5 years in all asymptomatic individuals beginning at 50 years old.[52] In the United

States, the US Preventive Services Task Force recommends periodic screening for colorectal cancer in men and women ≥50 years old.[53] Medicare, the national health insurance plan for the elderly, began to pay for periodic screening tests for colorectal cancer effective January 1, 1998. Screening FOBT is covered at a frequency of every 12 months, and screening flexible sigmoidoscopy is covered at a frequency of once every 48 months, for individuals ≥50 years old who have Medicare insurance. Screening colonoscopy is included at a frequency of once every 24 months for individuals at high risk for colorectal cancer (positive family history, prior colorectal cancer or precursor neoplastic polyps, history of inflammatory bowel disease, the presence of any appropriate gene markers for colorectal cancer, or other predisposing factors). Recently, screening colonoscopy has been made available for the average-risk Medicare population once every 10 years. Screening barium enema may be substituted for either a screening flexible sigmoidoscopy or a screening colonoscopy.[54] This screening policy for average- and high-risk groups has been adopted for many of the major United States medical insurance companies such as Aetna, Cigna Health Care, Humana, Kaiser Permanente, and PacifiCare.

An overview of colorectal screening internationally is given in Chapter 1 (see Table 1.7). Specifically, in Japan, a yearly 2-day immunochemical FOBT screen is offered to individuals over 40 years old.[55] They are now examining the possibility of adding colonoscopic screening.[56] Whereas the European Group for Colorectal Cancer Screening strongly recommends the implementation of repeated FOBT screening for asymptomatic individuals ≥50 years old, health policy on this issue varies by country within Europe (see Table 1.7).[56,57] Many countries, such as Germany, the Czech Republic, and Israel, have for some time promoted FOBT colorectal cancer screening in asymptomatic individuals, beginning at age 50 years. The UK has now decided to implement such a recommendation as a national policy, following a demonstration pilot FOBT screening project that was implemented successfully in five defined geographic areas of the UK in the year 2000.[58] The UK large-scale flexible sigmoidoscopy and polypectomy program has completed enrollment and the investigators are awaiting follow-up results on cancer incidence and mortality (see Chapter 8). Norway does not yet recommend population colorectal cancer screening, despite a cost-effectiveness analysis of a one-time sigmoidoscopy examination at age 60 years, modeled on Norwegian data, which showed a favorable marginal cost-effectiveness ratio.[59] However, the original study has been extended to defined geographic areas, and the populations at risk are offered flexible sigmoidoscopy and an immunochemical FOBT (interestingly, they found that adding an FOBT reduced compliance for screening sigmoidoscopy). In Italy, a 5-yearly screening colonoscopic examination is now being offered to the average-risk population; however, the uptake is low and requires more public education.[56] In Australia, the Health Technology Advisory Committee of the National Health and Medical Research Council, based on successful pilot and feasibility studies, recently recommended the introduction of population screening by FOBT for the average-risk population over age 50 years.[60]

In New Zealand, the National Advisory Committee on Health and Disability Working Party on Population Screening for Colorectal Cancer[61] recently recommended against population-based screening for colorectal cancer because of the costs. They do perform breast cancer screening. The Canadian Task Force on Preventive Health Care[62] concludes that there is good evidence to recommend biennial or annual FOBT screening, and fair evidence to recommend flexible sigmoidoscopy screening for colorectal cancer screening.

Why do such discrepancies exist in colorectal cancer screening policies between developed countries? Although cost-effective compared with other healthcare interventions, colorectal cancer screening may not be viewed as affordable by health policymakers in some countries. Initiation of such a program will generate an immediate increase in healthcare costs. Furthermore, implementation of screening needs to be feasible in the context of existing medical and financial resources. Whynes[63] has estimated that the incremental cost to the UK National Health Service for implementing a biennial FOBT screening program in individuals aged 45–74 years old, would be £40 million per year. This figure does not include the extra costs of treatment, and the investment necessary to establish the national screening infrastructure, including the provision of additional capacity for evaluating positive FOBTs, manpower training, and the development of call–recall systems for the invitation of subjects. The addition of such a screening program would require either an overall increase in healthcare expenditures, which some countries are not prepared to incur, or the shifting of resources away from some other, established, healthcare intervention to the new screening program. In a healthcare system with finite resources, there is an opportunity cost to implementing a new program, which means the loss of opportunity to continue some other, established, intervention.[64] Some countries are awaiting the results of randomized clinical trials testing other methods of colorectal cancer screening, or the results of pilot programs implemented within the country on a trial basis.

To help promote colorectal cancer screening internationally, the International Digestive Cancer Alliance (IDCA) was formed by the major gastroenterology societies. They are active in providing a format for the interchange of experience and interactions with countries wanting to introduce screening.[65]

How will the family physician manage?

Primary care-givers are subject to numerous competing demands: not only do they have to manage the medical problems that brought patients to their attention but they are also expected to provide a battery of preventive health recommendations for patients—examine for hypertension, hyperlipidemia, mammography, deal with tobacco smoking and obesity, and now to add colorectal cancer screening.[66]

Although cost-effectiveness analysis data may be useful to healthcare policymakers trying to decide how to allocate healthcare resources, they may be less useful to the physician faced with trying to implement several preventive interventions with his patients, and to the patient, who has to decide with which of those interventions he will choose to comply with. If the patient's health insurance covers the proposed preventive interventions, then the 'scarce' resources which necessitate prioritization are the physician's time and energy, and the patient's willingness to undergo the screening intervention, or, in the case of primary prevention, to change health habits and lifestyle. How are the physician and the patient to prioritize among potential preventive interventions? One option is to prioritize based on the effectiveness of the potential interventions. Wright and Weinstein[67] have compiled effectiveness data, in terms of average gains in life expectancy, for several medical interventions, based on a number of decision and cost-effectiveness analyses. Table 10.9 summarizes some of the findings of their study, and may be useful to

Table 10.9 Effectiveness of various preventive interventions by gain in life expectancy[a]

Disease/intervention[b]	Target population	Average gain in life expectancy (months)	
		Males	Females
Breast cancer/ 10 years of biennial mammograms	50-year-old women	—	0.8
Cervical cancer/ Pap smear every 3 years for 55 years[30]	20-year-old women	—	3.1
Colon cancer/ Annual FOBT and flexible sigmoidoscopy every 5 years for 25 years[26]	50 year-olds	1.6	1.5
Reduction of diastolic BP to 88 mmHg	35 year-olds with hypertension, diastolic blood pressure BP 90–94 mmHg	13	11
Reduction of cholesterol to 200 mg/dl (5.2 mmol/l)	35 year-olds with hypercholesterolemia of 200–239 mg/dl (5.2–6.2 mmol/L)	6	5

[a]Adapted from reference 67.
[b]FOBT, fecal occult blood test; BP, blood pressure.

physicians and patients in prioritizing among potential preventive interventions. The incremental life expectancy estimates reflect the average increase in life expectancy gained by every individual participating in the specific intervention. An individual who develops a cancer and is diagnosed at an early asymptomatic stage will benefit by an increase in life expectancy that is much greater than the estimated average, whereas an individual who never develops a cancer will receive no benefit from the screening in terms of increased life expectancy. The goal is not just to prevent mortality from colorectal cancer, but to lengthen quality life expectancy.[68]

Are there legal obligations to promote colorectal cancer screening?

There are now precedents where the treating physician has been successfully sued for negligence for not recommending preventive medical examinations to family members at risk and having a defined inherited risk for cancer (see Chapter 6). At present, there are various national recommendations or screening guidelines for the average-risk population. What are the medicolegal implications of national (or international) policies or guidelines for colorectal cancer screening? What liability does a physician assume if he doesn't recommend FOBT screening on an annual basis, and flexible sigmoidoscopy screening on an every 5-year basis to a 55-year-old patient at average risk, who is later diagnosed with an advanced stage colorectal carcinoma, in a country with a national colorectal cancer screening policy? Will the courts consider this an act of medical negligence by omission? Although there is no substantial case law on this subject at this time, we can only speculate that this could eventually become an important cause for litigation. Whereas physicians should base their practice on the best available evidence and doing what is best for their patients, the specter of malpractice litigation can be a powerful force in shaping physician behavior. It would seem prudent for treating physicians to offer the screening standard of care accepted in their particular community or medical insurance group.

Conclusions

In conclusion, a strong case can be made for the primary and secondary prevention of colorectal cancer. The potential benefits of prevention significantly outweigh the potential risks. Colorectal cancer screening has been shown to be of comparable cost-effectiveness to other common preventive healthcare interventions. There are significant medicolegal reasons why physicians should encourage their patients to participate in colorectal cancer screening programs. And there are a number of proven methods for increasing both physician/practice compliance and patient compliance with screening recommendations.

References (*Reviews and general articles)

1. *Rozen P, Cancer of the gastrointestinal tract: early detection or early prevention? Eur J Cancer Prev 2004; 13: 71–5.
2. Tosteson AN, Weinstein MC, Hunink MG et al, Cost-effectiveness of population wide educational approaches to reduce serum cholesterol levels. Circulation 1997; 95: 24–30.
3. *Ferlay J, Bray F, Pisani P et al, GLOBOCAN 2002: Cancer Incidence, Mortality and Prevalence Worldwide, Version 2.0. IARC Cancer Base No. 5. Lyon: IARC Press, 2004. http://www-depdb.iarc.fr/globocan/GLOBOframe.htm
4. *Lieberman D. Mass screening: North American perspective. In: Prevention and Early Detection of Colorectal Cancer. (Young GP, Rozen P, Levin B, eds). WB Saunders, London: 1996: 289–300.
5. Ramsey SD, Mandelson MT, Berry K, et al, Cancer-attributable costs of diagnosis and care for persons with screen-detected versus symptom-detected colorectal cancer. Gastroenterology 2003; 125: 1645–50.
6. Lindfors KK, Rosenquist CJ, The cost-effectiveness of mammographic screening strategies. JAMA 1995; 274: 881–4.
7. *Wagner JL, Tunis S, Brown M et al, Cost-effectiveness of colorectal cancer screening in average-risk adults. In: (Young GP, Rozen P, Levin B, eds) Prevention and Early Detection of Colorectal Cancer WB Saunders, London: 1996; 321–41.
8. Pignone M, Rich M, Teutsch SM et al, Screening for colorectal cancer in adults at average risk: a summary of the evidence for the U.S. Preventive Services Task Force. Ann Intern Med 2002; 137: 132–41.
9. *Vernon SW, Participation in colorectal cancer screening: a review. J Natl Cancer Inst 1997; 89: 1406–21.
10. Centers for Disease Control and Prevention, Colorectal cancer test use among persons aged ≥50 years-United States. 2001, MMWR 2003; 52: 193–6.

11. Etzioni DA, Ponce NA, Babey SH, A population-based study of colorectal cancer test use. Results from the 2001 California Health Interview Survey. Cancer 2004; 101: 2523–32.
12. *Mandel JS, Church TR, Bond JH et al, The effect of fecal occult-blood screening on the incidence of colorectal cancer. N Engl J Med 2000; 343: 1603–7.
13. Blom J, Liden A, Jeppsson B et al, Compliance and findings in a Swedish population screened for colorectal cancer with sigmoidoscopy. Eur J Surg Oncol 2002; 28: 827–31.
14. Subramanian S, Klosterman M, Amonkar MM et al, Adherence with colorectal screening guidelines: a review. Prev Med 2004; 38: 536–50.
15. Pasick RJ, Hiatt RA, Paskett ED, Lessons learned from community-based cancer screening intervention research. Cancer 2004; 101: 1146–64.
16. Zapka JG, Lemon SC, Interventions for patients, providers, and health care organizations. Cancer 2004; 101: 1165–87.
17. Miles A, Cockburn J, Smith RA et al, A perspective from countries using organized screening programs. Cancer 2004; 101: 1201–13.
18. *Levin B, Smith RA, Feldman GE et al, Promoting early detection tests for colorectal carcinoma and adenomatous polyps. A framework for action: the strategic plan of the National Colorectal Roundtable. Cancer 2002; 95: 1618–28.
19. Cram P, Fendrick AM, Inadomi J et al, The impact of a celebrity promotional campaign on the use of colon cancer screening. The Katie Couric Effect. Arch Intern Med 2003; 163: 1601–5.
20. Peterson SK, Vernon SW, A review of patient and physician adherence to colorectal cancer screening guidelines. Semin Colon Rectal Surg 2000; 11: 58–72.
21. *Rozen P, Blanchard J, Campbell D et al, Implementing colorectal cancer screening: Group 2 report. ESGE/UEGF Colorectal Cancer–Public Awareness Campaign. The Public/Professional Interface Workshop: Oslo, Norway, June 20–22, 2003. Endoscopy 2004; 36: 354–8.
22. Yarnall KS, Rimer BK, Hynes D et al, Computerized prompts for cancer screening in a community health center. J Am Board Fam Pract 1998; 11: 96–104.
23. http: //www.ncqa.org/Programs/HEDIS/HEDIS%202005%20Summary.pdf.
24. McCarthy BD, Yood MU, Bolton MB et al, Redesigning primary care processes to improve the offering of mammography. The use of clinic protocols by non-physicians. J Gen Intern Med 1997; 12: 357–63.
25. Molina L, Carlos RC, Fendrick AM et al, Completion of colorectal cancer screening in women attending screening mammography. Acad Radiol 2004; 11: 1237–41.
26. Leard LE, Savides TJ, Ganiats TG, Patient preferences for colorectal cancer screening. J Fam Pract 1997; 45: 211–18.
27. Pignone M, Bucholtz D, Harris R, Patient preferences for colon cancer screening. J Gen Intern Med 1999; 14: 432–7.
28. Dominitz JA, Provenzale D, Patient preferences and quality of life associated with colorectal cancer screening. Am J Gastroenterol 1997; 92: 2171–8.
29. Ling BS, Moskowitz MA, Wachs D et al, Attitudes toward colorectal cancer screening tests. A survey of patients and physicians. J Gen Intern Med 2001; 16: 822–30.
30. McCarthy BD, Moskowitz MA, Screening flexible sigmoidoscopy: patient attitudes and compliance. J Gen Intern Med 1993; 8: 120–5.
31. Cockburn J, Thomas RJS, McLaughlin SJ et al, Acceptance of screening for colorectal cancer by flexible sigmoidoscopy. J Med Screen 1995; 2: 79–83.
32. Rimer BK, Briss PA, Zeller PK et al, Informed decision making: what is its role in cancer screening? Cancer 2004; 101: 1214–28.
33. Pignone M, Harris R, Kininger L, Videotape-based decision aid for colon cancer screening. Ann Intern Med 2000; 133: 761–9.
34. www.med.unc.edu/medicine/edursrc/colon.htm.
35. Dolan JG, Frisina S, Randomized controlled trial of a patient decision aid for colorectal cancer screening. Med Decis Making 2002; 22: 125–39.
36. Wolf AMD, Schorling JB, Does informed consent alter elderly patients' preferences for colorectal cancer screening? Results of a randomized trial. J Gen Intern Med 2000; 15: 24–30.
37. *Weinstein MC, Stason WB, Foundations of cost-effectiveness analysis for health and medical practices. N Engl J Med 1977; 296: 716–21.
38. Brown ML, Knopf KB, Is colorectal cancer screening really cost-effective? Desk Reference/Prim Care Cancer 1999; 19: 15–21.
39. Pignone M, Saha S, Hoerger T et al, Cost-effectiveness analyses of colorectal cancer screening: a systematic review for the U.S. Preventive Services Task Force. Ann Intern Med 2002; 137: 96–104.
40. Frazier AL, Colditz GA, Fuchs CS et al, Cost-effectiveness of screening for colorectal cancer in the general population. JAMA 2000; 284: 1954–61.
41. Khandker RK, Dulski JD, Kilpatrick JB et al, A decision model and cost-effectiveness analysis of colorectal cancer screening and surveillance guidelines for average-risk adults. Int J Technol Assess Health Care 2000; 16: 799–810.
42. Sonnenberg A, Delco F, Inadomi JM, Cost-effectiveness of colonoscopy in screening for colorectal cancer. Ann Intern Med 2000; 133: 573–84.
43. Vijan S, Hwang EW, Hofer TP et al, Which colon cancer screening test? A comparison of costs, effectiveness, and compliance. Am J Med 2001; 111: 593–601.
44. Whynes DK, Neilson AR, Robinson MH et al, Colorectal cancer screening and quality of life. Qual Life Res 1994; 3: 191–8.

45. Whynes DK, Cost-effectiveness of screening for colorectal cancer: evidence from the Nottingham faecal occult blood trial. J Med Screen 2004; 11: 11–15.
46. Gyrd-Hansen D, Sogaard J, Kronborg O, Colorectal cancer screening: efficiency and effectiveness. Health Econ 1998; 7: 9–20.
47. Eddy DM, Screening for cervical cancer. Ann Intern Med 1990; 113: 214–26.
48. Edelson JT, Weinstein MC, Tosteson AN, et al, Long-term cost-effectiveness of various initial monotherapies for mild to moderate hypertension. JAMA 1990; 263: 407–13.
49. Goldman L, Weinstein MC, Goldman PA et al, Cost-effectiveness of HMG-CoA reductase inhibition for primary and secondary prevention of coronary heart disease, JAMA 1991; 265: 1145–51.
50. Leshno M, Halpern Z, Arber N, Cost-effectiveness of colorectal cancer screening in the average risk population. Health Care Manag Sci 2003; 6: 165–74.
51. Griffith GL, Edwards RT, Gray J, Cancer genetics services: a systematic review of the economic evidence and issues. Br J Cancer 2004; 90: 1697–703.
52. Winawer SJ, St John DJ, Bond JH et al, Prevention of colorectal cancer: guidelines based on new data. WHO Collaborating Center for the Prevention of Colorectal Cancer. Bull World Health Organ 1995; 73: 7–10.
53. *U.S. Preventive Services Task Force, Screening for colorectal cancer: recommendation and rationale. Ann Intern Med 2002; 137: 129–31.
54. Colorectal cancer screening, Medicare, http: //www.hcfa.gov. news/pr2001/pr010414.htm
55. Saito H, Yoshida Y, Mass screening: Japanese perspective. In: Prevention and Early Detection of Colorectal Cancer. (Young GP, Rozen P, Levin B, eds). WB Saunders, London: 1996: 301–11.
56. *Rozen P, Winawer SJ, Report of the OMED Colorectal Cancer Screening Committee Meeting, New Orleans, 2004—in collaboration with the IDCA. Eur J Cancer Prev 2004; 13: 461–4.
57. The European Group for Colorectal Cancer Screening, Recommendation to include colorectal cancer screening in public health policy. J Med Screen 1999; 6: 80–1.
58. UK Colorectal Cancer Screening Pilot Group, Results of the first round of a demonstration pilot of screening for colorectal cancer in the United Kingdom. BMJ 2004; 329: 133. doi:110.1136/bmj. 38153.491887.7c.
59. Norum J, Prevention of colorectal cancer: a cost-effectiveness approach to a screening model employing sigmoidoscopy. Ann Oncol 1998; 9: 613–18.
60. Gow J, Costs of screening for colorectal cancer: an Australian programme. Health Econ 1999; 8: 531–40.
61. Members of the National Health Committee Working Party on Population Screening for Colorectal Cancer, Recommendations on population screening for colorectal cancer in New Zealand. N Z Med J 1999; 112: 4–6.
62. Colorectal cancer screening, Recommendation statement from the Canadian Task Force on Preventive Health Care. CMAJ 2001; 165: 206–8.
63. Whynes DK, Cost-effectiveness of faecal occult blood screening for colorectal cancer: results of the Nottingham trial. Crit Rev Oncol Hematol 1999; 32: 155–65.
64. Ganiats TG, A spectrum of health policy methods: lessons from the British. J Fam Pract 1997; 45: 391–3.
65. Winawer SJ, Classen M, Rozen P, Report of the International Digestive Disease Alliance, New Orleans, 2004—in collaboration with the OMED Colorectal Cancer Screening Committee. Eur J Cancer Prev 2004; 13: 457–9.
66. *Smith RA, Wender RC, Cancer screening and the periodic health examination. Cancer 2004; 100: 1553–7.
67. Wright JC, Weinstein MC, Gains in life expectancy from medical interventions—standardizing data on outcomes. N Engl J Med 1998; 339: 380–6.
68. Correspondence. J Natl Cancer Inst 2002; 94: 861–6.

Index

N.B. Page numbers in *italic* denote figures and tables.